D0903861

NASM's Essentials of Corrective Exercise Training

Micheal A. Clark, DPT, MS, PES, CES
Chief Executive Officer
National Academy of Sports Medicine
Mesa, AZ

Scott C. Lucett, MS, PES, CES, NASM—CPT
Director of Education
National Academy of Sports Medicine
Mesa, AZ

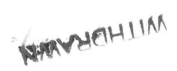

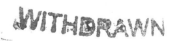

Wolters Kluwer | Lippincott Williams & Wilkins
Health
Philadelphia • Baltimore • New York • London
Buenos Aires • Hong Kong • Sydney • Tokyo

Acquisitions Editor: Emily Lupash
Product Manager: Andrea Klingler
Marketing Manager: Christen Murphy
Designer: Teresa Mallon
Compositor: SPi Technologies

First Edition

Library of Congress Cataloging-in-Publication Data
NASM essentials of corrective exercise training/[edited by] Micheal A. Clark, Scott C. Lucett. — 1st ed.
      p. ; cm.
   Other title: Essentials of corrective exercise training
   Includes bibliographical references and index.
   ISBN 978-0-7817-6802-3 (alk. paper)
  1. Exercise therapy. I. Clark, Micheal. II. Lucett, Scott. III. National Academy of Sports Medicine. IV. Title: Essentials of corrective exercise training.
   [DNLM: 1. Athletic Injuries—rehabilitation. 2. Athletic Injuries—diagnosis. 3. Athletic Injuries—prevention & control. 4. Exercise Movement Techniques. 5. Exercise Therapy—methods. 6. Sports Medicine. QT 261 N255 2011]
   RM725.N373   2011
   615.8′2—dc22

                                                                                2010023998

NASM's Essentials of Corrective Exercise Training Mission

To provide health and fitness professionals with the best evidence-based
injury prevention education, systems, and solutions

THE following code of ethics is designed to assist certified and non-certified members of the National Academy of Sports Medicine (NASM) to uphold (both as individuals and as an industry) the highest levels of professional and ethical conduct. This Code of Ethics reflects the level of commitment and integrity necessary to ensure that all NASM members provide the highest level of service and respect for all colleagues, allied professionals and the general public.

Professionalism

Each certified or non-certified member must provide optimal professional service and demonstrate excellent client care in his/her practice. Each member shall:

1. Abide fully by the NASM Code of Ethics.
2. Conduct themselves in a manner that merits the respect of the public, other colleagues and NASM.
3. Treat each colleague and/or client with the utmost respect and dignity.
4. Not make false or derogatory assumptions concerning the practices of colleagues and/or clients.
5. Use appropriate professional communication in all verbal, non-verbal and written transactions.
6. Provide and maintain an environment that ensures client safety that, at minimum, requires that the certified or non-certified member:
   a. Shall not diagnose or treat illness or injury (except for basic first aid) unless the certified or non-certified member is legally licensed to do so and is working in that capacity, at that time.
   b. Shall not train clients with a diagnosed health condition unless the certified or non-certified member has been specifically trained to do so, is following procedures prescribed and supervised by a valid licensed medical professional, or unless the certified or non-certified member is legally licensed to do so and is working in that capacity at that time.
   c. Shall not begin to train a client prior to receiving and reviewing a current health-history questionnaire signed by the client.
   d. Shall hold a CPR certification at all times.
7. Refer the client to the appropriate medical practitioner when, at minimum, the certified or non-certified member:
   a. Becomes aware of any change in the client's health status or medication
   b. Becomes aware of an undiagnosed illness, injury or risk factor
   c. Becomes aware of any unusual client pain and/or discomfort during the course the training session that warrants professional care after the session has been discontinued and assessed

8. Refer the client to other healthcare professionals when nutritional and supplemental advice is requested unless the certified or non-certified member has been specifically trained to do so or holds a credential to do so and is acting in that capacity at the time.
9. Maintain a level of personal hygiene appropriate for a health and fitness setting.
10. Wear clothing that is clean, modest and professional.
11. If certified, remain in good standing and maintain current certification status by acquiring all necessary continuing-education requirements (see NASM Recertification Information).

Confidentiality

Each certified and non-certified member shall respect the confidentiality of all client information. In his/her professional role, the certified or non-certified member:

1. Protect the client's confidentiality in conversations, advertisements and any other arena, unless otherwise agreed upon by the client in writing, or due to medical and/or legal necessity.
2. Protect the interest of clients who are minors by law, or who are unable to give voluntary consent by securing the legal permission of the appropriate third party or guardian.
3. Store and dispose of client records in secure manner.

Legal and Ethical

Each certified or non-certified member must comply with all legal requirements within the applicable jurisdiction. In his/her professional role, the certified or non-certified member must:

1. Obey all local, state, providence and/or federal laws.
2. Accept complete responsibility for his/her actions.
3. Maintain accurate and truthful records.
4. Respect and uphold all existing publishing and copyright laws.

Business Practice

Each certified or non-certified member must practice with honesty, integrity and lawfulness. In his/her professional role, the certified or non-certified member shall:

1. Maintain adequate liability insurance.
2. Maintain adequate and truthful progress notes for each client.
3. Accurately and truthfully inform the public of services rendered.
4. Honestly and truthfully represent all professional qualifications and affiliations.
5. Advertise in a manner that is honest, dignified and representative of services that can be delivered without the use of provocative and/or sexual language and/or pictures.
6. Maintain accurate financial, contract, appointment and tax records including original receipts for a minimum of four years.
7. Comply with all local, state, federal or providence laws regarding sexual harassment.

NASM expects each member to uphold the Code of Ethics in its entirety. Failure to comply with the NASM Code of Ethics may result in disciplinary actions including but not limited to suspension or termination of membership and/or certification. All members are obligated to report any unethical behavior or violation of the Code of Ethics by other NASM members.

Preface

THE NASM Corrective Exercise Continuum has been a facet in both the fitness and sports performance training arenas for years and as such, has benefited many professionals and top-notch athletes along the way. From top-level trainers, executives owning and managing professional teams, to the athletes themselves, the reach of the Corrective Exercise Continuum is beyond compare as noted by the following friends of NASM, who have been instrumental in the success of the best performance and injury prevention training system in the field.

"NASM OPT-Training is a huge benefit. It has a cumulative effect on your body. If your body is more receptive every night, it's going to help you over the long term."

—*Steve Nash, Phoenix Suns, Two-Time NBA MVP*

"NASM's Corrective Exercise Training course is by far the best continuing education I have taken. The systematic process, the redefining of preventative care, and the hands-on focus has allowed me to do my job better."

—*Fred Tedeschi, Head Athletic Trainer, Chicago Bulls*

"I felt like I didn't have the competitive edge to make a lasting impact in the personal training industry. I would struggle to see what other trainers were doing and what I wasn't doing. I finally realized that the one major thing that NASM offered, that most other certifications didn't offer, was Corrective Exercise as well as Optimum Performance Training. Keep up the great work NASM as you continue to lead the fitness industry and change the lives of many for years to come!"

—*Ralph Arellanes, NASM CPT, CES, Personal Trainer, New Mexico*

"The health and wellness of professional athletes has an intangible value—sickness or injury can devastate an organization, team, and athlete. As a medical professional, I understand the importance of keeping each athlete healthy and I rely on the best science and techniques to do just that. NASM's unique programming model and integrated training techniques exemplify their commitment to cutting-edge performance training methods. Too often we dedicate our resources to rehabilitating an athlete and neglect to focus on injury prevention, but NASM's programs combine the latest science, research and clinical applications available to help athletes reduce injuries and reach their performance potential. NASM's evidence-based approach systematically progresses athletes through a solid foundation punctuated with preventative measures and works to ensure a physically sound athlete throughout their career."

—*Dr. Thomas Carter, Team Physician, Phoenix Suns and Emeritus Head of Orthopedic Surgery, Arizona State University*

"I feel like I'm contributing. As long as I feel like that, I'll keep playing . . . I feel like I found the fountain of youth."

—*Grant Hill, Phoenix Suns*

"As an athletic trainer with the Chicago Cubs, I applied the information and principles from NASM's Sports Performance and Corrective Exercise programs with great results. These courses made me an even better athletic trainer and the players respected me even more."

—*Esteban Melendez, MS, ATC, LAT, NASM PES, CES, Florida*

"NASM has given me more avenues to explore what a player is going through. Watching his movements, seeing what he's lacking, then assessing and stretching the asymmetries in players. The more you have in your toolbox, the better you'll be professionally, and the better you'll be for your players."

—*Ben Potenziano, ATC, CES. Strength and Conditioning Coach, San Francisco Giants*

"NASM has been an unparalleled education provider to myself and my staff. They have helped us provide our athletes with the best possible training and corrective strategies to keep them on the court."

—*Aaron Nelson, Head Athletic Trainer, Phoenix Suns*

"I had been a trainer and in the business for approximately 13 years and carried three other certifications . . . They were helpful, but I knew I needed something to augment and enhance my knowledge . . . NASM provided this. Because of the educational opportunities and leadership provided by NASM, I have been greatly enhanced as a trainer, simply because it is effective and builds upon itself."

—*Dan Cordell, NASM CPT, PES, CES, Georgia*

"I've obtained numerous certifications from nationally recognized organizations, but NASM is simply the best. NASM has given me scientific, progressive knowledge that I apply to all of my client programs."

—*Patrick Murphy, NASM CPT, CES, PES*

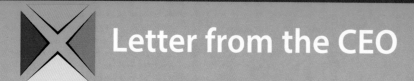

Letter from the CEO

I applaud you on your dedication to helping athletes achieve the height of their physical skill, and thank you for entrusting the National Academy of Sports Medicine (NASM) with your education. By following the techniques in this book, *NASM's Essentials of Corrective Exercise Training*, you will gain the information, insight, and inspiration you need to change the world as a health and fitness professional.

Since 1987, NASM has been the leading authority in certification, continuing education, solutions and tools for health and fitness, sports performance and sports medicine professionals. Our systematic and scientific approach to both fitness and performance continues to raise the bar as the "gold standard" in the industry. Today, we serve as the global authority in more than 80 countries, serving more than 100,000 members! Tomorrow, our possibilities are endless.

The health and fitness and sports performance industries are prime for a convergence of the latest science with cutting-edge technological solutions for maximizing the human potential. With the advances in research and application techniques, exercise and sports performance training will shift upward, drawing on traditional approaches while embracing new ideologies for enhancing the abilities of gym enthusiast and athletes alike. These industry shifts will continue to provide unlimited opportunities for you as an elite NASM professional.

Today's gym member and athlete have an increasingly high level of expectations. They demand the best and the brightest who can provide unparalleled results. To meet these expectations and better deliver quality, innovation, and evidence-based performance enhancement solutions to the world, NASM has developed new and exciting solutions with best-in-class partners from the education, healthcare, sports and entertainment, and technology industries. With the help of our best-in-class partnerships—and top professionals like you—we will continue to live up to the expectations placed upon us and strive to raise the bar in our pursuit of excellence!

Innovation is important in performance and the new NASM reflects our ability to stay ground-breaking in an ever evolving world. Amidst all of the change, we will always stay true to our mission and values: delivering evidence-based solutions driven by excellence, innovation and results. This is essential to our long-term success as a company, and to your individual career success as a health and fitness professional.

Scientific research and techniques also continue to advance and, as a result, you must remain on the cutting edge in order to remain competitive. The NASM education continuum—certification, specializations, continuing and higher education—is based on a foundation of comprehensive, scientific research supported by leading institutes and universities. As a result, NASM offers scientifically-validated education, evidence-based solutions and user-friendly tools that can be applied immediately.

The tools and solutions in the Corrective Exercise Continuum is an innovative, systemic approach, used by thousands of health and fitness and sports performance professionals worldwide to help decrease the risk of injury and maximize results. NASM's techniques work, creating a dramatic difference in training programs and their results.

One of the most influential people of the twentieth century told us "a life is not important except for the impact it has on other lives."[1] For us as health and fitness professionals in the twenty-first century, the truth behind this wisdom has never been greater.

There is no quick fix to a healthy lifestyle. However, NASM's education, solutions, and tools can positively impact behavior by allowing the masses to participate in practical, customized, evidence-based exercise.

The future of fitness and sports performance is upon us all, and there is much work to be done. With that, I welcome you to the NASM community of health and fitness professionals. If you ever need assistance from one of our subject matter experts, or simply want to learn more about our new partnerships and evidence-based health and fitness solutions, please call us at 800-460-NASM or visit us online at www.nasm.org.

We look forward to working with you to impact the performance world.
Now let's go out together and empower our athletes to achieve their potential!

Micheal A. Clark, DPT, MS, PT, PES, CES
CEO

---

1. Jackie Robinson, Hall of Fame baseball player and civil rights leader (1919–1972)

New Content

BASED upon feedback from past students and health and professionals, this new textbook includes several new updates in comparison to the previous corrective exercise materials:

1. **The Corrective Exercise Continuum.** The NASM OPT model™ has been simplified to include the most commonly used phases of training for health and fitness as well as sports performance goals. One of the phases of training that is no longer included in the updated version of the OPT™ model is Corrective Exercise Training. Corrective Exercise Training would be used for individuals who posses muscle imbalances or who've come off an injury and *prepares* that individual to enter into the OPT model™. This form of training is covered exclusively in this book and introduces the health and fitness professional to the Corrective Exercise Continuum, a system of training that uses corrective exercise strategies to help improve muscle imbalance, movement capabilities and decrease the risk of injury.

2. **Additional Content Areas.** This textbook includes several new chapters not included in the previous corrective exercise materials. These additional chapter topics will assist in creating a more well-round health and fitness professional and thus creating more value in you as a professional. These additional chapters include:

   - The Rationale for Corrective Exercise Training
   - Health Risk Assessments
   - Static Postural Assessments
   - Range of Motion Assessments (Goniometric Assessments)
   - Strength Assessments (Manual Muscle Testing)
   - Corrective Strategies for the Cervical Spine, Elbow and Wrist

3. **Updated Chapter Content.** All of the chapter topics in this textbook have been updated to include new information and the most up to date research provided and reviewed by some of the most well respected professionals in the industry. Some of the new content update highlights include:
   A. A variety of both transitional and dynamic movement assessments
   B. Updated content for all components of the Corrective Exercise Continuum

   - Inhibitory techniques
   - Lengthening techniques
   - Activation techniques
   - Integration techniques

   C. Advanced corrective exercise applications

   - Neuromuscular stretching
   - Positional isometrics

D. More than 100 corrective exercise techniques in the categories of self-myofascial release, static stretching, neuromuscular stretching, isolated strength training, positional isometrics, and integrated dynamic movements.

E. Step-by-step assessment and corrective exercise strategies for common movement impairments seen in each segment of the body:

- Foot and ankle complex
- Knee
- Lumbo-pelvic-hip complex
- Shoulder, elbow, and wrist
- Cervical spine

4. **Glossary.** We've included a Glossary to include a number of important terms and definitions. We've also included an index for easy navigation when searching for topics, concepts or programming strategies.

5. **Appendix.** We've also included an Appendix that includes example corrective exercise programs for common impairments seen in each segment of the body as well as a guide to common myofascial dysfunction.

New Pedagoligical Features

The new textbook comes with a variety of new educational features. These features include:

- New illustrations
- Updated tables
- New anatomical images
- Sidebars to emphasize key terms and concepts
- Updated photos
- Sample programs

Additional Resources

NASM Essentials of Corrective Exercise Training includes additional resources for students and instructors that are available on the book's companion website at thePoint.lww.com/NASMCES.

- PowerPoint lecture outlines
- Image Bank
- Test Bank
- Quiz Bank
- Lab Activities

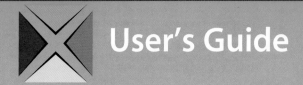

User's Guide

NASM Essentials of Corrective Exercise Training was created and developed by the National Academy of Sports Medicine to introduce health and fitness professionals to NASM's proprietary Corrective Exercise Continuum, a system of training that uses corrective exercise strategies to help improve muscle imbalances and movement efficiency to decrease the risk of injury. Please take a few moments to look through this User's Guide, which will introduce you to the tools and features that will enhance your learning experience.

Objectives open each chapter and present learning goals to help you focus on and retain the crucial topics discussed.

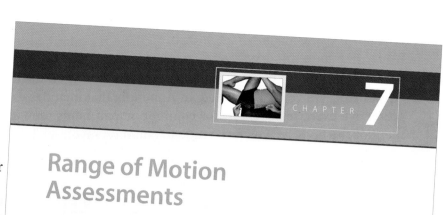

CHAPTER 7

Range of Motion Assessments

OBJECTIVES — Upon completion of this chapter, you will be able to:

➤ Identify the importance of achieving optimal range of motion in human movement.

➤ Explain how the integrated function of the muscular, skeletal, and nervous systems collectively influences the ability to move through a full range of motion.

➤ Discuss how a goniometer and an inclinometer can be used to measure joint range of motion and why it is important for the health and fitness professional to develop skill in taking these measures.

➤ Discuss the various components of a goniometer and specifically explain how to use this instrument to measure joint range of motion.

➤ Demonstrate the ability to measure joint range of motion at the foot, knee, hip, and shoulder joints.

➤ Explain how optimal range of motion at these joints correlates to the overhead squat and single-leg squat assessments.

➤ For each joint movement identified, discuss the muscles being assessed, the antagonist muscles, positioning of the client, the execution of the goniometric measurement, common errors in measurement, and the movement compensations to look for.

Sidebars, set in the margins, highlight the definitions of key terms that are presented in the chapter. The key terms are bolded throughout the chapter for easy reference.

In other words, although a muscle may not be as resistant to being stretched (allowing for better extensibility), it still maintains the rate of increase in stiffness in response to stimuli (the ability to respond to a stretch force).

Neurologically, static stretching of neuromyofascial tissue to the end ROM appears to decrease motor neuron excitability, possibly through the inhibitory effects from the Golgi tendon organs (autogenic inhibition) as well as possible contributions from the Renshaw recurrent loop (**recurrent inhibition**) (6). Recurrent inhibition is a feedback circuit that can decrease the excitability of motor neurons via the interneuron called the Renshaw cell (11) (Figure 10-2). Collectively, these may decrease the responsiveness of the **stretch reflex** (Figure 10-3) and increase the tolerance a person has to stretch and thus allow for increased ROM.

> Recurrent inhibition: a feedback circuit that can decrease the excitability of motor neurons via the interneuron called the Renshaw cell.

> Stretch reflex: a muscle contraction in response to stretching within the muscle.

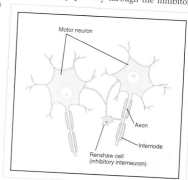

Figure 10.2 Renshaw cells and recurrent inhibition.

In general, it is thought that static stretching of 20 to 30 seconds causes an acute viscoelastic stress relaxation response, allowing for an immediate increase in ROM. Long-term, the increases in maximal joint ROM may be caused by increased tolerance to stretch and not necessarily changes in the viscoelastic properties of myofascial tissue (5,12) or a possible increase in muscle mass and added sarcomeres in series (4).

Table 2.3	MUSCLE ACTION SPECTRUM
Concentric	Developing tension while a muscle is shortening; when developed tension overcomes resistive force
Eccentric	Developing tension while a muscle is lengthening; when resistive force overcomes developed tension
Isometric	When the contractile force is equal to the resistive force

the muscles must decelerate or reduce the forces acting on the body (or force reduction). This is a critical aspect of all forms of movement because the weight of the body must be decelerated and then stabilized to properly accelerate during movement.

Getting Your Facts Straight boxes emphasize key concepts and findings from current research.

GETTING YOUR FACTS STRAIGHT

Gravity and Its Effect on Movement

Gravity is a constant downward-directed force that we are influenced by every second of every day. This increases the eccentric demand that our muscles are placed under, which must therefore be trained for accordingly, making the eccentric action of training just as important (if not more important) as the concentric action.

Movement Assessment sections discuss the purpose and procedures of various techniques that can be used in corrective exercise.

Overhead Squat Views

| Anterior | Lateral | Posterior |

Compensations: Anterior View

1. Feet:
   a. Do the feet flatten and/or turn out?
2. Knees:
   a. Do the knees move inward (adduct and internally rotate)?
   b. Do the knees move outward (abduct and externally rotate)?

High-quality, four-color photographs and artwork throughout the text help to draw attention to important concepts in a visually stimulating and intriguing manner. They help to clarify the text and are particularly helpful for visual learners.

Overhead Squat Compensations, Anterior View

| Feet Flatten | Feet Turn Out | Knees Move Inward | Knees Move Outward |

Student Resources

Inside the front cover of your textbook, you'll find your personal access code. Use it to log on to http://thePoint.lww.com/NASMCES—the companion website for this textbook. On the website, you can access various supplemental materials available to help enhance and further your learning. These assets include the fully searchable online text, a quiz bank, and lab activities.

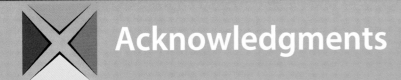

Acknowledgments

Photography:
Ben Bercovici
President
In Sync Productions
Calabasas, CA

Anton Polygalov
Photographer
In Sync Productions
Calabasas, CA

Models:
Joey Metz
Monica Munson
Allie Shira
Cameron Klippsten
Zack Miller
Paul Terek

Photo Shoot Sites:
National Academy of Sports Medicine Headquarters
26632 Agoura Rd
Calabasas, CA 91302

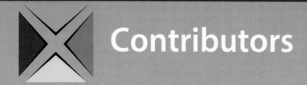
Contributors

Micheal A. Clark, DPT, MS, PES, CES
CEO
National Academy of Sports Medicine
Calabasas, CA

Scott C. Lucett, MS, PES, CES, NASM – CPT
Director of Education
National Academy of Sports Medicine
Mesa, AZ

Cathleen N. Brown, PhD, ATC
University of Georgia
Department of Kinesiology
Athens, GA

Chuck Thigpen, PhD, PT, ATC
Assistant Professor
Department of Athletic Training & Physical Therapy
Brooks College of Health
University of North Florida
Jacksonville, FL

Marjorie A. King, PhD, ATC, PT
Director of Graduate Athletic Training Education
Plymouth State University
Plymouth, NH

William Prentice, PhD, PT, ATC, FNATA
Associate Professor
Coordinator, Sports Medicine Program
Department of Exercise and Sports Science
University of North Carolina at Chapel Hill
Chapel Hill, NC

Kim D. Christensen, DC, DACRB, CSCS, CES, PES
Peacehealth Medical Group
Chiropractic Physician
Longview, WA

Jeffrey Tucker, DC
Diplomate American Chiropractic Rehabilitation Board
Certified in Chiropractic Spinal Trauma
Post Graduate Rehab Instructor
NASM Instructor
Private Practice
Los Angeles, CA

Russell D. Fiore, MEd, ATC
Head Athletic Trainer
Brown University
Providence, RI

Gregory D. Myer, PhD, CSCS
Sports Biomechanist
Cincinnati Children's Hospital Medical Center
Cincinnati, OH

Melanie McGrath, PhD, ATC
Assistant Professor
Health, Physical Education, & Recreation Department
Program Director
Athletic Training Education Program
University of Nebraska at Omaha
Omaha, NE

Lindsay J. DiStefano, PhD, ATC, PES
Assistant Professor
University of Connecticut
Storrs, CT

Michael Rosenberg, MEd, PT, ATC-L, PES, CES
Lead Physical Therapist
Presbyterian Rehabilitation Center
Charlotte, NC

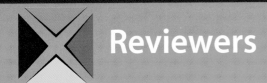

Reviewers

George J. Davies, DPT, MEd, PT, SCS, ATC, LAT, CSCS, FAPTA
Professor – Physical Therapy
Armstrong Atlantic State University
Sports Physical Therapist - Coastal Therapy
Savannah, GA
and
Professor Emeritus
UW-LaCrosse
Sports Physical Therapist and Consultant
Sports Physical Therapy Residency Program
Gundersen Lutheran Sports Medicine
LaCrosse, WI

Darin A. Padua, PhD, ATC
Associate Professor
Director, Sports Medicine Research Laboratory
Department of Exercise and Sport Science
University of North Carolina at Chapel Hill
Chapel Hill, NC

Table of Contents

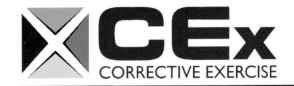

SECTION 1 INTRODUCTION TO CORRECTIVE EXERCISE TRAINING

CHAPTER 1

The Rationale for Corrective Exercises

OBJECTIVES *Upon completion of this chapter, you will be able to:*

- ➤ Understand the state of today's typical client.
- ➤ Be familiar with injury rates of today and rationalize the need for corrective exercise.
- ➤ Understand and describe the Corrective Exercise Continuum.

INTRODUCTION

FROM the mid-1980s to the present, the wealth of technology and automation in the United States has begun to take a toll on public health. The work and home environments are inundated with automation, personal computers, cell phones, and other technology that are more prevalent today than ever before. Housekeepers, gardeners, remote controls, and video games now run a household. People are less active and are no longer spending as much of their free time engaged in physical activity (1). Physical education and after-school sports programs are being cut from school budgets, further decreasing the amount of physical activity in children's lives. Today, approximately one third (33.8%) of adults are estimated to be obese (2). This also carries over to the adolescent population, with 18% of adolescents and teenagers considered overweight (3). This new environment is producing more inactive, less healthy, and nonfunctional people (4) who are more prone to injury.

RATIONALE FOR CORRECTIVE EXERCISE

Research suggests that musculoskeletal pain is more common now than it was 40 years ago (5). This lends support to the concept that decreased activity may lead to muscular dysfunction and, ultimately, injury.

Foot and Ankle Injuries

In the general population, plantar fasciitis accounted for more than 1 million ambulatory care (doctor) visits per year (6). Ankle sprains are reported to be the most common sports-related injury (7). Individuals who suffer a lateral ankle sprain are at risk for developing chronic ankle instability (8). It has also been shown that individuals may experience hip weakness after an ankle sprain (9).

Low-Back Pain

Low-back pain is one of the major forms of musculoskeletal degeneration seen in the adult population, affecting nearly 80% of all adults (10, 11). Research has shown low-back pain to be predominant among workers in enclosed workspaces (such as offices) (12, 13), as well as in people engaged in manual labor (farming) (14), in people who sit for periods greater than 3 hours (13), and in people who have altered lumbar lordosis (curve in the lumbar spine) (15). More than one third of all work-related injuries involve the trunk, and of these, more than 60% involve the low back (16). These work-related injuries cost workers approximately 9 days per back episode or, combined, more than 39 million days of restricted activity. It has been estimated that the annual costs attributable to low-back pain in the United States are greater than $26 billion (16). In addition, 6 to 15% of athletes experience low-back pain in a given year (17, 18).

Knee Injuries

The incidence of knee injuries is also a concern. An estimated 80,000 to 100,000 anterior cruciate ligament (ACL) injuries occur annually in the general U.S. population. Approximately 70 to 75% of these are noncontact injuries (19–25). In addition, ACL injuries have a strong correlation to acquiring arthritis in the affected knee (26). Most ACL injuries occur between 15 and 25 years of age (19). This comes as no surprise when considering the lack of activity and increased obesity occurring in this age group owing to the abundance of automation and technology, combined with a lack of mandatory physical education in schools (4).

Shoulder Injuries

Shoulder pain is reported to occur in up to 21% of the general population (27, 28), with 40% persisting for at least 1 year (29) at an estimated annual cost of $39 billion (30). Shoulder impingement is the most prevalent diagnosis, accounting for 40 to 65% of reported shoulder pain. The persistent nature of shoulder pain may be the result of degenerative changes to the shoulder's capsuloligamentous structures, articular cartilage, and tendons as the result of altered shoulder mechanics.

With this growing population of untrained or undertrained individuals, it is important to ensure that all components of their bodies are properly prepared for the stress that will be placed on them both inside and outside of the gym.

Unfortunately, many training programs for conditioning the musculoskeletal system often neglect proper training guidelines and do not address potential muscle imbalances one may possess from a sedentary lifestyle. This can result in a weakened structure and lead to injury.

Simply put, the extent to which we condition our musculoskeletal system directly influences our risk of injury. The less conditioned our musculoskeletal systems are, the higher the risk of injury (31). Therefore, as our daily lives include less physical activity, the less prepared we are to partake in recreational and leisure activities such as resistance training, weekend sports, or simply playing on the playground.

THE FUTURE

There is a general inability to meet the needs of today's client and athlete. The health and fitness industry has only recently recognized the trend toward nonfunctional living. Health and fitness professionals are now noticing a decrease in the physical functionality of their clients and athletes and are beginning to address it.

This is a new state of training, in which the client has been physically molded by furniture, gravity, and inactivity. The continual decrease in everyday activity has contributed to many of the postural deficiencies seen in people (32). Today's client is not ready to begin physical activity at the same level that a typical client could 20 years ago. Therefore, today's training programs cannot stay the same as programs of the past.

> Corrective exercise: a term used to describe the systematic process of identifying a neuromusculoskeletal dysfunction, developing a plan of action, and implementing an integrated corrective strategy.

The new mindset in fitness should cater to creating programs that address functional capacity as part of a safe program designed especially for each individual person. In other words, training programs must consider each person, their environment, and the tasks that will be performed. It will also be important to address any potential muscle imbalances and movement deficiencies that one may possess to improve function and decrease the risk of injury. This is best achieved by introducing an integrated approach to program design. It is on this premise that the National Academy of Sports Medicine (NASM) presents the rationale for the Corrective Exercise Continuum and its importance to integrate into today's exercise programs.

THE CORRECTIVE EXERCISE CONTINUUM

> Corrective Exercise Continuum: the systematic programming process used to address neuromusculoskeletal dysfunction through the use of inhibitory, lengthening, activation, and integration techniques.

Corrective exercise is a term used to describe the systematic process of identifying a neuromusculoskeletal dysfunction, developing a plan of action and implementing an integrated corrective strategy. This process requires knowledge and application of an integrated assessment process, corrective program design, and exercise technique. Collectively, the three-step process is to:

1. Identify the problem (integrated assessment)
2. Solve the problem (corrective program design)
3. Implement the solution (exercise technique)

Solving the identified neuromusculoskeletal problems will require a systematic plan. This plan is known as the **Corrective Exercise Continuum**

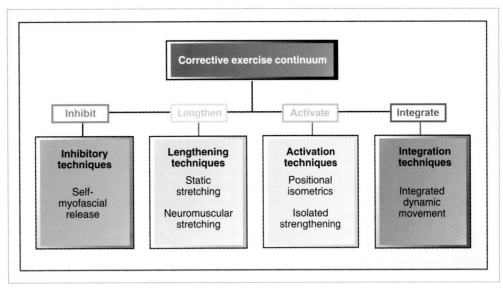

Figure 1.1 The corrective exercise continuum.

Inhibitory techniques: corrective exercise techniques used to release tension or decrease activity of overactive neuromyofascial tissues in the body.

Lengthening technique: corrective exercise techniques used to increase the extensibility, length, and range of motion (ROM) of neuromyofascial tissues in the body.

Activation techniques: corrective exercise techniques used to reeducate or increase activation of underactive tissues.

Integration techniques: corrective exercise techniques used to retrain the collective synergistic function of all muscles through functionally progressive movements.

(Figure 1-1) and will specifically outline the necessary steps needed to properly structure a corrective exercise program.

The Corrective Exercise Continuum includes four primary phases (Figure 1-1). The first phase is the *Inhibit* phase using **inhibitory techniques**. Inhibitory techniques are used to release tension or decrease activity of overactive neuromyofascial tissues in the body. This can be accomplished through the use of self-myofascial release techniques (e.g., foam roller). This phase will be covered in more detail in chapter nine of the textbook. The second phase is the *Lengthen* phase using **lengthening techniques**. Lengthening techniques are used to increase the extensibility, length, and range of motion (ROM) of neuromyofascial tissues in the body. This can be accomplished through the use of static stretching and neuromuscular stretching. This phase will be covered in more detail in chapter ten of the textbook. The third phase is the *Activate* phase using **activation techniques**. Activation techniques are used to reeducate or increase activation of underactive tissues. This can be accomplished through the use of isolated strengthening exercises and positional isometric techniques. This phase will be covered in more detail in chapter eleven of the textbook. The fourth and final phase is the *Integrate* phase using **integration techniques**. Integration techniques are used to retrain the collective synergistic function of all muscles through functionally progressive movements through the use of integrated dynamic movements. This will be covered in more detail in chapter eleven of the textbook.

Before implementing the Corrective Exercise Continuum, an integrated assessment process must be done to determine dysfunction and ultimately the design of the corrective exercise program. This assessment process should include (but not be limited to) movement assessments, range of motion assessments, and muscle strength assessments. This integrated assessment process will help in determining which tissues need to be inhibited and lengthened and which tissues need to be activated and strengthening through the use of the Corrective Exercise Continuum. These assessments will be covered in greater detail in the Assessment section of this textbook.

SUMMARY • Today, more people work in offices, have longer work hours, use better technology and automation, and are required to move less on a daily basis. This new environment produces more inactive and nonfunctional people and leads to dysfunction and increased incidents of injury including low-back pain, knee injuries, and other musculoskeletal injuries.

In working with today's typical client and athlete, who more than likely possesses muscle imbalances, health and fitness professionals must take special consideration when designing programs. An integrated approach should be used to create safe programs that consider the functional capacity for each individual person. They must address factors such as appropriate forms of flexibility, increasing strength and neuromuscular control, training in different types of environments (stable to unstable), and training in different planes of motion. These are the basis for the use of corrective exercise and NASM's Corrective Exercise Continuum model. All of the phases included in the model have been specifically designed to follow biomechanical, physiologic, and functional principles of the human movement system. They should provide an easy-to-follow systematic process that will help improve muscle imbalances, minimize injury, and maximize results.

References

1. Centers for Disease Control and Prevention. Prevalence of physical activity, including lifestyle activities among adults—United States, 2000-2001. *Morbid Mortal Wkly Rep* 2003;52:764-9.
2. Flegal KM, Carroll MD, Ogden CL, Curtin LR. Prevalence and trends in obesity among US adults, 1999-2008. *JAMA* 2010;303:235-41. Epub 2010 Jan 13.
3. Ogden CL, Carroll MD, Curtin LR, Lamb MM, Flegal KM. Prevalence of high body mass index in US children and adolescents, 2007-2008. *JAMA* 2010;303:242-9. Epub 2010 Jan 13.
4. Centers for Disease Control and Prevention. The burden of obesity in the United States: a problem of massive proportions. *Chronic Dis Notes Rep* 2005;17:4-9.
5. Harkness EF, Macfarlane GJ, Silman AJ, McBeth J. Is musculoskeletal pain more common now than 40 years ago?: two population-based cross-sectional studies. *Rheumatology (Oxford)* 2005;44:890-5.
6. Riddle DL, Schappert SM. Volume of ambulatory care visits and patterns of care for patients diagnosed with plantar fasciitis: a national study of medical doctors. *Foot Ankle Int* 2004;25:303-10.
7. McKay GD, Goldie PA, Payne WR, Oakes BW. Ankle injuries in basketball: injury rate and risk factors. *Br J Sports Med* 2001;35:103-8.
8. Garrick JG. The frequency of injury, mechanism of injury, and epidemiology of ankle sprains. *Am J Sports Med* 1977;5:241-2.
9. Hosea TM, Carrey CC, Harrer MF. The gender issue: epidemiology of knee and ankle injuries in high school and college players. *Clin Orthop Relat Res* 2000;372:45-9.
10. Walker BF, Muller R, Grant WD. Low back pain in Australian adults: prevalence and associated disability. *J Manipulative Physiol Ther* 2004;27:238-44.
11. Cassidy JD, Carroll LJ, Cote P. The Saskatchewan health and back pain survey. The prevalence of low back pain and related disability in Saskatchewan adults. *Spine* 1998;23:1860-6.
12. Volinn E. The epidemiology of low back pain in the rest of the world. A review of surveys in low- and middle-income countries. *Spine* 1997;22:1747-54.
13. Omokhodion FO, Sanya AO. Risk factors for low back pain among office workers in Ibadan, Southwest Nigeria. *Occup Med (Lond)* 2003;53:287-9.
14. Omokhodion FO. Low back pain in a rural community in South West Nigeria. West *Afr J Med* 2002; 21:87-90.
15. Tsuji T, Matsuyama Y, Sato K, Hasegawa Y, Yimin Y, Iwata H. Epidemiology of low back pain in the elderly: correlation with lumbar lordosis. *J Orthop Sci* 2001;6:307-11.
16. Luo X, Pietrobon R, Sun SX, Liu GG, Hey L. Estimates and patterns of direct health care expenditures among individuals with back pain in the United States. *Spine* 2004;29:79-86.
17. Nadler SF, Malanga GA, DePrince M, Stitik TP, Feinberg JH. The relationship between lower extremity injury, low back pain, and hip muscle strength in male and female collegiate athletes. *Clin J Sport Med* 2000;10:89-97.
18. Nadler SF, Malanga GA, Feinberg JH, Rubanni M, Moley P, Foye P. Functional performance deficits in athletes with previous lower extremity injury. *Clin J Sport Med* 2002;12:73-8.
19. Griffin LY, Agel J, Albohm MJ, et al. Noncontact anterior cruciate ligament injuries: risk factors and prevention strategies. *J Am Acad Orthop Surg* 2000;8: 141-50.
20. Noyes FR, Mooar PA, Matthews DS, Butler DL. The symptomatic anterior cruciate deficient knee. Part I: the long-term functional disability in athletically active individuals. *J Bone Joint Surg Am* 1983;65:154-62.

21. Arendt E, Dick R. Knee injury patterns among men and women in collegiate basketball and soccer. NCAA data and review of literature. *Am J Sports Med* 1995;23:694–701.

22. Arendt EA, Agel J, Dick R. Anterior cruciate ligament injury patterns among collegiate men and women. *J Athl Train* 1999;34:86–92.

23. Boden BP, Dean GS, Feagin JA, Garrett WE. Mechanisms of anterior cruciate ligament injury. *Orthopedics* 2000;23:573–8.

24. Engstrom B, Johansson C, Tornkvist H. Soccer injuries among elite female players. *Am J Sports Med* 1991;19:372–5.

25. Ireland ML, Wall C. Epidemiology and comparison of knee injuries in elite male and female United States basketball athletes. *Med Sci Sports Exerc* 1990;22:S82.

26. Hill CL, Seo GS, Gale D, Totterman S, Gale ME, Felson DT. Cruciate ligament integrity in osteoarthritis of the knee. *Arthritis Rheum* 2005;52:3:794–9.

27. Bongers PM. The cost of shoulder pain at work. *BMJ* 2001;322:64–5.

28. Urwin M, Symmons D, Allison T, et al. Estimating the burden of musculoskeletal disorders in the community: the comparative prevalence of symptoms at different anatomical sites, and the relation to social deprivation. *Ann Rheum Dis* 1998;57:649–55.

29. Van der Heijden G. Shoulder disorders: a state of the art review. *Baillieres Best Pract Res Clin Rheumatol* 1999;13:287–309.

30. Johnson M, Crosley K, O'Neil M, Al Zakwani I. Estimates of direct health care expenditures among individuals with shoulder dysfunction in the United States. *J Orthop Sports Phys Ther* 2005;35:A4–PL8.

31. Barr KP, Griggs M, Cadby T. Lumbar stabilization: core concepts and current literature, part 1. *Am J Phys Med Rehabil* 2005;84:473–80.

32. Hammer WI. Chapter 12. Muscle Imbalance and Postfacilitation Stretch. In: Hammer WI, ed. Functional Soft Tissue Examination and Treatment by Manual Methods. 2nd ed. Gaithersburg, MD: Aspen Publishers; 1999:415–446.

Introduction to Human Movement Science

INTRODUCTION

HUMAN movement science is the study of how the human movement system (HMS) functions in an interdependent, interrelated scheme. The HMS consists of the muscular system (functional anatomy), the skeletal system (functional biomechanics), and the nervous system (motor behavior) (1–3). Although they appear separate, each system and its components must collaborate to form interdependent links. In turn, this entire interdependent system must be aware of its relationship to internal and external environments while gathering necessary information to produce the appropriate movement patterns. This process ensures optimum functioning of the HMS and optimum human movement. This chapter will review the pertinent aspects of each component of the HMS as it relates to function and human movement (Figure 2-1).

BIOMECHANICS

Biomechanics: a study that uses principles of physics to quantitatively study how forces interact within a living body.

Biomechanics applies the principles of physics to quantitatively study how forces interact within a living body (4–7). For purposes of this text, the specific focus will be on the motions that the HMS produces (kinematics) and the forces (kinetics) that act on it. This includes basic understanding of anatomic terminology, planes of motion, joint motions, muscle action, force-couples, leverage, and basic muscle mechanics.

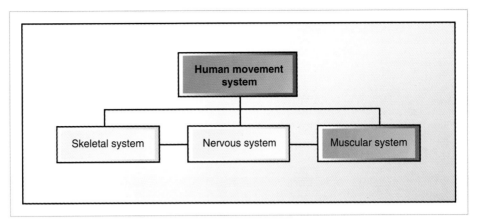

Figure 2.1   Components of the human movement system.

ANATOMIC TERMINOLOGY

All professions have language that is specific to their needs. The health and fitness professional needs to understand the basic anatomic terminology for effective communication.

Planes of Motion and Axes, and Combined Joint Motions

Human movement occurs in three dimensions and is universally discussed in a system of planes and axes (Figure 2-2). Three imaginary planes are positioned through the body at right angles so they intersect at the body's center of mass. These planes are termed the sagittal, frontal, and transverse planes. Movement is said to occur predominantly in a specific plane when that movement occurs along or parallel to the plane. Although movements can be dominant in one plane, no motion occurs strictly in one plane of motion. Movement in a plane occurs around an axis running perpendicular to that plane—much like the axle that a car wheel revolves around. This is known as joint motion. Joint motions are termed for their action in each of the three planes of motion (Table 2-1).

THE SAGITTAL PLANE

The sagittal plane bisects the body into right and left halves. Sagittal plane motion occurs around a frontal axis (4,5,8). Movements in the sagittal plane include flexion and extension (Figure 2-3). Flexion occurs when the relative angle between two adjacent segments decreases (5,9). Extension occurs when the relative angle between two adjacent segments increases (5,9) (Table 2-1). Flexion and extension occur in many joints in the body including vertebral, shoulder, elbow, wrist, hip, knee, foot, and hand. The ankle is unique and includes special terms for movement in the sagittal plane. "Flexion" is more accurately termed dorsiflexion and "extension" is referred to as plantarflexion (4,5,9). Examples of predominantly sagittal plane movements include biceps curls, triceps pushdowns, squats, front lunges, calf raises, walking, running, and climbing stairs (Table 2-1).

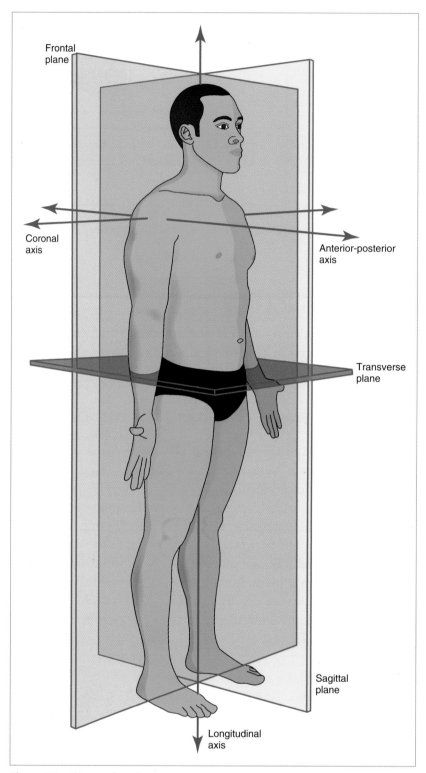

Figure 2.2   Planes of motion.

THE FRONTAL PLANE

The frontal plane bisects the body into front and back halves with frontal plane motion occurring around an anterior-posterior axis (4,5,9). Movements in the frontal plane include abduction and adduction of the limbs (relative to the trunk), lateral flexion in the spine, and eversion and inversion of the foot and ankle complex (Figure 2-4) (4,5,8,9). Abduction is a movement away

Table 2.1   **EXAMPLES OF PLANES OF MOTION, MOTIONS, AND AXES**

Plane	Motion	Axis	Example
Sagittal	Flexion/Extension	Coronal	• Bicep curls
			• Tricep pushdowns
			• Squats
			• Front lunges
			• Calf raises
			• Walking
			• Running
			• Vertical jumping
			• Climbing stairs
Frontal	Adduction/Abduction	Anterior-Posterior	• Lateral shoulder raises
	Lateral Flexion		• Side lunges
	Eversion/Inversion		• Side shuffling
Transverse	Internal/External Rotation	Longitudinal	• Cable rotations
	Left/Right Spinal Rotation		• Transverse plane lunges
	Horizontal Add/Abduction		• Throwing
			• Golfing
			• Swinging a bat

from the midline of the body or, similar to extension, an increase in the angle between two adjoining segments only in the frontal plane (4,5,8,9). Adduction is a movement of the segment toward the midline of the body or, like flexion, a decrease in the angle between two adjoining segments only in the frontal plane (4,5,8,9). Lateral flexion is the bending of the spine (cervical, thoracic, lumbar) from side to side or simply side-bending (4,5). Eversion and inversion relate specifically to the movement of the calcaneus and tarsals in the frontal plane during functional movements of pronation and supination (discussed later) (4,5,8,9). Examples of frontal plane movements include lateral shoulder raises, side lunges, and side shuffling (Table 2-1).

THE TRANSVERSE PLANE

The transverse plane bisects the body to create upper and lower halves. Transverse plane motion occurs around a longitudinal or a vertical axis (4,5,8). Movements in the transverse plane include internal rotation and external rotation for the limbs, right and left rotation for the head and trunk, and radioulnar pronation and supination (4,5,8) (Figure 2-5). The transverse plane motions of the foot are termed abduction (toes pointing outward, externally rotated) and adduction (toes pointing inward, internally rotated) (5). Examples of transverse plane movements include cable rotations, turning lunges, throwing a ball, and swinging a bat (Table 2-1).

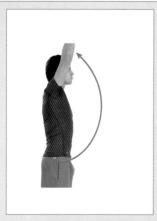

Figure 2.3A Shoulder flexion

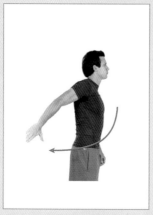

Figure 2.3B Shoulder extension

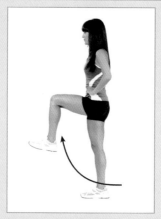

Figure 2.3C Hip flexion

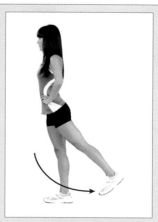

Figure 2.3D Hip extension

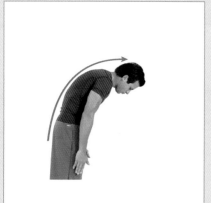

Figure 2.3E Spinal flexion

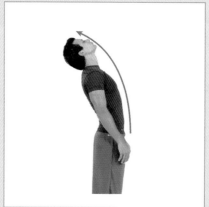

Figure 2.3F Spinal extension

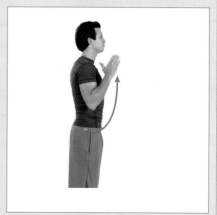

Figure 2.3G Elbow flexion

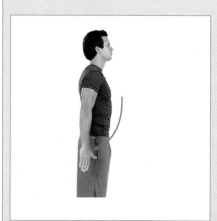

Figure 2.3H Elbow extension

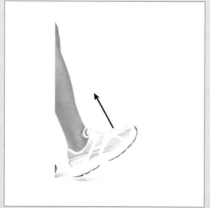

Figure 2.3I Dorsiflexion

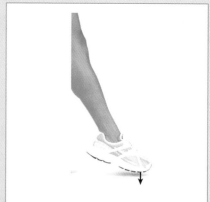

Figure 2.3J Plantarflexion

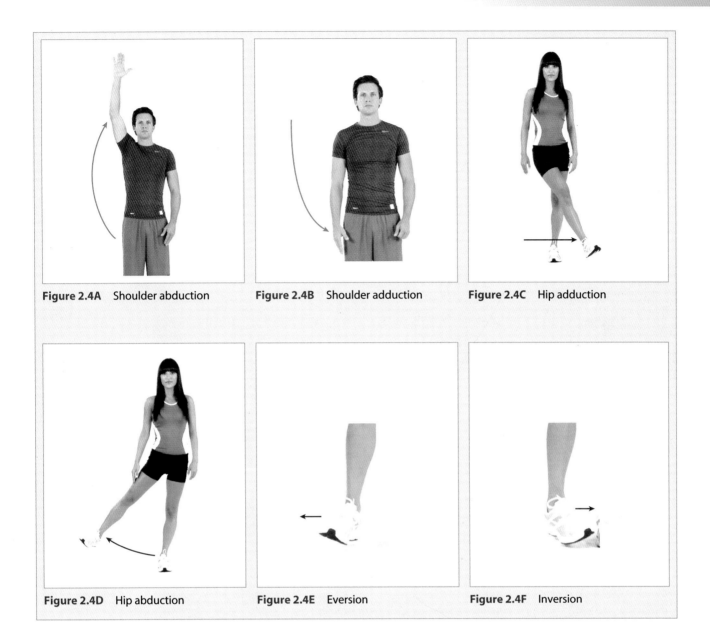

Figure 2.4A Shoulder abduction

Figure 2.4B Shoulder adduction

Figure 2.4C Hip adduction

Figure 2.4D Hip abduction

Figure 2.4E Eversion

Figure 2.4F Inversion

COMBINED JOINT MOTIONS

During movement, the body must maintain its center of gravity aligned over a constantly changing base of support. If a change in alignment occurs at one joint, changes in alignment of other joints must occur. For example, when individuals stand and turn their patella inward, then outward, you will notice obligatory effects from the subtalar joint to the pelvis. When the patella is turned inward (tibial and femoral internal rotation), pronation occurs at the subtalar joint (Figure 2-6). When the patella is turned outward (tibial and femoral external rotation), subtalar joint supination occurs (Figure 2-6).

Even though a joint has a predominant plane of movement, all freely moveable joints can display some movement in all three planes of motion. Functional multiplanar biomechanics of the subtalar joint can be simplified into pronation and supination (10). In reality, subtalar pronation with obligatory tibial and femoral internal rotation is a multiplanar, synchronized joint motion that occurs with eccentric muscle function. Thus, subtalar supination

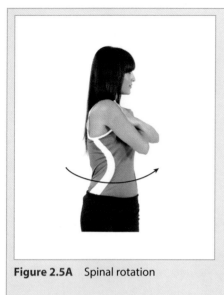

Figure 2.5A   Spinal rotation

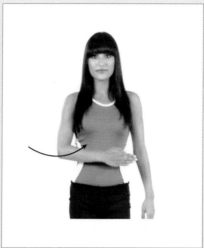

Figure 2.5B   Shoulder internal rotation

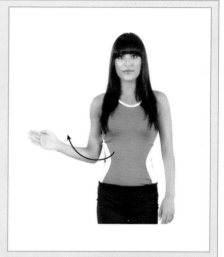

Figure 2.5C   Shoulder external rotation

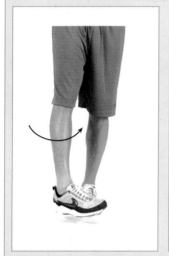

Figure 2.5D   Hip internal rotation

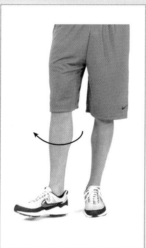

Figure 2.5E   Hip external rotation

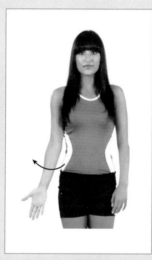

Figure 2.5F   Radioulnar supination

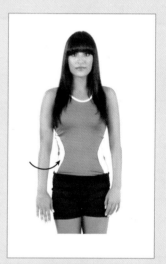

Figure 2.5G   Radioulnar pronation

with obligatory tibial and femoral external rotation is also a multiplanar, synchronized joint motion that occurs with concentric muscle function (Table 2-2).

The gait cycle will be used to briefly describe functional biomechanics to show the interdependence of joint and muscle actions on each other (11,12). During the initial contact phase of gait, the subtalar joint pronates creating obligatory internal rotation of the tibia, femur, and pelvis. At mid-stance, the subtalar joint supinates leading to obligatory external rotation of the tibia, femur, and pelvis (Figure 2-7). The health and fitness professional should remember that these linkages are bidirectional: pelvic motion can create lower extremity motion and lower extremity motion can create pelvic motion (Figure 2-8) (10,13).

Poor control of subtalar joint pronation along with tibial and femoral internal rotation decreases the ability to eccentrically decelerate multisegmental

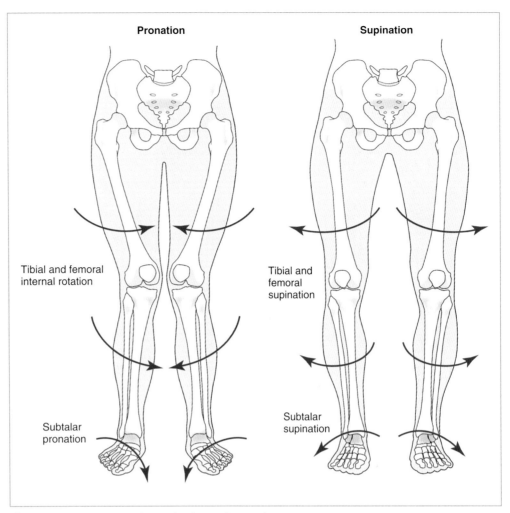

Figure 2.6   Lower extremity supination and pronation.

motion that can lead to muscle imbalances, joint dysfunction, and injury. Poor production of subtalar joint supination along with tibial and femoral external rotation decreases the ability of the human movement system to concentrically produce the appropriate force for push-off that can lead to synergistic dominance (which will be explained in greater detail in chapter 3).

Table 2.2	FUNCTIONAL BIOMECHANICS
During Pronation	
The foot	Dorsiflexes, everts, abducts
The ankle	Dorsiflexes, everts, abducts
The knee	Flexes, adducts, internally rotates
The hip	Flexes, adducts, internally rotates
During Supination	
The foot	Plantarflexes, inverts, adducts
The ankle	Plantarflexes, inverts, adducts
The knee	Extends, abducts, externally rotates
The hip	Extends, abducts, externally rotates

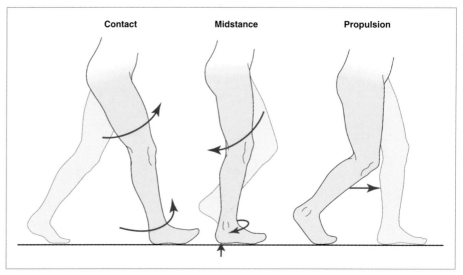

Figure 2.7 Supination and pronation during gait.

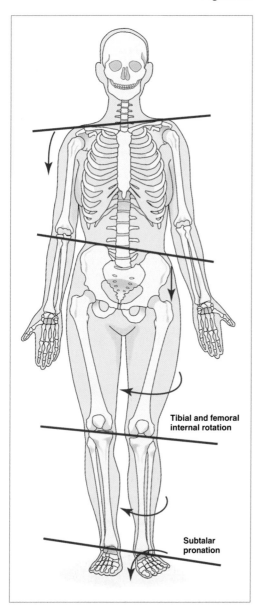

Tibial and femoral internal rotation

Subtalar pronation

Figure 2.8 Pronations effect on the entire kinetic chain.

During functional movement patterns, almost every muscle has the same synergistic function: to eccentrically decelerate pronation or to concentrically accelerate supination. When an articular structure is out of alignment, abnormal distorting forces are placed on the articular surfaces. Poor alignment also changes the mechanical function of muscle and force-couple relationships of all of the muscles that cross that joint. This leads to altered movement patterns, altered reciprocal inhibition, synergistic dominance, and ultimately, decreased neuromuscular efficiency; these concepts will be developed throughout this book.

Muscle Actions

Muscles produce tension through a variety of means to effectively manipulate gravity, ground reaction forces, momentum, and external resistance. There are three different muscle actions: eccentric, isometric, and concentric (Table 2-3).

ECCENTRIC

An eccentric action occurs when a muscle develops tension while lengthening; the muscle lengthens because the contractile force is less than the resistive force. The overall tension within the muscle is less than the external forces trying to lengthen the muscle. During resistance training, an eccentric muscle action is also known as "a negative." This occurs during the lowering phase of any resistance exercise. During integrated resistance training, the eccentric action exerted by the muscle(s) prevents the weight/resistance/implement from accelerating in an uncontrolled manner downward as a result of gravitational force.

In all activities, muscles work as much eccentrically as they do concentrically or isometrically (14,15). Eccentrically,

Table 2.3	MUSCLE ACTION SPECTRUM
Concentric	Developing tension while a muscle is shortening; when developed tension overcomes resistive force
Eccentric	Developing tension while a muscle is lengthening; when resistive force overcomes developed tension
Isometric	When the contractile force is equal to the resistive force

the muscles must decelerate or reduce the forces acting on the body (or force reduction). This is a critical aspect of all forms of movement because the weight of the body must be decelerated and then stabilized to properly accelerate during movement.

GETTING YOUR FACTS STRAIGHT

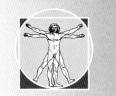

Gravity and Its Effect on Movement

Gravity is a constant downward-directed force that we are influenced by every second of every day. This increases the eccentric demand that our muscles are placed under, which must therefore be trained for accordingly, making the eccentric action of training just as important (if not more important) as the concentric action.

ISOMETRIC

An isometric muscle action occurs when the contractile force is equal to the resistive force, leading to no visible change in the muscle length (5,9). As the muscle shortens, elastic components of the muscle lengthen. The muscle is shortening; however, there is no movement of the joint.

In all activities, isometric actions dynamically stabilize the body. This can be seen when stabilizers isometrically contract to restrict a limb from moving in an unwanted direction. For example, when walking, the hip adductors and abductors will dynamically stabilize the leg and pelvis from excessive movements in the frontal and transverse planes (Figure 2-9) (4,9,15).

CONCENTRIC

A concentric muscle action occurs when the contractile force is greater than the resistive force, resulting in

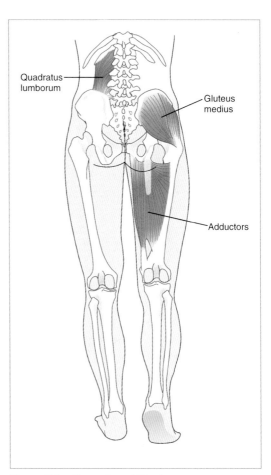

Figure 2.9 Dynamic stabilization.

shortening of the muscle and visible joint movement. This is referred to as the "positive" during integrated resistance training (5,11). All movements require concentric muscle actions.

Muscular Force

Force: an influence applied by one object to another, which results in an acceleration or deceleration of the second object.

A **force** is defined as the interaction between two entities or bodies that result in either the acceleration or deceleration of an object (1,4,5,7). Forces are characterized by both magnitude (how strong) and direction (which way they are moving) (1,5). The HMS manipulates variable forces from a multitude of directions to effectively produce movement. As such, the health and fitness professional must gain an understanding of some of the more pertinent mechanical factors that affect force development that the HMS must deal with and how motion is affected.

GETTING YOUR FACTS STRAIGHT

Forces and Their Effect on the HMS

Every time one takes a step, gravity and momentum forces the body down onto the ground. The ground then exerts an opposite and equal force back onto the body up through the foot. This is known as ground reaction force (1). Ground reaction force places further stresses through the HMS. Not only do we have gravity pushing us downward, but also we have ground reaction force pushing from below back up through the body. As the speed and amplitude of movement increases so does the ground reaction force (2). While walking, ground reaction force can be *1 to 1.5 times* one's body weight (3), *2 to 5 times* one's body weight during running (3) and *4 to 11 times* one's body weight when jumping (4). This is important for a health and fitness professional to note when designing a proper program. Think of a 150-pound person who goes jogging or a person walking up and down stairs. They must withstand approximately 300 to 600 pounds of force on one leg, each and every step, in an unstable, unpredictable environment. Thus, a program must be designed to help individuals be able to control themselves (decelerate and dynamically stabilize) against these forces and decrease their risk of injury.

1. Hamill J, Knutzen JM. Biomechanical Basis of Human Movement. Baltimore, MD: Williams & Wilkins; 1995.
2. Voloshin A. The influence of walking speed on dynamic loading on the human musculoskeletal system. *Med Sci Sports Exerc* 2000;32:1156–9.
3. Brett GA, Whalen RT. Prediction of human gait parameters from temporal measures of foot-ground contact. *Med Sci Sports Exerc* 1997;29:540–7.
4. Witzke KA, Snow CM. Effects of plyometric jumping on bone mass in adolescent girls. *Med Sci Sports Exerc* 2000;32:1051–7.

LENGTH-TENSION RELATIONSHIPS

Length-tension relationship: the resting length of a muscle and the tension the muscle can produce at this resting length.

Length-tension relationship refers to the resting length of a muscle and the tension the muscle can produce at this resting length (1,6,16,17). There is an optimal muscle length at which the actin and myosin filaments in the sarcomere have the greatest degree of overlap (Figure 2-10). The thick myosin filament is able to make the maximal amount of connections with active sites on the thin actin filament, leading to maximal tension development of that muscle. When the muscle is stimulated at lengths greater than or less than this optimal length, the resulting tension is less because there are fewer interactions of the myosin cross-bridges and actin active sites (1,5,6,16-18).

This concept is important to the health and fitness professional and coincides with the previously discussed concept of joint alignment. The starting point for a lift, the proper posture, the ability (or inability) to develop tension when reacting or correcting a movement are all impacted by the length of the muscle when stimulated. Just as the position of one joint can drastically affect other joints, a change in joint angle can affect the tension produced by muscles that surround the joint. If muscle length is altered as a result of misalignment (i.e., poor posture), then tension development will be reduced and the muscle will be unable to generate proper force for efficient movement. With movement at one joint being interdependent on movement or preparation for movement of other joints, any dysfunction in the chain of events producing movement will have direct effects elsewhere (2,10).

FORCE-VELOCITY CURVE AND FORCE-COUPLE RELATIONSHIPS

Force-velocity curve: the relationship of a muscle's ability to produce tension at differing shortening velocities.

The **force-velocity curve** refers to the relationship of a muscle's ability to produce tension at differing shortening velocities. This hyperbolic relationship shows that as the velocity of a concentric contraction increases, the developed tension decreases (Figure 2-11). The velocity of shortening appears to be related to the maximum rate at which the cross-bridges can cycle and be influenced by the external load (17). Conversely, with eccentric muscle action, as the velocity of muscle action increases, the ability to develop force increases. This is believed to be the result of the use of the elastic component of the connective tissue surrounding and within the muscle (1,4–6,16–18).

Force-couple: the synergistic action of muscles to produce movement around a joint.

Muscles produce a force that is transmitted to bones through elastic and connective tissues (tendons). Because muscles are recruited as groups, many muscles will transmit force onto their respective bones, creating movement at the joints (1,5,8). This synergistic action of muscles to produce movement around a joint is also known as a **force-couple** (1,5,8). Muscles in a force-couple provide divergent tension to the bone or bones to which they attach. Because each muscle has different attachment sites and lever systems, the tension at different angles creates a different force on that joint. The motion that results from these forces depends on the structure of the joint, the intrinsic properties of each fiber, and the collective pull of each muscle involved (Figure 2-12).

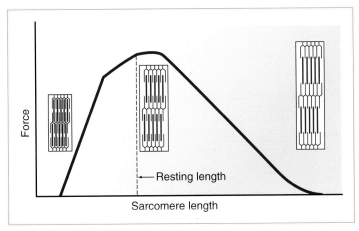

Figure 2.10 Length-tension relationships.

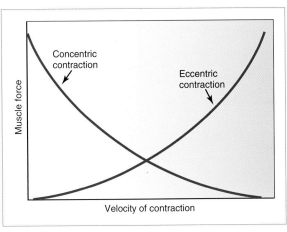

Figure 2.11 Force-velocity curves.

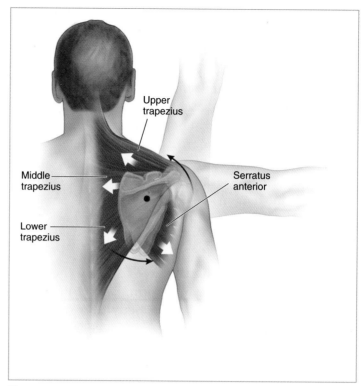

Figure 2.12   Force-couple relationships.

In reality, however, every movement we produce must involve all muscle actions (eccentric, isometric, concentric) and functions (agonists, synergists, stabilizers, and antagonists) to ensure proper joint motion as well as minimize

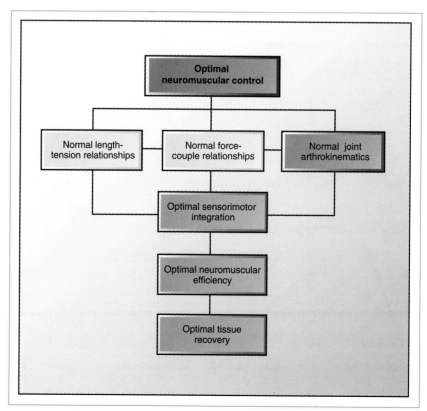

Figure 2.13   Efficient human movement.

unwanted motion. Therefore, all muscles working together for the production of proper movement are working in a force-couple (1,5,8). Proper force-couple relationships are needed so that the HMS moves in the desired manner. This can only happen if the muscles are at the optimal length-tension relationships and the joints have proper arthrokinematics (or joint motion). Collectively, optimal length-tension relationships, force-couple relationships, and arthrokinematics produce ideal sensorimotor integration and ultimately proper and efficient movement (2,3) (Figure 2-13).

Muscular Leverage and Arthrokinematics

The amount of force that the human movement system can produce depends not only on motor unit recruitment and muscle size but also on the lever system of the joint (1,4). A lever system is composed of some force (muscles), a resistance (load to be moved), lever arms (bones), and a fulcrum (the pivot point). Three classes of levers are present in the body (Figure 2-14). A first class lever has the fulcrum between the force/effort(E) and the load/resistance(R). A second class lever has the load between the force and the fulcrum. Third class levers, the most common in the body, have the pull between the load and the fulcrum.

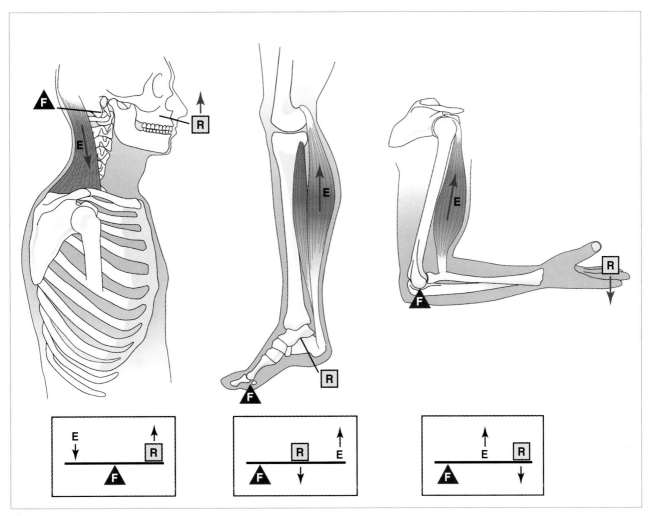

Figure 2.14   Levers.

Rotary motion: movement of the bones around the joints.

Torque: a force that produces rotation. Common unit of torque is the newton-meter or N·m.

In the HMS, the bones act as lever arms that move a load from the force applied by the muscles. This movement around an axis can be termed **rotary motion** and implies that the levers (bones) rotate around the axis (joints) (4,5,9). This "turning" effect of the joint is often referred to as **torque** (10,19).

In resistance training, torque (distance from the load to the center of the axis of rotation X the force) is applied so we can move our joints. Because the neuromuscular system is ultimately responsible for manipulating force, the amount of leverage the HMS will have (for any given movement) depends on the leverage of the muscles in relation to the resistance. The difference between the distance that the weight is from the center of the joint, the muscle's attachment and it's line of pull (direction through which tension is applied through the tendon) will determine the efficiency with which the muscles manipulate the movement (1,4,5,9). Because we cannot alter the attachment sites or the line of pull of our muscles through the tendon, the easiest way to alter the amount of torque generated at a joint is to move the resistance. In other words, the closer the weight is to the point of rotation (the joint), the less torque it creates (Figure 2-15). The farther away the weight is from the point of rotation, the more torque it creates.

For example, to hold a dumbbell straight out to the side at arm's length (shoulder abduction), the weight may be approximately 24 inches from the center of the shoulder joint. The prime mover for shoulder abduction is the deltoid muscle. Let's say its attachment is approximately two inches from the joint center. That is a disparity of 22 inches (or roughly 12 times the difference). If the weight is moved closer to the joint center, let's say to the

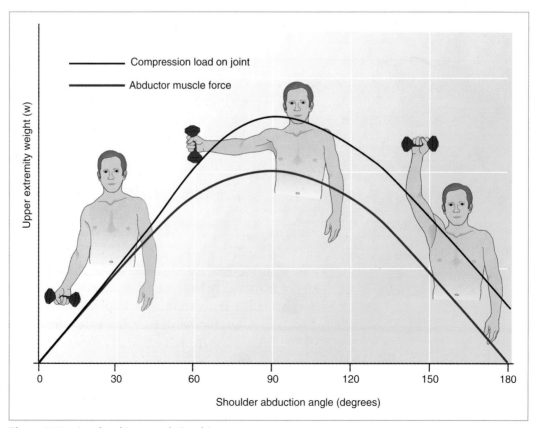

Figure 2.15 Load and torque relationship.

elbow, the resistance is only approximately 12 inches from the joint center. Now the difference is only 10 inches or five times greater. Essentially, the torque required to hold the weight was reduced by half. Many people performing side lateral raises with dumbbells (laterally raising dumbbells to the side) do this inadvertently by flexing their elbow, bringing the weight closer to the shoulder joint and effectively reducing the required torque. Health and fitness professionals can use this principle as a regression for exercises that are too demanding, reducing the torque placed on the HMS, or as a progression to increase the torque and place a greater demand on the HMS.

FUNCTIONAL ANATOMY

Traditionally, anatomy has been taught in isolated, fragmented components. The traditional approach mapped the body, provided simplistic answers about the structures, and categorized each component. Looking at each muscle as an isolated structure fails to answer complex questions, such as "How does the human movement system function as an integrated system?" Or even more simply, "What do our muscles do when we move?" The everyday functioning of the human body is an integrated and multidimensional system, not a series of isolated, independent pieces. During the last 25 years, traditional training has focused on training specific body parts, often in single, fixed planes of motion. The new paradigm is to present anatomy from a functional, integrated perspective. The health and fitness professional armed with a thorough understanding of functional anatomy will be better equipped to select exercises and design programs.

Although muscles have the ability to dominate a certain plane of motion, the central nervous system optimizes the selection of muscle synergies (1,20–25), not simply the selection of individual muscles. The central nervous system coordinates deceleration, stabilization, and acceleration at every joint in the HMS in all three planes of motion. Muscles must also react proprioceptively to gravity, momentum, ground reaction forces, and forces created by other functioning muscles. Depending on the load, the direction of resistance, body position, and the movement being performed, muscles will participate as an agonist, antagonist, synergist, or stabilizer. Although they may have different characteristics, all muscles work in concert with one another to produce efficient motion (1,23,24,26,27). **Agonists** are muscles that act as prime movers. For example, the gluteus maximus is the prime mover for hip extension. **Antagonists** are muscles that act in direct opposition to prime movers. For example, the psoas (hip flexor) is antagonistic to the gluteus maximus. **Synergists** are muscles that assist prime movers during functional movement patterns. For example, the hamstring complex and the erector spinae are synergists to the gluteus maximus during hip extension. **Stabilizer** muscles support or stabilize the body while the prime movers and the synergists perform the movement patterns. For example, the transversus abdominus, internal oblique, multifidus, and deep erector spinae muscles stabilize the lumbo-pelvic-hip complex (LPHC) during functional movements while the prime movers and synergists perform functional activities.

Agonists: muscles that act as prime movers.

Antagonists: muscles that act in direct opposition to prime movers.

Synergists: muscles that assist prime movers during functional movement patterns.

Stabilizers: muscles that support or stabilize the body while the prime movers and the synergists perform the movement patterns.

Traditional training has focused almost exclusively on uniplanar, concentric force production. But this is a shortsighted approach as muscles function synergistically in force-couples to produce force, reduce force, and dynamically stabilize the entire HMS; they function in integrated groups to provide control during functional movements (5,8,9,28). Realizing this allows one to view muscles functioning in all planes of motion throughout the full spectrum of muscle action (eccentric, concentric, isometric).

Current Concepts in Functional Anatomy

It has been proposed that there are two distinct, yet interdependent, muscular systems that enable our bodies to maintain proper stabilization and ensure efficient distribution of forces for the production of movement (28–30). Muscles that are located more centrally to the spine provide intersegmental stability (support from vertebra to vertebra), whereas the more lateral muscles support the spine as a whole (30). Bergmark (28) categorized these different systems in relation to the trunk into local and global muscular systems.

JOINT SUPPORT SYSTEM

The Local Muscular System (Stabilization System)

Local musculature system: muscles that are predominantly involved in joint support or stabilization.

The **local musculature system** consists of muscles that are predominantly involved in joint support or stabilization (3,28–31) (Figure 2-16). It is important to note, however, that joint support systems are not confined to the spine and are evident in peripheral joints as well. Joint support systems consist of muscles that are not movement specific, rather they provide stability to allow movement of a joint. They are usually located in close proximity to the joint with a broad spectrum of attachments to the joint's passive elements that make them ideal for increasing joint stiffness and stability (3,31). A common example of a peripheral joint support system is the rotator cuff that provides dynamic stabilization for the humeral head in relation to the glenoid fossa (32–35). Other joint support systems include the posterior fibers of the gluteus medius and the external rotators of the hip that provide pelvofemoral stabilization (1,36–39) and the oblique fibers of the vastus medialis that provides patellar stabilization at the knee (1,40,41).

The joint support system of the core or LPHC includes muscles that either originate or insert (or both) into the lumbar spine (28,31). The major muscles include the transversus abdominis, multifidus, internal oblique, diaphragm, and the muscles of the pelvic floor (13,28,30,31).

THE GLOBAL MUSCULAR SYSTEMS (MOVEMENT SYSTEMS)

Global muscular systems: muscles responsible predominantly for movement and consisting of more superficial musculature that originates from the pelvis to the rib cage, the lower extremities, or both.

The **global muscular systems** are responsible predominantly for movement and consist of more superficial musculature that originate from the pelvis to the rib cage, the lower extremities, or both (1,23,24,28,30,31,42) (Figure 2-17). Some of these major muscles include the rectus abdominis, external obliques, erector spinae, hamstring complex, gluteus maximus, latissimus dorsi, adductors, quadriceps, and gastrocnemius. The movement system muscles are predominantly larger and associated with movements of the trunk and limbs that equalize external loads placed on the body. These muscles are also important in transferring and absorbing forces from the upper and lower extremities

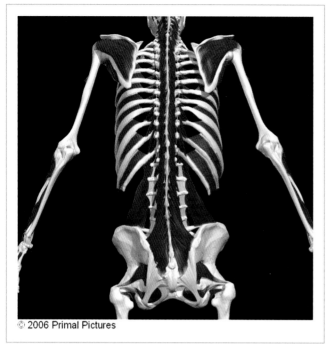

© 2006 Primal Pictures

Figure 2.16   Local muscular system.

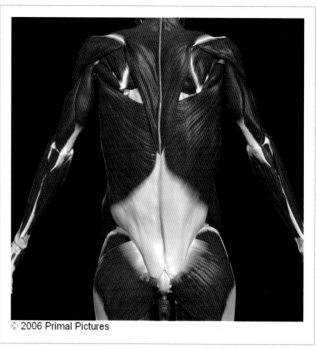

© 2006 Primal Pictures

Figure 2.17   Global muscular system.

to the pelvis. The movement system muscles have been broken down and described as force-couples working in four distinct subsystems (1,29,43,44):

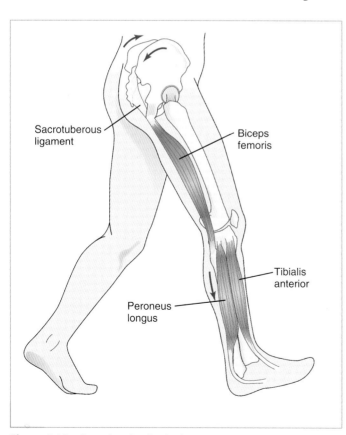

Sacrotuberous ligament

Biceps femoris

Tibialis anterior

Peroneus longus

Figure 2.18   Deep longitudinal sub-system.

the deep longitudinal, posterior oblique, anterior oblique, and lateral subsystems. This distinction allows for an easier description and review of functional anatomy. It is crucial for health and fitness professionals to think of these subsystems operating as an integrated functional unit. Remember, the central nervous system optimizes the selection of muscle synergies, not isolated muscles (23,24,45,46).

The Deep Longitudinal Subsystem (DLS)
The major soft tissue contributors to the deep longitudinal subsystem are the erector spinae, thoracolumbar fascia, sacrotuberous ligament biceps femoris, and peroneus longus (Figure 2-18). Some experts suggest that the DLS provides a longitudinal means of reciprocal force transmission from the trunk to the ground (13,23,24,43,44). As illustrated in Figure 2-18, the long head of the biceps femoris attaches in part to the sacrotuberous ligament at the ischium. The sacrotuberous ligament in turn attaches from the ischium to the sacrum. The erector spinae attach from the sacrum and

ilium up the ribs to the cervical spine. Thus, activation of the biceps femoris increases tension in the sacrotuberous ligament, which in turn transmits force across the sacrum, stabilizing the sacroiliac joint, then up the trunk through the erector spinae (43,44) (Figure 2-18).

As illustrated in Figure 2-18, this transference of force is apparent during normal gait. Before heel strike, the biceps femoris activates to eccentrically decelerate hip flexion and knee extension. Just after heel strike, the biceps femoris is further loaded through the lower leg via posterior movement of the fibula. This tension from the lower leg, up through the biceps femoris, into the sacrotuberous ligament, and up the erector spinae creates a force that assists in stabilizing the sacroiliac joint (SIJ) (12).

Another force-couple not often mentioned in this subsystem consists of the superficial erector spinae, the psoas, and the intrinsic core stabilizers (transverses abdominus, multifidus). Although the erector spinae and psoas create lumbar extension and an anterior shear force at L4 through S1, during functional movements the local muscular system provides intersegmental stabilization and a posterior shear force (29,31,43,44,47,48). Dysfunction in any of these structures can lead to SIJ instability and low-back pain (LBP) (44).

The Posterior Oblique Subsystem (POS)

The posterior oblique subsystem works synergistically with the DLS. As illustrated in Figure 2-19, both the gluteus maximus and latissimus dorsi have attachments to the thoracolumbar fascia, which connects to the sacrum, whose fibers run perpendicular to the SIJ. Thus, when the contralateral gluteus maximus and latissimus dorsi contract, a stabilizing force is transmitted across the SIJ (force closure) (44). Just before heel strike, the latissimus dorsi and the contralateral gluteus maximus are eccentrically loaded. At heel strike, each muscle accelerates its respective limb (through its concentric action) and creates tension across the thoracolumbar fascia. This tension also assists in stabilizing the SIJ. Thus, when an individual walks or runs, the POS transfers forces that are summated from the muscle's transverse plane orientation to propulsion in the

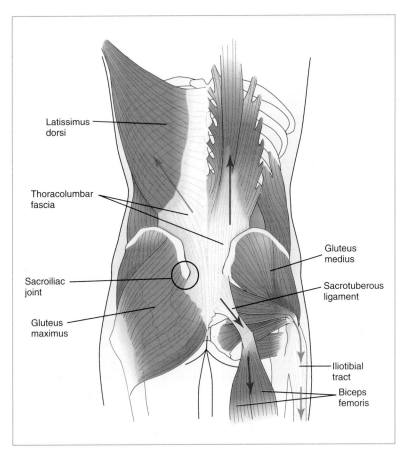

Latissimus dorsi

Thoracolumbar fascia

Sacroiliac joint

Gluteus maximus

Gluteus medius

Sacrotuberous ligament

Iliotibial tract

Biceps femoris

Figure 2.19   Posterior oblique sub-system.

sagittal plane. The POS is also of prime importance for rotational activities such as swinging a golf club or a baseball bat, or throwing a ball (29,43,47). Dysfunction of any structure in the POS can lead to SIJ instability and LBP. The weakening of the gluteus maximus, the latissimus dorsi, or both can lead to increased tension in the hamstring complex—a factor in recurrent hamstring strains (42,44,47). If performed in isolation, squats for the gluteus maximus and pulldowns/pull-ups for the latissimus dorsi will not adequately prepare the POS to perform optimally during functional activities.

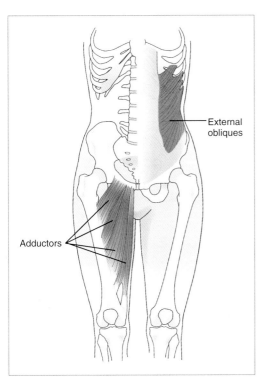

Figure 2.20 Anterior oblique sub-system.

The Anterior Oblique Subsystem (AOS)

The anterior oblique subsystem (Figure 2-20) is similar to the POS in that it also functions in a transverse plane orientation, mostly in the anterior portion of the body. The prime contributors are the internal and external oblique muscles, the adductor complex, and hip external rotators. Electromyography of these AOS muscles show that they aid in pelvic stability and rotation as well as contributing to leg swing (11,12,14). The AOS is also a factor in the stabilization of the SIJ (48).

When we walk, our pelvis rotates in the transverse plane to create a swinging motion for the legs (43). The POS (posteriorly) and the AOS (anteriorly) contribute to this rotation. Knowing the fiber arrangements of the muscles involved (latissimus dorsi, gluteus maximus, internal and external obliques, adductors, and hip rotators) emphasizes this point. The AOS is also necessary for functional activities involving the trunk and upper and lower extremities. The obliques, in concert with the adductor complex, not only produce rotational and flexion movements, but are also instrumental in stabilizing the lumbo-pelvic-hip complex (29,48).

The Lateral Subsystem (LS)

The lateral subsystem is composed of the gluteus medius, tensor fascia latae, adductor complex, and the quadratus lumborum, all of which participate in frontal plane (13) and pelvofemoral stability (10,49). Figure 2-21 shows how the ipsilateral gluteus medius, tensor fascia latae, and adductors combine with the contralateral quadratus lumborum to control the pelvis and femur in the frontal plane during single leg functional movements such as in gait, lunges, or stair climbing (42). Dysfunction in the LS is evident during increased subtalar joint pronation in conjunction with increased tibial and femoral adduction and internal rotation during functional activities (10). Unwanted frontal plane movement is characterized by decreased strength and decreased neuromuscular control in the LS (10,49–51).

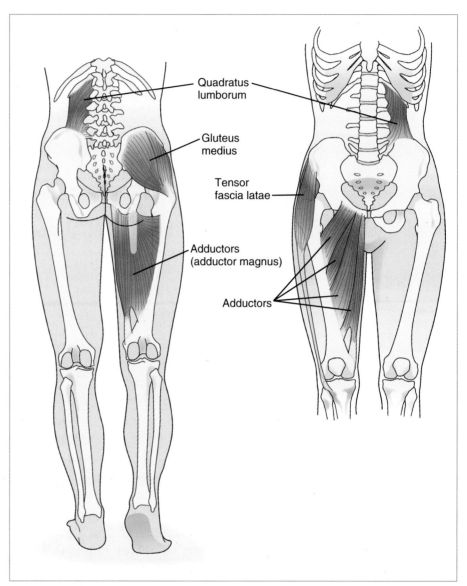

Quadratus lumborum

Gluteus medius

Tensor fascia latae

Adductors (adductor magnus)

Adductors

Figure 2.21 Lateral sub-system.

The descriptions of these four systems have been simplified, but realize that the human body simultaneously coordinates these subsystems during activity. Each system individually and collectively contributes to the production of efficient movement by accelerating, decelerating, and dynamically stabilizing the HMS during motion.

Functional Anatomy of the Major Muscles

The traditional, simplistic explanation of skeletal muscles is that they work concentrically and predominantly in one plane of motion. However, muscles should be viewed as functioning in all planes of motion, throughout the full muscle action spectrum. The following section lists attachments and innervations as well as the isolated and integrated functions of the major muscles of the human movement system (1,6,52).

LEG COMPLEX

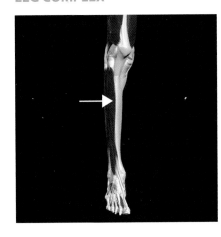

ANTERIOR TIBIALIS

ORIGIN
- Lateral condyle and proximal two-thirds of the lateral surface of the tibia

INSERTION
- Medial and plantar aspects of the medial cuneiform and the base of the first metatarsal

ISOLATED FUNCTION
Concentric Action
- Ankle dorsiflexion and inversion

INTEGRATED FUNCTION
Eccentric Action
- Ankle plantar flexion and eversion

Isometric Action
- Stabilizes the arch of the foot

INNERVATION
- Deep peroneal nerve

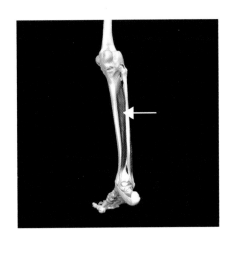

POSTERIOR TIBIALIS

ORIGIN
- Proximal two-thirds of posterior surface of the tibia and fibula

INSERTION
- Every tarsal bone (navicular, cuneiform, cuboid) but the talus plus the bases of the second through the fourth metatarsal bones. The main insertion is on the navicular tuberosity and the medial cuneiform bone

ISOLATED FUNCTION
Concentric Action
- Ankle plantar flexion and inversion of the foot

INTEGRATED FUNCTION
Eccentric Action
- Ankle dorsiflexion and eversion

Isometric Action
- Stabilizes the arch of the foot

INNERVATION
- Tibial nerve

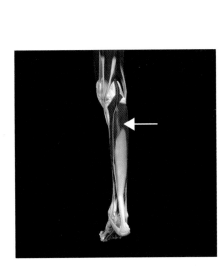

SOLEUS

ORIGIN
- Posterior surface of the fibular head and proximal one-third of its shaft and from the posterior side of the tibia

INSERTION
- Calcaneus via the Achilles tendon

ISOLATED FUNCTION
Concentric Action
- Accelerates plantar flexion

INTEGRATED FUNCTION
Eccentric Action
- Decelerates ankle dorsiflexion

Isometric Action
- Stabilizes the foot and ankle complex

INNERVATION
- Tibial nerve

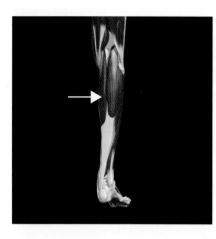

GASTROCNEMIUS

ORIGIN
- Posterior aspect of the lateral and medial femoral condyles

INSERTION
- Calcaneus via the Achilles tendon

ISOLATED FUNCTION

Concentric Action
- Accelerates plantar flexion

INTEGRATED FUNCTION

Eccentric Action
- Decelerates ankle dorsiflexion

Isometric Action
- Isometrically stabilizes the foot and ankle complex

INNERVATION
- Tibial nerve

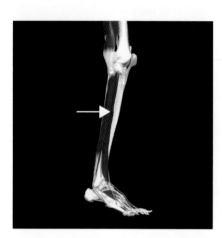

PERONEUS LONGUS

ORIGIN
- Lateral condyle of tibia, head and proximal two-thirds of the lateral surface of the fibula

INSERTION
- Lateral surface of the medial cuneiform and lateral side of the base of the first metatarsal

ISOLATED FUNCTION

Concentric Action
- Plantar flexes and everts the foot

INTEGRATED FUNCTION

Eccentric Action
- Decelerates ankle dorsiflexion and inversion

Isometric Action
- Stabilizes the foot and ankle complex

INNERVATION
- Superficial peroneal nerve

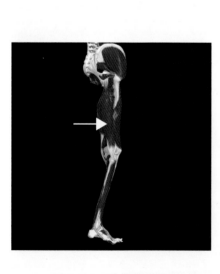

BICEPS FEMORIS-LONG HEAD

ORIGIN
- Ischial tuberosity of the pelvis, part of the sacrotuberous ligament

INSERTION
- Head of the fibula

ISOLATED FUNCTION

Concentric Action
- Accelerates knee flexion and hip extension, tibial external rotation

INTEGRATED FUNCTION

Eccentric Action
- Decelerates knee extension, hip flexion, and tibial internal rotation

Isometric Action
- Stabilizes the lumbo-pelvic-hip complex and knee

INNERVATION
- Tibial nerve

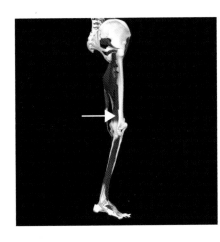

BICEPS FEMORIS-SHORT HEAD

ORIGIN
- Lower one-third of the posterior aspect of the femur

INSERTION
- Head of the fibula

ISOLATED FUNCTION
Concentric Action
- Accelerates knee flexion and tibial external rotation

INTEGRATED FUNCTION
Eccentric Action
- Decelerates knee extension and tibial internal rotation

Isometric Action
- Stabilizes the knee

INNERVATION
- Common peroneal nerve

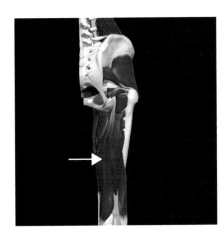

SEMIMEMBRANOSUS

ORIGIN
- Ischial tuberosity of the pelvis

INSERTION
- Posterior aspect of the medial tibial condyle of the tibia

ISOLATED FUNCTION
Concentric Action
- Accelerates knee flexion, hip extension and tibial internal rotation

INTEGRATED FUNCTION
Eccentric Action
- Decelerates knee extension, hip flexion and tibial external rotation

Isometric Action
- Stabilizes the lumbo-pelvic-hip complex and knee

INNERVATION
- Tibial nerve

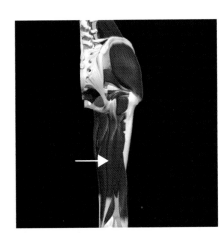

SEMITENDINOSUS

ORIGIN
- Ischial tuberosity of the pelvis and part of the sacrotuberous ligament

INSERTION
- Proximal aspect of the medial tibial condyle of the tibia (pes anserine)

ISOLATED FUNCTION
Concentric Action
- Accelerates knee flexion, hip extension and tibial internal rotation

INTEGRATED FUNCTION
Eccentric Action
- Decelerates knee extension, hip flexion and tibial external rotation

Isometric Action
- Stabilizes the lumbo-pelvic-hip complex and knee

INNERVATION
- Tibial nerve

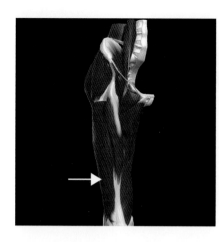

VASTUS LATERALIS

ORIGIN
- Anterior and inferior border of the greater trochanter, lateral region of the gluteal tuberosity, lateral lip of the linea aspera of the femur

INSERTION
- Base of patella and tibial tuberosity of the tibia

ISOLATED FUNCTION

Concentric Action
- Accelerates knee extension

INTEGRATED FUNCTION

Eccentric Action
- Decelerates knee flexion

Isometric Action
- Stabilizes the knee

INNERVATION
- Femoral nerve

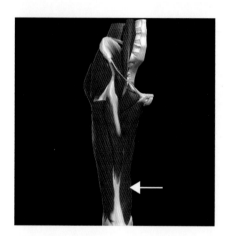

VASTUS MEDIALIS

ORIGIN
- Lower region of intertrochanteric line, medial lip of linea aspera, proximal medial supracondylar line of the femur

INSERTION
- Base of patella, tibial tuberosity of the tibia

ISOLATED FUNCTION

Concentric Action
- Accelerates knee extension

INTEGRATED FUNCTION

Eccentric Action
- Decelerates knee flexion

Isometric Action
- Stabilizes the knee

INNERVATION
- Femoral nerve

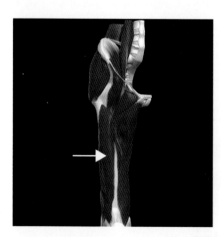

VASTUS INTERMEDIUS

ORIGIN
- Anterior-lateral regions of the upper two-thirds of the femur

INSERTION
- Base of patella, tibial tuberosity of the tibia

ISOLATED FUNCTION

Concentric Action
- Accelerates knee extension

INTEGRATED FUNCTION

Eccentric Action
- Decelerates knee flexion

Isometric Action
- Stabilizes the knee

INNERVATION
- Femoral nerve

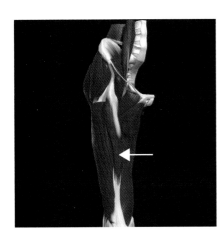

RECTUS FEMORIS

ORIGIN
- Anterior-inferior iliac spine of the pelvis

INSERTION
- Base of patella, tibial tuberosity of the tibia

ISOLATED FUNCTION

Concentric Action
- Accelerates knee extension and hip flexion

INTEGRATED FUNCTION

Eccentric Action
- Decelerates knee flexion and hip extension

Isometric Action
- Stabilizes the lumbo-pelvic-hip complex and knee

INNERVATION
- Femoral nerve

HIP COMPLEX

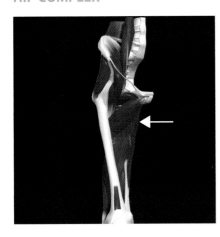

ADDUCTOR LONGUS

ORIGIN
- Anterior surface of the inferior pubic ramus of the pelvis

INSERTION
- Proximal one-third of the linea aspera of the femur

ISOLATED FUNCTION

Concentric Action
- Accelerates hip adduction, flexion and internal rotation

INTEGRATED FUNCTION

Eccentric Action
- Decelerates hip abduction, extension and external rotation

Isometric Action
- Stabilizes the lumbo-pelvic-hip complex

INNERVATION
- Obturator nerve

ADDUCTOR MAGNUS, ANTERIOR FIBERS

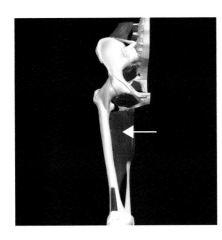

ORIGIN
- Ischial ramus of the pelvis

INSERTION
- Linea aspera of the femur

ISOLATED FUNCTION

Concentric Action
- Accelerates hip adduction, flexion and internal rotation

INTEGRATED FUNCTION

Eccentric Action
- Decelerates hip abduction, extension and external rotation

Isometric Action
- Stabilizes the lumbo-pelvic-hip complex

INNERVATION
- Obturator nerve

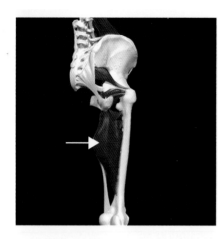

ADDUCTOR MAGNUS, POSTERIOR FIBERS

ORIGIN
- Ischial tuberosity of the pelvis

INSERTION
- Adductor tubercle on femur

ISOLATED FUNCTION
Concentric Action
- Accelerates hip adduction, extension and external rotation

INTEGRATED FUNCTION
Eccentric Action
- Decelerates hip abduction, flexion and internal rotation
Isometric Action
- Stabilizes the lumbo-pelvic-hip complex

INNERVATION
- Sciatic nerve

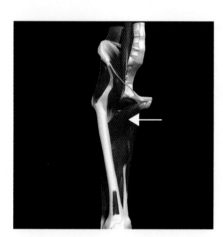

ADDUCTOR BREVIS

ORIGIN
- Anterior surface of the inferior pubic ramus of the pelvis

INSERTION
- Proximal one-third of the linea aspera of the femur

ISOLATED FUNCTION
Concentric Action
- Accelerates hip adduction, flexion and internal rotation

INTEGRATED FUNCTION
Eccentric Action
- Decelerates hip abduction, extension and external rotation
Isometric Action
- Stabilizes the lumbo-pelvic-hip complex

INNERVATION
- Obturator nerve

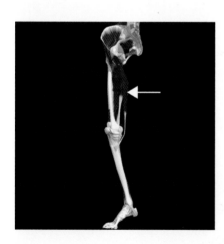

GRACILIS

ORIGIN
- Anterior aspect of lower body of pubis

INSERTION
- Proximal medial surface of the tibia (pes anserine)

ISOLATED FUNCTION
Concentric Action
- Accelerates hip adduction, flexion and internal rotation; assists in tibial internal rotation

INTEGRATED FUNCTION
Eccentric Action
- Decelerates hip abduction, extension and external rotation
Isometric Action
- Stabilizes the lumbo-pelvic-hip complex and knee

INNERVATION
- Obturator nerve

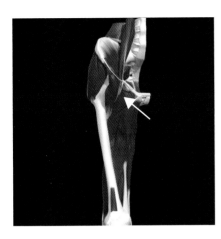

PECTINEUS

ORIGIN
- Pectineal line on the superior pubic ramus of the pelvis

INSERTION
- Pectineal line on the posterior surface of the upper femur

ISOLATED FUNCTION

Concentric Action
- Accelerates hip adduction, flexion and internal rotation

INTEGRATED FUNCTION

Eccentric Action
- Decelerates hip abduction, extension and external rotation

Isometric Action
- Stabilizes the lumbo-pelvic-hip complex

INNERVATION
- Obturator nerve

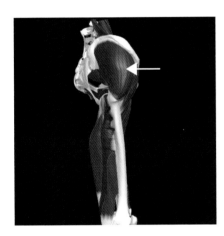

GLUTEUS MEDIUS, ANTERIOR FIBERS

ORIGIN
- Outer surface of the ilium

INSERTION
- Lateral surface of the greater trochanter on the femur

ISOLATED FUNCTION

Concentric Action
- Accelerates hip abduction and internal rotation

INTEGRATED FUNCTION

Eccentric Action
- Decelerates hip adduction and external rotation

Isometric Action
- Dynamically stabilizes the lumbo-pelvic-hip complex

INNERVATION
- Superior gluteal nerve

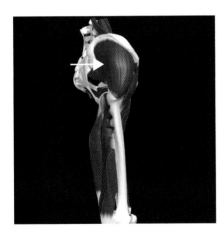

GLUTEUS MEDIUS, POSTERIOR FIBERS

ORIGIN
- Outer surface of the ilium

INSERTION
- Lateral surface of the greater trochanter on the femur

ISOLATED FUNCTION

Concentric Action
- Accelerates hip abduction and external rotation

INTEGRATED FUNCTION

Eccentric Action
- Decelerates hip adduction and internal rotation

Isometric Action
- Stabilizes the lumbo-pelvic-hip complex

INNERVATION
- Superior gluteal nerve

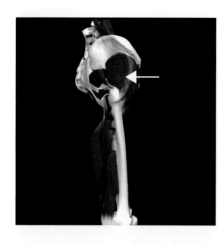

GLUTEUS MINIMUS

ORIGIN
- Ilium between the anterior and inferior gluteal line

INSERTION
- Greater trochanter of the femur

ISOLATED FUNCTION
Concentric Action
- Accelerates hip abduction, flexion, and internal rotation

INTEGRATED FUNCTION
Eccentric Action
- Decelerates frontal plane hip adduction, extension, and external rotation

Isometric Action
- Stabilizes the lumbo-pelvic-hip complex

INNERVATION
- Superior gluteal nerve

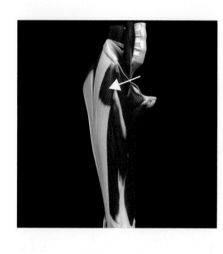

TENSOR FASCIA LATAE

ORIGIN
- Outer surface of the iliac crest just posterior to the anterior-superior iliac spine of the pelvis

INSERTION
- Proximal one-third of the iliotibial band

ISOLATED FUNCTION
Concentric Action
- Accelerates hip flexion, abduction and internal rotation

INTEGRATED FUNCTION
Eccentric Action
- Decelerates hip extension, adduction and external rotation
Isometric Action
- Stabilizes the lumbo-pelvic-hip complex

INNERVATION
- Superior gluteal nerve

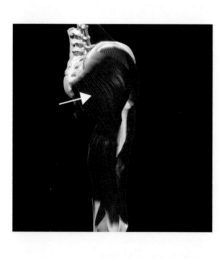

GLUTEUS MAXIMUS

ORIGIN
- Outer ilium, posterior side of sacrum and coccyx and part of the sacrotuberous and posterior sacroiliac ligament

INSERTION
- Gluteal tuberosity of the femur and iliotibial tract

ISOLATED FUNCTION
Concentric Action
- Accelerates hip extension and external rotation

INTEGRATED FUNCTION
Eccentric Action
- Decelerates hip flexion, internal rotation, and tibial internal rotation via the iliotibial band
Isometric Action
- Stabilizes the lumbo-pelvic-hip complex

INNERVATION
- Inferior gluteal nerve

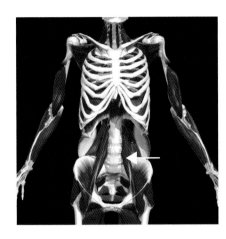

PSOAS

ORIGIN
- Transverse processes and lateral bodies of the last thoracic and all lumbar vertebrae including intervertebral discs

INSERTION
- Lesser trochanter of the femur

ISOLATED FUNCTION
Concentric Action
- Accelerates hip flexion and external rotation, extends and rotates lumbar spine

INTEGRATED FUNCTION
Eccentric Action
- Decelerates hip internal rotation and decelerates hip extension
Isometric Action
- Stabilizes the lumbo-pelvic-hip complex

INNERVATION
- Spinal nerve branches of L2-L4

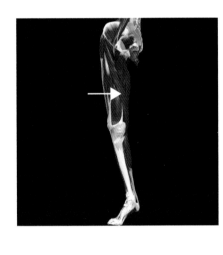

SARTORIUS

ORIGIN
- Anterior-superior iliac spine of the pelvis

INSERTION
- Proximal medial surface of the tibia

ISOLATED FUNCTION
Concentric Action
- Accelerates hip flexion, external rotation and abduction, accelerates knee flexion and internal rotation

INTEGRATED FUNCTION
Eccentric Action
- Decelerates hip extension, external rotation, knee extension and external rotation
Isometric Action
- Stabilizes the lumbo-pelvic-hip complex and knee

INNERVATION
- Femoral nerve

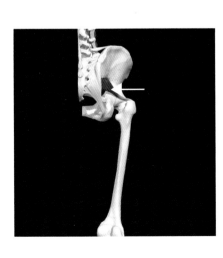

PIRIFORMIS

ORIGIN
- Anterior surface of the sacrum

INSERTION
- The greater trochanter of the femur

ISOLATED FUNCTION
Concentric Action
- Accelerates hip external rotation, abduction and extension

INTEGRATED FUNCTION
Eccentric Action
- Decelerates hip internal rotation, adduction and flexion
Isometric Action
- Stabilizes the hip and sacroiliac joints

INNERVATION
- Sciatic nerve

ABDOMINAL MUSCULATURE

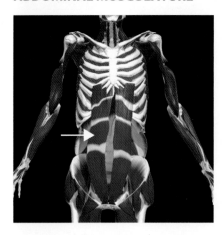

RECTUS ABDOMINIS

ORIGIN
- Pubic symphysis of the pelvis

INSERTION
- Ribs 5-7

ISOLATED FUNCTION
Concentric Action
- Spinal flexion, lateral flexion and rotation

INTEGRATED FUNCTION
Eccentric Action
- Spinal extension, lateral flexion and rotation
Isometric Action
- Stabilizes the lumbo-pelvic-hip complex

INNERVATION
- Intercostal nerve T7-T12

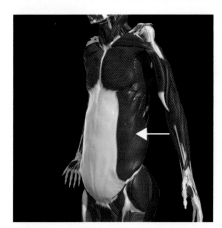

EXTERNAL OBLIQUE

ORIGIN
- External surface of ribs 4-12

INSERTION
- Anterior iliac crest of the pelvis, linea alba and contralateral rectus sheaths

ISOLATED FUNCTION
Concentric Action
- Spinal flexion, lateral flexion and contralateral rotation

INTEGRATED FUNCTION
Eccentric Action
- Spinal extension, lateral flexion and rotation
Isometric Action
- Stabilizes the lumbo-pelvic-hip complex

INNERVATION
- Intercostal nerves (T8-T12), iliohypogastric (L1), ilioinguinal (L1)

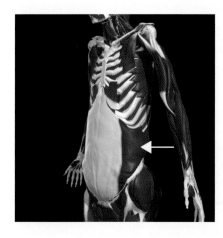

INTERNAL OBLIQUE

ORIGIN
- Anterior two-thirds of the iliac crest of the pelvis and thoracolumbar fascia

INSERTION
- Ribs 9-12, linea alba and contralateral rectus sheaths

ISOLATED FUNCTION
Concentric Action
- Spinal flexion (bilateral), lateral flexion and ipsilateral rotation

INTEGRATED FUNCTION
Eccentric Action
- Spinal extension, rotation and lateral flexion
Isometric Action
- Stabilizes the lumbo-pelvic-hip complex

INNERVATION
- Intercostal nerves (T8-T12), iliohypogastric (L1), ilioinguinal (L1)

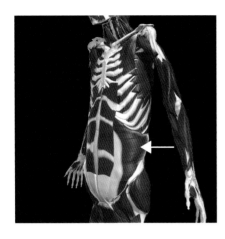

TRANSVERSE ABDOMINIS

ORIGIN
- Ribs 7-12, anterior two-thirds of the iliac crest of the pelvis and thoracolumbar fascia

INSERTION
- Lineae alba and contralateral rectus sheaths

ISOLATED FUNCTION

Concentric Action
- Increases intra-abdominal pressure. Supports the abdominal viscera.

INTEGRATED FUNCTION

Isometric Action
- Synergistically with the internal oblique, multifidus and deep erector spinae to stabilize the lumbo-pelvic-hip complex

INNERVATION
- Intercostal nerves (T7-T12), iliohypogastric (L1), ilioinguinal (L1)

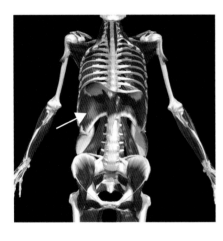

DIAPHRAGM

ORIGIN
- Costal part: inner surfaces of the cartilages and adjacent bony regions of ribs 6-12. Sternal part: posterior side of the xiphoid process. Crural (lumbar) part: (1) two aponeurotic arches covering the external surfaces of the quadratus lumborum and psoas major; (2) right and left crus, originating from the bodies of L1-L3 and their intervertebral discs

INSERTION
- Central tendon

ISOLATED FUNCTION

Concentric Action
- Pulls the central tendon inferiorly, increasing the volume in the thoracic cavity

INTEGRATED FUNCTION

Isometric Action
- Stabilization of the lumbo-pelvic-hip complex

INNERVATION
- Phrenic nerve (C3-C5)

BACK MUSCULATURE

SUPERFICIAL ERECTOR SPINAE

ORIGIN
- Common origin: iliac crest of the pelvis, sacrum, spinous and transverse processes of T1-L5

ILIOCOSTALIS: LUMBORUM DIVISION

ORIGIN
- Common origin

INSERTION
- Inferior border of ribs 7-12

ISOLATED FUNCTION

Concentric Action
- Spinal extension, rotation and lateral flexion

INTEGRATED FUNCTION

Eccentric Action
- Spinal flexion, rotation and lateral flexion

Isometric Action
- Stabilizes the spine during functional movements

INNERVATION
- Dorsal rami of thoracic and lumbar nerves

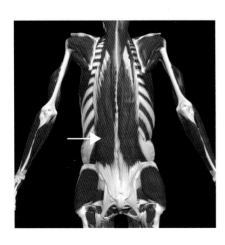

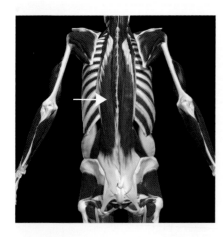

ILIOCOSTALIS: THORACIS DIVISION

ORIGIN
- Common origin

INSERTION
- Superior border of ribs 1-6

ISOLATED FUNCTION

Concentric Action
- Spinal extension, rotation and lateral flexion

INTEGRATED FUNCTION

Eccentric Action
- Spinal flexion, rotation and lateral flexion

Isometric Action
- Stabilizes the spine during functional movements

INNERVATION
- Dorsal rami of thoracic nerves

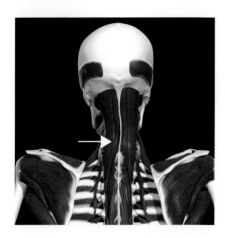

ILIOCOSTALIS: CERVICUS DIVISION

ORIGIN
- Common origin

INSERTION
- Transverse process of C4-C6

ISOLATED FUNCTION

Concentric Action
- Spinal extension, rotation and lateral flexion

INTEGRATED FUNCTION

Eccentric Action
- Spinal flexion, rotation and lateral flexion.

Isometric Action
- Stabilizes the spine during functional movements

INNERVATION
- Dorsal rami of thoracic nerves

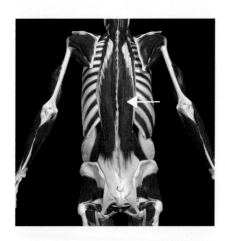

LONGISSIMUS: THORACIS DIVISION

ORIGIN
- Common origin

INSERTION
- Transverse process T1-T12; Ribs 2-12

ISOLATED FUNCTION

Concentric Action
- Spinal extension, rotation and lateral flexion

INTEGRATED FUNCTION

Eccentric Action
- Spinal flexion, rotation and lateral flexion

Isometric Action
- Stabilizes the spine during functional movements

INNERVATION
- Dorsal rami of thoracic and lumbar nerves

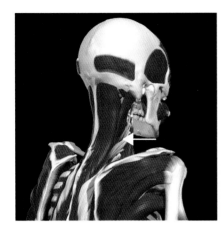

LONGISSIMUS: CERVICUS DIVISION

ORIGIN
- Common origin

INSERTION
- Transverse process of C6-C2

ISOLATED FUNCTION
Concentric Action
- Spinal extension, rotation and lateral flexion

INTEGRATED FUNCTION
Eccentric Action
- Spinal flexion, rotation and lateral flexion
Isometric Action
- Stabilizes the spine during functional movements

INNERVATION
- Dorsal rami of cervical nerves

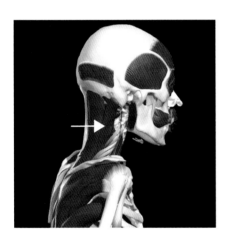

LONGISSIMUS: CAPITIS DIVISION

ORIGIN
- Common origin

INSERTION
- Mastoid process of the skull

ISOLATED FUNCTION
Concentric Action
- Spinal extension, rotation and lateral flexion

INTEGRATED FUNCTION
Eccentric Action
- Spinal flexion, rotation and lateral flexion
Isometric Action
- Stabilizes the spine during functional movements

INNERVATION
- Dorsal rami of cervical nerves

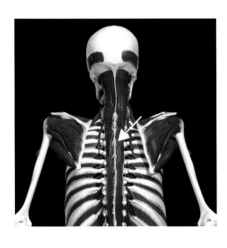

SPINALIS: THORACIS DIVISION

ORIGIN
- Common origin

INSERTION
- Spinous process of T7-T4

ISOLATED FUNCTION
Concentric Action
- Spinal extension, rotation and lateral flexion

INTEGRATED FUNCTION
Eccentric Action
- Spinal flexion, rotation and lateral flexion
Isometric Action
- Stabilizes the spine during functional movements

INNERVATION
- Dorsal rami of thoracic nerves

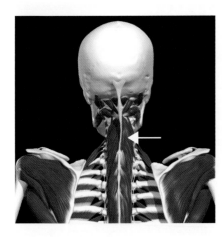

SPINALIS: CERVICUS DIVISION

ORIGIN
- Common origin

INSERTION
- Spinous process of C3-C2

ISOLATED FUNCTION
Concentric Action
- Spinal extension, rotation and lateral flexion

INTEGRATED FUNCTION
Eccentric Action
- Spinal flexion, rotation and lateral flexion
Isometric Action
- Stabilizes the spine during functional movements

INNERVATION
- Dorsal rami of cervical nerves

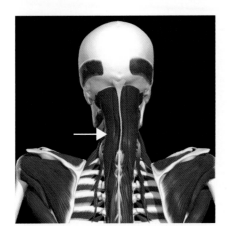

SPINALIS: CAPITIS DIVISION

ORIGIN
- Common origin

INSERTION
- Between the superior and inferior nuchal lines on occipital bone of the skull

ISOLATED FUNCTION
Concentric Action
- Spinal extension, rotation and lateral flexion

INTEGRATED FUNCTION
Eccentric Action
- Spinal flexion, rotation and lateral flexion
Isometric Action
- Stabilizes the spine during functional movements

INNERVATION
- Dorsal rami of cervical nerves

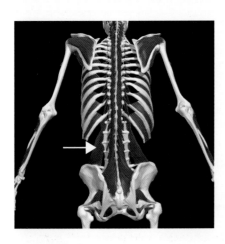

QUADRATUS LUMBORUM

ORIGIN
- Iliac crest of the pelvis

INSERTION
- 12th rib, transverse processes L2-L5

ISOLATED FUNCTION
Concentric Action
- Spinal lateral flexion

INTEGRATED FUNCTION
Eccentric Action
- Decelerates contralateral lateral spinal flexion
Isometric Action
- Stabilizes the lumbo-pelvic-hip complex

INNERVATION
- Spinal nerves (T12-L3)

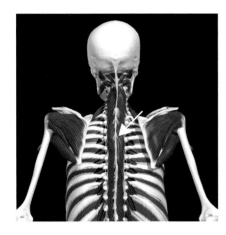

TRANSVERSOSPINALIS: THORACIS DIVISION

ORIGIN
- Transverse process T12-T7

INSERTION
- Spinous process T4-C6

ISOLATED FUNCTION
Concentric Action
- Produces spinal extension and lateral flexion; extension and contralateral rotation of the head

INTEGRATED FUNCTION
Eccentric Action
- Decelerates lateral flexion of the spine, flexion and contralateral rotation of the head

Isometric Action
- Stabilizes the spine

INNERVATION
- Dorsal rami C1-T6 spinal nerves

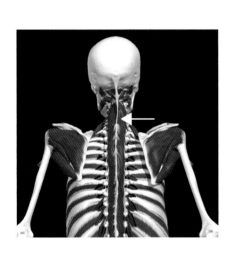

TRANSVERSOSPINALIS: CERVICIS DIVISION

ORIGIN
- Transverse process T6-C4

INSERTION
- Spinous process C5-C2

ISOLATED FUNCTION
Concentric Action
- Produces spinal extension and lateral flexion; extension and contralateral rotation of the head

INTEGRATED FUNCTION
Eccentric Action
- Decelerates lateral flexion of the spine, flexion and contralateral rotation of the head

Isometric Action
- Stabilizes the spine

INNERVATION
- Dorsal rami C1-T6 spinal nerves

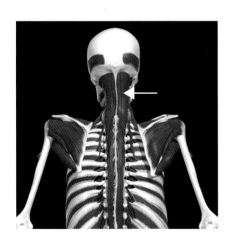

TRANSVERSOSPINALIS: CAPITUS DIVISION

ORIGIN
- Transverse process T6-C7
- Articular process C6-C4

INSERTION
- Nuchal line of occipital bone of the skull

ISOLATED FUNCTION
Concentric Action
- Produces spinal extension and lateral flexion; extension and contralateral rotation of the head

INTEGRATED FUNCTION
Eccentric Action
- Decelerates lateral flexion of the spine, flexion and contralateral rotation of the head

Isometric Action
- Stabilizes the spine

INNERVATION
- Dorsal rami C1-T6 spinal nerves

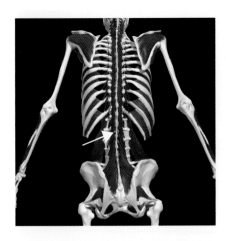

MULTIFIDUS

ORIGIN
- Posterior aspect of the sacrum; Processes of the lumbar, thoracic and cervical spine

INSERTION
- Spinous processes 1 to 4 segments above the origin

ISOLATED FUNCTION

Concentric Action
- Spinal extension and contralateral rotation

INTEGRATED FUNCTION

Eccentric Action
- Spinal flexion and rotation

Isometric Action
- Stabilizes the spine

INNERVATION
- Corresponding spinal nerves

SHOULDER MUSCULATURE

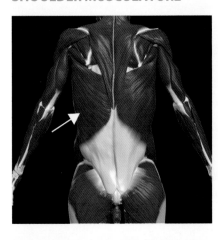

LATISSIMUS DORSI

ORIGIN
- Spinous processes of T7-T12; Iliac crest of the pelvis; Thoracolumbar fascia; Ribs 9-12

INSERTION
- Inferior angle of the scapula; Intertubecular groove of the humerus

ISOLATED FUNCTION

Concentric Action
- Shoulder extension, adduction and internal rotation

INTEGRATED FUNCTION

Eccentric Action
- Shoulder flexion, abduction and external rotation and spinal flexion

Isometric Action
- Stabilizes the lumbo-pelvic-hip complex and shoulder

INNERVATION
- Thoracodorsal nerve (C6-C8)

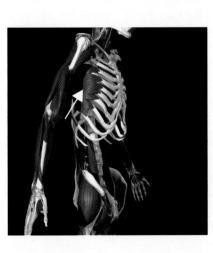

SERRATUS ANTERIOR

ORIGIN
- Ribs 4-12

INSERTION
- Medial border of the scapula

ISOLATED FUNCTION

Concentric Action
- Scapular protraction

INTEGRATED FUNCTION

Eccentric Action
- Scapular retraction

Isometric Action
- Stabilizes the scapula

INNERVATION
- Long thoracic nerve (C5-C7)

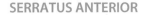

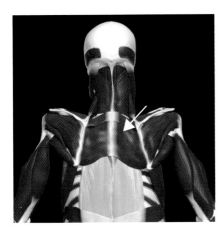

RHOMBOIDS

ORIGIN
- Spinous processes of C7-T5

INSERTION
- Medial border of the scapula

ISOLATED FUNCTION

Concentric Action
- Produces scapular retraction and downward rotation

INTEGRATED FUNCTION

Eccentric Action
- Scapular protraction and upward rotation

Isometric Action
- Stabilizes the scapula

INNERVATION
- Dorsal scapular nerve (C4-C5)

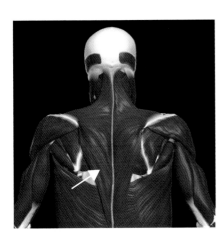

LOWER TRAPEZIUS

ORIGIN
- Spinous processes of T6-T12

INSERTION
- Spine of the scapula

ISOLATED FUNCTION

Concentric Action
- Scapular depression

INTEGRATED FUNCTION

Eccentric Action
- Scapular elevation

Isometric Action
- Stabilizes the scapula

INNERVATION
- Cranial nerve XI, ventral rami C2-C4

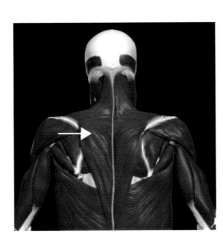

MIDDLE TRAPEZIUS

ORIGIN
- Spinous processes of T1-T5

INSERTION
- Acromion process of the scapula; Superior aspect of the spine of the scapula

ISOLATED FUNCTION

Concentric Action
- Scapular retraction

INTEGRATED FUNCTION

Eccentric Action
- Scapular protraction and elevation

Isometric Action
- Stabilizes scapula

INNERVATION
- Cranial nerve XI, ventral rami C2-C4

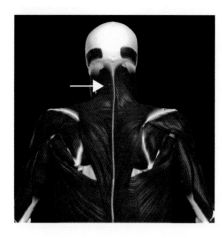

UPPER TRAPEZIUS

ORIGIN
- External occipital protuberance of the skull; Spinous process of C7

INSERTION
- Lateral third of the clavicle; Acromion process of the scapula

ISOLATED FUNCTION
Concentric Action
- Cervical extension, lateral flexion and rotation; scapular elevation

INTEGRATED FUNCTION
Eccentric Action
- Cervical flexion, lateral flexion, rotation, scapular depression

Isometric Action
- Stabilizes the cervical spine and scapula, stabilizes the medial border of the scapula creating a stable base for the prime movers during scapular abduction and upward rotation

INNERVATION
- Cranial nerve XI, ventral rami C2-C4

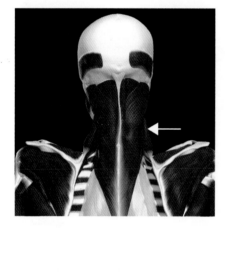

LEVATOR SCAPULAE

ORIGIN
- Transverse processes of C1-C4

INSERTION
- Superior vertebral border of the scapulae

ISOLATED FUNCTION
Concentric Action
- Cervical extension, lateral flexion and ipsilateral rotation when the scapulae is anchored; Assists in elevation and downward rotation of the scapulae

INTEGRATED FUNCTION
Eccentric Action
- Cervical flexion, contralateral cervical rotation, lateral flexion, scapular depression and upward rotation when the neck is stabilized

Isometric Action
- Stabilizes the cervical spine and scapulae

INNERVATION
- Ventral rami C3-C4, dorsal of subscapular nerve

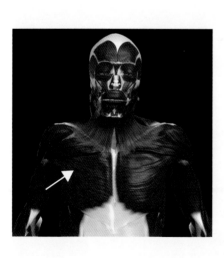

PECTORALIS MAJOR

ORIGIN
- Anterior surface of the clavicle; Anterior surface of the sternum, cartilage of ribs 1-7

INSERTION
- Greater tubercle of the humerus

ISOLATED FUNCTION
Concentric Action
- Shoulder flexion (clavicular fibers), horizontal adduction and internal rotation

INTEGRATED FUNCTION
Eccentric Action
- Shoulder extension horizontal abduction and external rotation

Isometric Action
- Stabilizes the shoulder girdle

INNERVATION
- Medial and lateral pectoral nerve (C5-C7)

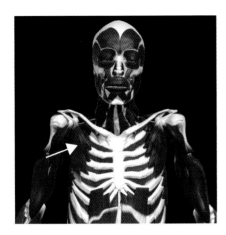

PECTORALIS MINOR

ORIGIN
- Ribs 3-5

INSERTION
- Coracoid process of the scapula

ISOLATED FUNCTION
Concentric Action
- Protracts the scapula

INTEGRATED FUNCTION
Eccentric Action
- Scapular retraction
Isometric Action
- Stabilizes the shoulder girdle

INNERVATION
- Medial pectoral nerve (C6-T1)

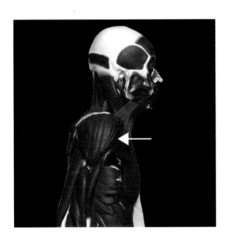

ANTERIOR DELTOID

ORIGIN
- Lateral third of the clavicle

INSERTION
- Deltoid tuberosity of the humerus

ISOLATED FUNCTION
Concentric Action
- Shoulder flexion and internal rotation

INTEGRATED FUNCTION
Eccentric Action
- Shoulder extension and external rotation
Isometric Action
- Stabilizes the shoulder girdle

INNERVATION
- Axillary nerve (C5-C6)

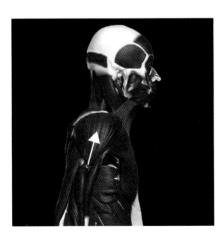

MEDIAL DELTOID

ORIGIN
- Acromion process of the scapula

INSERTION
- Deltoid tuberosity of the humerus

ISOLATED FUNCTION
Concentric Action
- Shoulder abduction

INTEGRATED FUNCTION
Eccentric Action
- Shoulder adduction
Isometric Action
- Stabilizes the shoulder girdle

INNERVATION
- Axillary nerve (C5-C6)

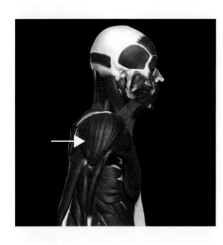

POSTERIOR DELTOID

ORIGIN
- Spine of the scapula

INSERTION
- Deltoid tuberosity of the humerus

ISOLATED FUNCTION
Concentric Action
- Shoulder extension and external rotation

INTEGRATED FUNCTION
Eccentric Action
- Shoulder flexion and internal rotation
Isometric Action
- Stabilizes the shoulder girdle

INNERVATION
- Axillary nerve (C5-C6)

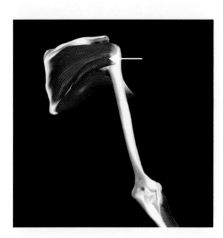

TERES MINOR

ORIGIN
- Lateral border of the scapula

INSERTION
- Greater tubercle of the humerus

ISOLATED FUNCTION
Concentric Action
- Shoulder external rotation

INTEGRATED FUNCTION
Eccentric Action
- Shoulder internal rotation
Isometric Action
- Stabilizes the shoulder girdle

INNERVATION
- Axillary nerve (C5-C6)

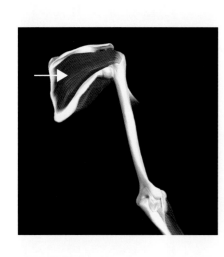

INFRASPINATUS

ORIGIN
- Infraspinous fossa of the scapula

INSERTION
- Middle facet of the greater tubercle of the humerus

ISOLATED FUNCTION
Concentric Action
- Shoulder external rotation

INTEGRATED FUNCTION
Eccentric Action
- Shoulder internal rotation
Isometric Action
- Stabilizes the shoulder girdle

INNERVATION
- Suprascapular nerve (C5-C6)

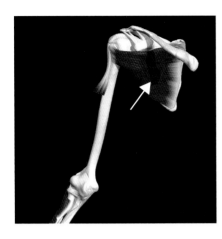

SUBSCAPULARIS

ORIGIN
- Subscapular fossa of the scapula

INSERTION
- Lesser tubercle of the humerus

ISOLATED FUNCTION
Concentric Action
- Shoulder internal rotation

INTEGRATED FUNCTION
Eccentric Action
- Shoulder external rotation
Isometric Action
- Stabilizes the shoulder girdle

INNERVATION
- Upper and lower subscapular nerve (C5-C6)

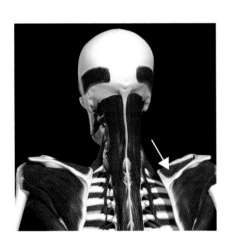

SUPRASPINATUS

ORIGIN
- Supraspinous fossa of the scapula

INSERTION
- Superior facet of the greater tubercle of the humerus

ISOLATED FUNCTION
Concentric Action
- Abduction of the arm

INTEGRATED FUNCTION
Eccentric Action
- Adduction of the arm
Isometric Action
- Stabilizes the shoulder girdle

INNERVATION
- Suprascapular nerve (C5-C6)

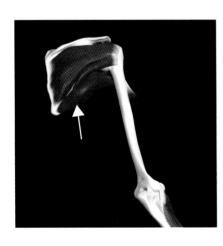

TERES MAJOR

ORIGIN
- Inferior angle of the scapula

INSERTION
- Lesser tubercle of the humerus

ISOLATED FUNCTION
Concentric Action
- Shoulder internal rotation, adduction and extension

INTEGRATED FUNCTION
Eccentric Action
- Shoulder external rotation, abduction and flexion
Isometric Action
- Stabilizes the shoulder girdle

INNERVATION
- Lower subscapular nerve

ARM MUSCULATURE

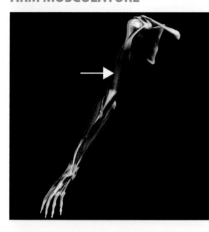

BICEPS BRACHII

ORIGIN
- Short head: Corocoid process; Long head: Tubercle above glenoid cavity on the humerus

INSERTION
- Radial tuberosity of the radius

ISOLATED FUNCTION

Concentric Action
- Elbow flexion, supination of the radioulnar joint, shoulder flexion

INTEGRATED FUNCTION

Eccentric Action
- Elbow extension, pronation of the radioulnar joint, shoulder extension

Isometric Action
- Stabilizes the elbow and shoulder girdle

INNERVATION
- Musculocutaneous nerve

TRICEPS BRACHII

ORIGIN
- Long head: Infraglenoid tubercle of the scapula; Short head: Posterior humerus; Medial head: posterior humerus

INSERTION
- Olecranon process of the ulna

ISOLATED FUNCTION

Concentric Action
- Elbow extension, shoulder extension

INTEGRATED FUNCTION

Eccentric Action
- Elbow flexion, shoulder flexion

Isometric Action
- Stabilizes the elbow and shoulder girdle

INNERVATION
- Radial nerve

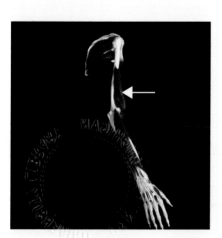

BRACHIALIS

ORIGIN
- Humerus

INSERTION
- Coronoid process of ulna

ISOLATED FUNCTION

Concentric Action
- Flexes elbow

INTEGRATED FUNCTION

Eccentric Action
- Elbow extension

Isometric Action
- Stabilizes the elbow

INNERVATION
- Musculocutaneous, radial nerve

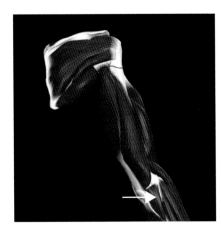

ANCONEUS

ORIGIN
- Lateral epicondyle of humerus

INSERTION
- Olecranon process, posterior ulna

ISOLATED FUNCTION
Concentric Action
- Extends elbow

INTEGRATED FUNCTION
Eccentric Action
- Elbow flexion
Isometric Action
- Stabilizes the elbow

INNERVATION
- Radial nerve

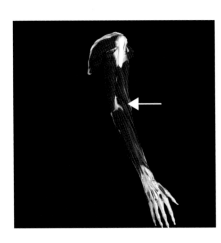

BRACHIORADIALIS

ORIGIN
- Lateral supracondylar ridge of humerus

INSERTION
- Styloid process of radius

ISOLATED FUNCTION
Concentric Action
- Flexes elbow

INTEGRATED FUNCTION
Eccentric Action
- Elbow extension
Isometric Action
- Stabilizes the elbow

INNERVATION
- Radial nerve

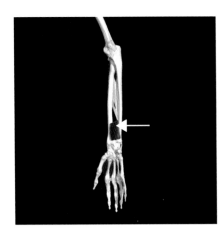

PRONATOR QUADRATUS

ORIGIN
- Distal ulna

INSERTION
- Distal radius

ISOLATED FUNCTION
Concentric Action
- Pronates forearm

INTEGRATED FUNCTION
Eccentric Action
- Forearm supination
Isometric Action
- Stabilizes distal radioulnar joint

INNERVATION
- Anterior interosseus nerve

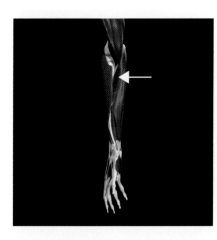

PRONATOR TERES

ORIGIN
- Medial epicondyle of humerus, coronoid process of ulna

INSERTION
- Radius

ISOLATED FUNCTION
Concentric Action
- Pronates forearm

INTEGRATED FUNCTION
Eccentric Action
- Forearm supination
Isometric Action
- Stabilizes proximal radioulnar joint and elbow

INNERVATION
- Median nerve

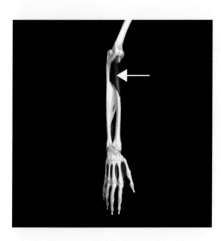

SUPINATOR

ORIGIN
- Lateral epicondyle of humerus

INSERTION
- Radius

ISOLATED FUNCTION
Concentric Action
- Supinates forearm

INTEGRATED FUNCTION
Eccentric Action
- Forearm pronation
Isometric Action
- Stabilizes proximal radioulnar joint and elbow

INNERVATION
- Radial nerve

NECK MUSCULATURE

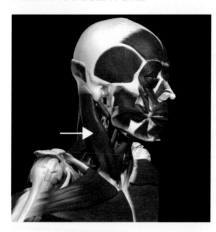

STERNOCLEIDOMASTOID

ORIGIN
- Sternal head: Top of Maubrium of the sternum; Clavicular head: Medial one-third of the clavicle

INSERTION
- Mastoid process, lateral superior nuchal line of the occiput of the skull

ISOLATED FUNCTION
Concentric Action
- Cervical flexion, rotation and lateral flexion

INTEGRATED FUNCTION
Eccentric Action
- Cervical extension, rotation and lateral flexion
Isometric Action
- Stabilizes the cervical spine and acromioclavicular joint

INNERVATION
- Cranial nerve XI

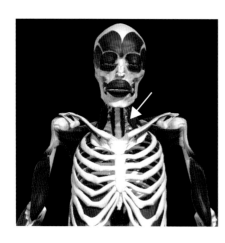

SCALENES

ORIGIN
- Transverse processes of C3-C7

INSERTION
- First and second ribs

ISOLATED FUNCTION
Concentric Action
- Cervical flexion, rotation and lateral flexion; Assists rib elevation during inhalation

INTEGRATED FUNCTION
Eccentric Action
- Cervical extension, rotation and lateral flexion
Isometric Action
- Stabilizes the cervical spine

INNERVATION
- Ventral rami (C3-C7)

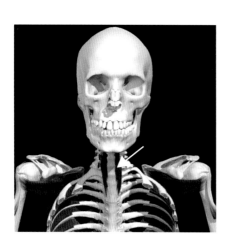

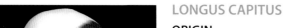

LONGUS COLLI

ORIGIN
- Anterior portion of T1-T3

INSERTION
- Anterior and lateral C1

ISOLATED FUNCTION
Concentric Action
- Cervical flexion, lateral flexion and ipsilateral rotation

INTEGRATED FUNCTION
Eccentric Action
- Cervical extension, lateral flexion and contralateral rotation
Isometric Action
- Stabilizes the cervical spine

INNERVATION
- Ventral rami (C2-C8)

LONGUS CAPITUS

ORIGIN
- Transverse processes of C3-C6

INSERTION
- Inferior occipital bone

ISOLATED FUNCTION
Concentric Action
- Cervical flexion and lateral flexion

INTEGRATED FUNCTION
Eccentric Action
- Cervical extension
Isometric Action
- Stabilizes the cervical spine

INNERVATION
- Ventral rami (C1-C3)

A review of the actions within this section of pertinent skeletal muscles should make it clear that muscles function in all three planes of motion (sagittal, frontal, and transverse) using the entire spectrum of muscle actions (eccentric, isometric, and concentric). In addition, the previous section shows which muscles work synergistically with each other to produce force, stabilize the body, reduce force, or all three.

Corrective exercise programs become more specific when there is a broader understanding of functional anatomy. A limited understanding of the synergistic functions of the HMS in all three planes of motion can lead to a lack of functional performance, the potential of developing muscle imbalances, and injury.

MOTOR BEHAVIOR

Motor behavior: the human movement systems response to internal and external environmental stimuli.

Sensory information: the data that the central nervous system receives from sensory receptors to determine such things as the body's position in space and limb orientation, as well as information about the environment, temperature, texture, etc.

Motor control: the study of posture and movements with the involved structures and mechanisms used by the central nervous system to assimilate and integrate sensory information with previous experiences.

Motor learning: the utilization of these processes through practice and experience leading to a relatively permanent change in one's capacity to produce skilled movements.

The functional anatomy and biomechanics portions of this chapter present information about how the different parts of the HMS operate as a synergistic, integrated functional unit in all three planes of motion. This is accomplished and retained using the concept of motor behavior. **Motor behavior** is the HMS response to internal and external environmental stimuli. The study of motor behavior examines the manner by which the nervous, skeletal, and muscular systems interact to produce skilled movement using **sensory information** from internal and external environments.

Motor behavior is the collective study of motor control, motor learning, and motor development (13,53) (Figure 2-22). **Motor control** is the study of posture and movements with the involved structures and mechanisms used by the central nervous system to assimilate and integrate sensory information with previous experiences (45,46). Motor control is concerned with what central nervous system structures are involved with motor behavior to produce movement (46). **Motor learning** is the utilization of these processes through practice and experience, leading to a relatively permanent change in one's capacity to produce skilled movements (21). Finally, **motor development** is defined as the change in motor behavior over time throughout one's lifespan (54). For the purposes of this text we will confine this section to a brief discussion of motor control and motor learning.

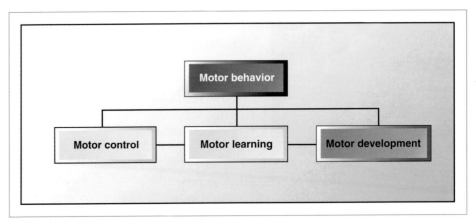

Figure 2.22 Components of motor behavior.

Motor development: the change in motor behavior over time throughout one's lifespan.

Motor Control

To move in an organized and efficient manner, the HMS must exhibit precise control over its collective segments. This segmental control is an integrated process involving neural, skeletal, and muscular components to produce appropriate motor responses. This process (and the study of these movements) is known as motor control and focuses on the involved structures and mechanisms used by the central nervous system to integrate internal and external sensory information with previous experiences to produce a skilled motor response. Essentially, motor control is concerned with the neural structures that are involved with motor behavior and how they produce movement (13,23,24,46).

One of the most important concepts in motor control and motor learning is how the central nervous system incorporates the information it receives to produce, refine, manipulate, and remember a movement pattern. The best place to start is with sensory information followed by proprioception, muscle synergies, and sensorimotor integration.

SENSORY INFORMATION

Sensory information is the data that the central nervous system receives from sensory receptors to determine such things as the body's position in space and limb orientation as well as information about the environment, temperature, texture, and so forth (45,46). This information allows the central nervous system to monitor the internal and external environments to modify motor behavior using adjustments ranging from simple reflexes to intricate movement patterns.

Sensory information is essential in protecting the body from harm. It also provides feedback about movement to acquire and refine new skills through sensory **sensations** and **perceptions**. A sensation is a process by which sensory information is received by the receptor and transferred either to the spinal cord for reflexive motor behavior, to higher cortical areas for processing, or both (45,46). Perception is the integration of sensory information with past experiences or memories (55).

The body uses sensory information in three ways:

Sensations: a process by which sensory information is received by the receptor and transferred either to the spinal cord for reflexive motor behavior, to higher cortical areas for processing, or both.

Perceptions: the integration of sensory information with past experiences or memories.

- Sensory information provides information about the body's spatial orientation to the environment and itself before, during, and after movement.
- It assists in planning and manipulating movement action plans. This may occur at the spinal level in the form of a reflex or at the cerebellum, where actual performance is compared.
- Sensory information facilitates learning new skills as well as relearning existing movement patterns that may have become dysfunctional (45,46).

PROPRIOCEPTION

Proprioception: the cumulative neural input from sensory afferents to the central nervous system.

Proprioception is one form of sensory (afferent) information that uses mechanoreceptors (from cutaneous, muscle, tendon, and joint receptors) to provide information about static and dynamic positions, movements, and sensations related to muscle force and movement (45). Lephart (53) defines proprioception as the cumulative neural input from sensory afferents to the central nervous system. This vital information ensures optimum motor behavior and neuromuscular efficiency (21,56). This afferent information is delivered to different levels of motor control within the central nervous system to use in monitoring and manipulating movement (53).

Proprioception is altered after injury (57–59). With many of the receptors being located in and around joints, any joint injury will likely also damage proprioceptive components that could be compromised for some time after an injury. When one considers the 85% of our population that experiences LBP, or the estimated 80,000 to 100,000+ anterior cruciate ligament (ACL) injuries annually, or the more than two million ankle sprains, individuals may have altered proprioception as a result of past injuries. A thorough rehabilitation program after a musculoskeletal injury will normally contain a proprioceptive component. Much of our movement is supported by the global muscular system, reinforcing the need for core and balance training to enhance one's proprioceptive capabilities, increase postural control, and decrease tissue overload (51,60,61).

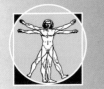

GETTING YOUR FACTS STRAIGHT

Rationale for Training in Unstable, Yet Controllable Environments

By placing the body in a multisensory environment (unstable, yet controllable), the brain is able to learn how to manipulate the musculoskeletal system to produce the movement with the right amount of force at the right time. If the structures of the brain are never challenged, they will never be forced to adapt and improve in their functional capabilities.

MUSCLE SYNERGIES

One of the most important concepts in motor control is that the central nervous system recruits muscles in groups or synergies (1,21,26). This simplifies movement by allowing muscles to operate as a functional unit (1,5). Through practice of proper movement patterns and technique, these synergies become more fluent and automated (Table 2-4).

SENSORIMOTOR INTEGRATION

Sensorimotor integration: the ability of the central nervous system to gather and interpret sensory information to execute the proper motor response.

Sensorimotor integration is the ability of the central nervous system to gather and interpret sensory information to execute the proper motor response (23,24,46,52,62). Sensorimotor integration is only as effective as the quality of the incoming sensory information (21,63). An individual who trains with improper form delivers improper sensory information to the central nervous system, which can lead to movement compensation and potential injury. Thus, programs need to be designed to train and to reinforce correct technique. For example, the individual who consistently performs a squat with an arched lower back and adducted femur will alter the length-tension relationships of muscles, force-couple relationships, and arthrokinematics. This can ultimately lead to back, knee, and hamstring problems (51,64–68).

Motor Learning

Motor learning is the integration of these motor control processes through practice and experience, leading to a relatively permanent change in the capacity to produce skilled movements (21,46). At its most basic, the study

Table 2.4	MUSCLE SYNERGIES
Bench Press	
Prime Mover	Pectoralis major
Synergists	Anterior deltoid
	Triceps
Stabilizers	Rotator cuff
	Biceps
Squats	
Prime Mover	Quadriceps
	Gluteus maximus
Synergists	Hamstrings complex
	Adductor magnus
	Gastrocnemius/soleus complex
	Posterior tibialis
Stabilizers	Lower extremity musculature
	◦ Flexor hallucis longus
	◦ Posterior tibialis
	◦ Anterior tibialis
	◦ Soleus
	◦ Gastrocnemius
	Lumbo-pelvic-hip complex
	◦ Adductor longus
	◦ Adductor brevis
	◦ Transverse abdominus
	◦ Gluteus medius
	Scapular stabilizes
	◦ Trapezius
	◦ Rhomboids
	Cervical stabilizers

Feedback: the utilization of sensory information and sensorimotor integration to aid in the development of permanent neural representations of motor patterns for efficient movement.

of motor learning looks at how movements are learned and retained for future use. Proper practice and experience will lead to a permanent change in an individual's ability to perform skilled movements effectively. For this to occur, feedback is necessary to ensure optimal development of these skilled movements.

FEEDBACK

Feedback is the utilization of sensory information and sensorimotor integration to aid in the development of permanent neural representations of motor patterns for efficient movement. This is achieved through internal (or sensory) feedback and external (or augmented) feedback (13,46,62).

Internal (or sensory) feedback is the process by which sensory information is used by the body via length-tension relationships, force-couple relationships, and arthrokinematics to monitor movement and the environment. Internal feedback acts as a guide, steering the human movement system to the proper force, speed, and amplitude of movement patterns. Proper form during movement ensures that the incoming internal (sensory) feedback is the correct information, allowing for optimal sensorimotor integration for ideal structural and functional efficiency (21).

External (or augmented) feedback is information provided by some external source, for example, a health and fitness professional, videotape, mirror, or heart rate monitor. This information is used to supplement internal feedback (46,62). External feedback provides another source of information that allows for the individual to associate the outcome of the achieved movement pattern ("good" or "bad") with what is felt internally.

Two major forms of external feedback are **knowledge of results** and **knowledge of performance** (21). Knowledge of results is used after the completion of a movement to inform individuals about the outcome of their performance. This can come from the health and fitness professional, the client, or some technological means. The health and fitness professional might inform individuals that their squats were "good" and ask clients whether they could "feel" or "see" their form. By getting clients involved with knowledge of results, they increase their own awareness and augment their impressions with multiple forms of feedback. This can be done after each repetition, after a few repetitions, or once the set is completed. As individuals become more familiar with the desired movement technique, knowledge of results from the health and fitness professional should be given less frequently. This improves neuromuscular efficiency (62).

Knowledge of performance provides information about the quality of the movement. An example would be noticing that, during a squat, the individual's feet were externally rotated, the femurs were excessively adducting, and then asking whether the individual felt or saw anything different about those repetitions. Or, to get individuals to absorb the shock of landing from a jump (and not landing with extended knees which places the ACL in a precarious position), telling them to listen to the impact and land quietly, effectively teaching the individual to absorb the shock of landing. These examples get the client involved in his or her own sensory process. Such feedback should be given less frequently as the client becomes more proficient (62).

These forms of external feedback identify performance errors. This feedback is also an important component in motivation. Further, feedback gives the client supplemental sensory input to help create an awareness of the desired action (21). It is important to state, however, that a client must not become too dependent on external feedback, especially from the health and fitness professional, as this may detract from the individual's own responsiveness to internal sensory input (21,46). This could alter sensorimotor integration and affect the learning by the client and the ultimate performance of new and skilled movement.

Internal (or sensory) feedback: the process by which sensory information is used by the body via length-tension relationships, force-couple relationships, and arthrokinematics to monitor movement and the environment.

External (or augmented) feedback: information provided by some external source, for example, a health and fitness professional, videotape, mirror, or heart rate monitor.

Knowledge of results: used after the completion of a movement to inform individuals about the outcome of their performance.

Knowledge of performance: provides information about the quality of the movement.

SUMMARY • In summary, each component of the HMS is interdependent. However, the HMS must work interdependently to gather information from internal and external environments to create, learn, and refine movements (or motor behavior) through proprioception, sensorimotor integration, and muscle synergies to create efficient movement (motor control). Then, repeated practice and incorporating internal and external feedback allows this efficient movement to be reproduced (motor learning).

References

1. Newmann D. Kinesiology of the Musculoskeletal System; Foundations for Physical Rehabilitation. St. Louis, MO: Mosby; 2002.
2. Sahrmann S. Diagnosis and Treatment of Movement Impairment Syndromes. St. Louis, MO: Mosby; 2002.
3. Panjabi MM. The stabilizing system of the spine. Part I. Function, dysfunction, adaptation, and enhancement. *J Spinal Disord* 1992;5:383–89; discussion 397.
4. Hamill J, Knutzen KM. Biomechanical Basis of Human Movement. 2nd ed. Philadelphia, PA: Lippincott Williams & Wilkins, 2003.
5. Levangle PK, Norkin CC. Joint Structure and Function: A Comprehensive Analysis. 3rd ed. Philadelphia, PA: FA Davis Company; 2001.
6. Watkins J. Structure and Function of the Musculoskeletal System. Champaign, IL: Human Kinetics; 1999.
7. Nordin M, Frankel VH. Basic Biomechanics of the Musculoskeletal System. 3rd ed. Philadelphia, PA: Lippincott Williams & Wilkins; 2001.
8. Kendall FP, McCreary EK, Provance PG. Muscles Testing and Function with Posture and Pain. 5th ed. Baltimore, MD: Lippincott Williams & Wilkins; 2005.
9. Luttgens K, Hamilton N. Kinesiology: Scientific Basis of Human Motion. 9th ed. Dubuque, IA: Brown & Benchmark Publishers; 1997.
10. Powers CM. The influence of altered lower-extremity kinematics on patellofemoral joint dysfunction: a theoretical perspective. *J Orthop Sports Phys Ther* 2003;33:639–46.
11. Inman VT, Ralston HJ, Todd F. Human Walking. Baltimore, MD: Williams & Wilkins; 1981.
12. Innes KA. The Effect of Gait on Extremity Evaluation. In: Hammer WI, ed. Functional Soft Tissue Examination and Treatment by Manual Methods. 2nd ed. Gaithersburg, MD: Aspen Publishers; 1999: 357-368.
13. Schmidt RA, Lee TD. Motor Control and Learning: A Behavioral Emphasis. 3rd ed. Champaign, IL: Human Kinetics; 1999.
14. Basmajian J: Muscles Alive: Their Functions Revealed by EMG. 5th ed. Baltimore, MD: Williams & Wilkins; 1985.
15. Clark MA. Integrated Core Stabilization Training. Thousand Oaks, CA: National Academy of Sports Medicine; 2000.
16. Aidley, DJ. Physiology of Excitable Cells. Cambridge, UK: Cambridge University Press; 1971.
17. Powers SK. Exercise Physiology: Theory and Application to Fitness and Performance. 5th ed. Dubuque, IA: McGraw-Hill; 2004.
18. Vander A, Sherman J, Luciano D. Human Physiology: The Mechanisms of Body Function. 8th ed. New York, NY: McGraw-Hill; 2001.
19. McArdle WD, Katch FI, Katch VL. Exercise Physiology: Energy, Nutrition and Human Performance. Philadelphia, PA: Lippincott Williams & Wilkins; 2007.
20. McClay I, Manal K. Three-dimensional kinetic analysis of running: significance of secondary planes of motion. *Med Sci Sports Exerc* 1999;31:1629–37.
21. Schmidt RA, Wrisberg CA. Motor Learning and Performance. 2nd ed. Champaign, IL: Human Kinetics; 2000.
22. Nyland J, Smith S, Beickman K, Armsey T, Caborn DN. Frontal plane knee angle affects dynamic postural control strategy during unilateral stance. *Med Sci Sports Exerc* 2002;34:1150–7.
23. Coker CA. Motor Learning and Control for Practitioners. Boston, MA: McGraw-Hill; 2004.
24. Magill RA. Motor Learning and Control: Concepts and Applications. Boston, MA: McGraw-Hill; 2007.
25. Grigg P. Peripheral neural mechanisms in proprioception. *J Sport Rehab* 1994;3:2–17.
26. Edgerton VR, Wolf SL, Levendowski DJ, Roy RR. Theoretical basis for patterning EMG amplitudes to assess muscle dysfunction. *Med Sci Sports Exerc* 1996;28:744–51.
27. Lieber RL. Skeletal Muscle Structure and Function: Implications for Rehabilitation. Baltimore, MD: Lippincott Williams & Wilkins; 2002.
28. Bergmark A. Stability of the lumbar spine. A study in mechanical engineering. *Acta Ortho Scand* 1989;230(Suppl):20–4.
29. Mooney V. Sacroiliac Joint Dysfunction. In: Vleeming A, Mooney V, Dorman T, Snijders C, Stoeckart R, eds. Movement, Stability and Low Back Pain. London, UK: Churchill Livingstone; 1997: 37–52.
30. Crisco JJ, Panjabi MM. The intersegmental and multisegmental muscles of the spine: a biomechanical model comparing lateral stabilizing potential. *Spine* 1991;7:793–9.
31. Richardson C, Jull G, Hodges P, Hides J. Therapeutic Exercise for Spinal Segmental Stabilization in Low Back Pain. London, UK: Churchill Livingstone; 1999.
32. Culham LC, Peat M. Functional anatomy of the shoulder complex. *J Ortho Sports Phys Ther* 1993;18:342–50.

33. Wilk KE, Reinold MM, Dugas JR, Arrigo CA, Moser MW, Andrews JR. Current concepts in the recognition and treatment of superior labral (SLAP) lesions. *J Orthop Sports Phys Ther* 2005;35:273–91.

34. Millett PJ, Wilcox RB 3rd, O'Holleran JD, Warner JJ. Rehabilitation of the rotator cuff: an evaluation-based approach. *J Am Acad Orthop Surg* 2006;14:599–609.

35. Kibler WB, Chandler TJ, Shapiro R, Conuel M. Muscle activation in coupled scapulohumeral motions in the high performance tennis serve. *Br J Sports Med* 2007;41:745–9.

36. Gottschalk F, Kourosh S, Leveau B. The functional anatomy of tensor fascia latae and gluteus medius and minimus. *J Anat* 1989;166:179–89.

37. Anderson FC, Pandy MG. Individual muscle contributions to support in normal walking. *Gait Posture* 2003;17:159–69.

38. Hossain M, Nokes LD. A model of dynamic sacro-iliac joint instability from malrecruitment of gluteus maximus and biceps femoris muscles resulting in low back pain. *Med Hypotheses* 2005;65:278–81.

39. Liu MQ, Anderson FC, Pandy MG, Delp SL. Muscles that support the body also modulate forward progression during walking. *J Biomech* 2006;39:2623–30.

40. Lieb FJ, Perry J. Quadriceps function. *J Bone Joint Surg* 1971;50A:1535–48.

41. Toumi H, Poumarat G, Benjamin M, Best T, F'Guyer S, Fairclough J. New insights into the function of the vastus medialis with clinical implications. *Med Sci Sports Exerc* 2007;39:1153–9.

42. Lee D. Instability of the Sacroiliac Joint and the Consequences for Gait. In: Vleeming A, Mooney V, Dorman T, Snijders C, Stoeckart R, eds. Movement, Stability and Low Back Pain. London, UK: Churchill Livingstone; 1997: 231-234.

43. Gracovetsky SA. Linking the Spinal Engine With the Legs: A Theory of Human Gait. In: Vleeming A, Mooney V, Dorman T, Snijders C, Stoeckart R, eds. Movement, Stability and Low Back Pain. London, UK: Churchill Livingstone; 1997: 243-252.

44. Vleeming A, Snijders CJ, Stoeckart R, Mens JMA. The Role of the Sacroiliac Joints in Coupling Between Spine, Pelvis, Legs and Arms. In: Vleeming A, Mooney V, Dorman T, Snijders C, Stoeckart R, eds. Movement, Stability and Low Back Pain. London, UK: Churchill Livingstone; 1997: 53-72.

45. Newton RA. Neural Systems Underlying Motor Control. In: Montgomery PC, Connoly BH, eds. Motor Control and Physical Therapy: Theoretical Framework and Practical Applications. Hixson, TN: Chattanooga Group; 1991.

46. Rose DJ. A Multi-level Approach to the Study of Motor Control and Learning. Needham Heights, MA: Allyn & Bacon; 1997.

47. Porterfield JA, DeRosa C. Mechanical Low Back Pain. Philadelphia, PA: WB Saunders; 1991.

48. Snijders CJ, Vleeming A, Stoeckart R, Mens JMA, Kleinrensink GJ. Biomechanics of the Interface Between Spine and Pelvis in Different Postures. In: Vleeming A, Mooney V, Dorman T, Snijders C, Stoeckart R, eds. Movement, Stability and Low Back Pain. London, UK: Churchill Livingstone; 1997: 103-114.

49. Fredericson M, Cookingham CL, Chaudhari AM, Dowdell BC, Oestreicher N, Sahrmann SA. Hip abductor weakness in distance runners with iliotibial band syndrome. *Clin J Sport Med* 2000;10:169–75.

50. Ireland ML, Wilson JD, Ballantyne BT, Davis IM. Hip strength in females with and without patellofemoral pain. *J Orthop Sports Phys Ther* 2003;33:671–6.

51. Hewett TE, Lindenfeld TN, Riccobene JV, Noyes FR. The effect of neuromuscular training on the incidence of knee injury in female athletes. A prospective study. *Am J Sports Med* 1999;27:699–706.

52. Seeley RR, Stephans TD, Tate P. Anatomy and Physiology. 6th ed. Boston, MA: McGraw-Hill; 2003.

53. Lephart SM, Fu FH. Proprioception and Neuromuscular Control in Joint Stability. Champaign, IL: Human Kinetics; 2000.

54. Gabbard C. Lifelong Motor Development. San Francisco, CA: Pearson Benjamin Cummings; 2008.

55. Sage GH. Introduction to Motor Behavior: A Neuropsychological Approach. 3rd ed. Dubuque, IA: WC Brown; 1984.

56. Ghez C. The Control of Movement. In: Kandel E, Schwartz J, Jessel T, eds. Principles of Neuroscience. New York, NY: Elsevier Science; 1991: 653-673.

57. Brown CN, Mynark R. Balance deficits in recreational athletes with chronic ankle instability. *J Athl Train* 2007;42:367–73.

58. Solomonow M, Barratta R, Zhou BH. The synergistic action of the anterior cruciate ligament and thigh muscles in maintaining joint stability. *Am J Sports Med* 1987;15:207–13.

59. Uremović M, Cvijetić S, Pasić MB, Serić V, Vidrih B, Demarin V. Impairment of proprioception after whiplash injury. *Coll Antropol* 2007;31:823–7.

60. Paterno MV, Myer GD, Ford KR, Hewett TE. Neuromuscular training improves single-limb stability in young female athletes. *J Orthop Sports Phys Ther* 2004;34:305–16.

61. Chmielewski TL, Hurd WJ, Rudolph KS, Axe MJ, Snyder-Mackler L. Perturbation training improves knee kinematics and reduces muscle co-contraction after complete unilateral anterior cruciate ligament rupture. *Phys Ther* 2005;85:740–9.

62. Swinnen SP. Information Feedback for Motor Skill Learning: A Review. In: Zelaznik HN, ed. Advances in Motor Learning and Control. Champaign, IL: Human Kinetics; 1996: 37-43.

63. Biedert RM. Contribution of the Three Levels of Nervous System Motor Control: Spinal Cord, Lower Brain, Cerebral Cortex. In: Lephart SM, Fu FH, eds. Proprioception and Neuromuscular Control in Joint Stability. Champaign, IL: Human Kinetics; 2000: 23-30.

64. Ford KR, Myer GD, Hewett TE. Valgus knee motion during landing in high school female and male basketball players. *Med Sci Sports Exerc* 2003;35:1745–50.

65. Nadler SF, Malanga GA, Bartoli LA, Feinberg JH, Prybicien M, Deprince M. Hip muscle imbalance and low back pain in athletes: influence of core strengthening. *Med Sci Sports Exerc* 2002;34:9–16.

66. Nadler SF, Malanga GA, Feinberg JH, Rubanni M, Moley P, Foye P. Functional performance deficits in athletes with previous lower extremity injury. *Clin J Sport Med* 2002;12:73–8.

67. Bullock-Saxton JE. Local sensation changes and altered hip muscle function following severe ankle sprain. *Phys Ther* 1994;74:17–28.

68. Knapik JJ, Bauman CL, Jones BH, Harris JM, Vaughan L. Preseason strength and flexibility imbalances associated with athletic injuries in female collegiate athletes. *Am J Sports Med* 1991;19:76–81.

CHAPTER 3

An Evidence-Based Approach to Understanding Human Movement Impairments

Upon completion of this chapter, you will be able to:

➤ Explain the importance that proper posture has on movement.

➤ Understand and explain common causes for movement dysfunction.

➤ Understand and explain common human movement system dysfunctions and potential causes for each.

Neuromuscular efficiency: the ability of the neuromuscular system to allow agonist, antagonists, synergists, and stabilizers to work synergistically to produce, reduce, and dynamically stabilize the HMS in all three planes of motion.

Posture: the independent and interdependent alignment (static posture) and function (transitional and dynamic posture) of all components of the HMS at any given moment, controlled by the central nervous system.

INTRODUCTION

As reviewed in the previous chapter, the human movement system (HMS) is a very complex, well-orchestrated system of interrelated and interdependent myofascial, neuromuscular, and articular components. The functional integration of each system allows for optimal **neuromuscular efficiency** during functional activities (Figure 3-1). Optimal alignment and functioning of all components (and segments of each component) result in optimum length-tension relationships, force-couple relationships, precise arthrokinematics (path of instantaneous center of rotation), and neuromuscular control (1–3). Optimum alignment and functioning of each component of the HMS depends on the structural and functional integrity of each of its interdependent systems. This structural alignment is known as posture. **Posture** is the independent and interdependent alignment (static posture) and function (transitional and dynamic posture) of all components of the HMS at any given moment, and is controlled by the central nervous system (4). Assessments for these different forms of posture will be covered in later chapters.

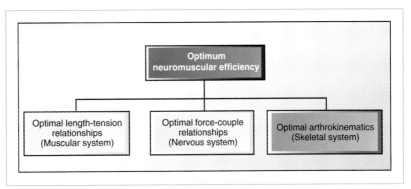

Figure 3.1   Optimal neuromuscular efficiency.

Efficiency and longevity of the HMS requires integration of all systems. **Structural efficiency** is the alignment of each segment of the HMS, which allows posture to be balanced in relation to one's center of gravity. This enables individuals to maintain their center of gravity over their constantly changing base of support during functional movements. **Functional efficiency** is the ability of the neuromuscular system to recruit correct muscle synergies, at the right time, with the appropriate amount of force to perform functional tasks with the least amount of energy and stress on the HMS. This helps prevent overtraining and the development of movement impairment syndromes.

Structural efficiency: the alignment of each segment of the HMS, which allows posture to be balanced in relation to one's center of gravity.

HUMAN MOVEMENT SYSTEM IMPAIRMENT

Impairment or injury to the HMS rarely involves one structure. Because the HMS is an integrated system, impairment in one system leads to compensations and adaptations in other systems. As outlined in Figure 3-2, if

Functional efficiency: the ability of the neuromuscular system to recruit correct muscle synergies, at the right time, with the appropriate amount of force to perform functional tasks with the least amount of energy and stress on the HMS.

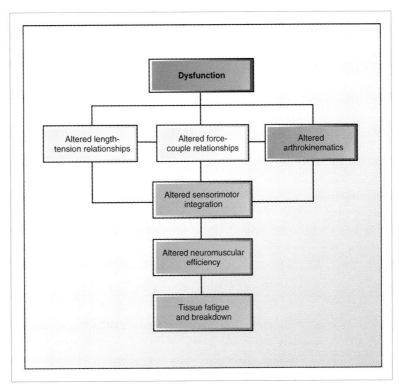

Figure 3.2   Human movement impairment.

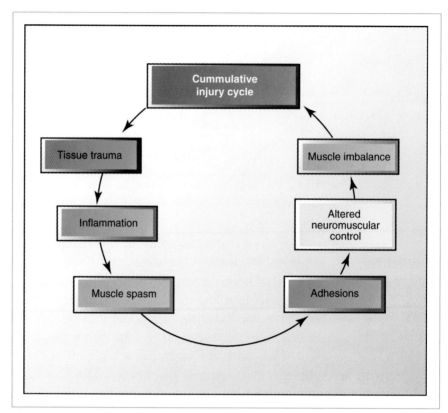

Figure 3.3 Cumulative injury cycle.

Cumulative injury
cycle: a cycle whereby
an injury will induce
inflammation, muscle
spasm, adhesion,
altered neuromuscular
control, and muscle
imbalances.

Movement impair-
ment syndromes: refer
to the state in which
the structural integrity
of the HMS is compro-
mised because the
components are out of
alignment.

one component in the HMS is out of alignment (muscle tightness, muscle weakness, altered joint arthrokinematics), it creates predictable patterns of tissue overload and dysfunction, which leads to decreased neuromuscular control and microtrauma, and initiates the **cumulative injury cycle** (Figure 3-3). The cumulative injury cycle causes decreased performance, myofascial adhesions (which further alter length-tension relationships and joint arthrokinematics), and eventually injury (5).

These predictable patterns of dysfunction are referred to as **movement impairment syndromes**. Movement impairment syndromes refer to the state in which the structural integrity of the HMS is compromised because the components are out of alignment (1). This places abnormal distorting forces on the structures in the HMS that are above and below the dysfunctional segment. If one segment in the HMS is out of alignment, then other movement segments have to compensate in attempts to balance the weight distribution of the dysfunctional segment. For example, if the gluteus medius is underactive, then the tensor fascia latae (TFL) may become synergistically dominant to produce the necessary force to accomplish frontal plane stability of the lumbo-pelvic-hip complex (LPHC). An overactive TFL can lead to tightness in the iliotibial band (ITB) and lead to patellofemoral joint pain, ITB tendonitis, and low-back pain (1,6–9). To avoid movement impairment syndromes and the chain reactions that one misaligned segment creates, the health and fitness professional must emphasize optimum static, transitional, and dynamic postural control to maintain the structural integrity of the HMS during functional activities. Optimum movement system balance and alignment helps prevent movement impairment syndromes and provides optimal shock absorption, weight acceptance, and transfer of force during functional movements.

STATIC MALALIGNMENTS

Static malalignments may alter normal length-tension relationships. Common static malalignments include joint hypomobility and myofascial adhesions that lead to or can be caused by poor static posture. Joint dysfunction (hypomobility) is one of the most common causes of pain in an individual (10,11). Once a joint has lost its normal arthrokinematics, the muscles around that joint may spasm and tighten in an attempt to minimize the stress at the involved segment (10,11). Certain muscles become tight (alters the length-tension relationship) or overactive (alters force-couple relationships) to prevent movement and further injury. This process initiates the cumulative injury cycle. Therefore, a joint dysfunction causes altered length-tension relationships. This alters normal force-couple relationships, which alters normal movement patterns and leads to structural and functional inefficiency (1,5,10–12) (Figure 3-4).

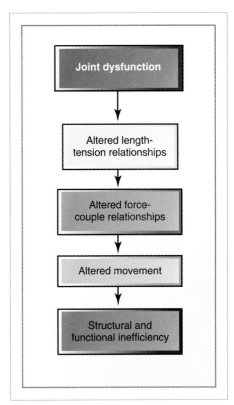

Figure 3.4 Joint dysfunction.

ALTERED MUSCLE RECRUITMENT

Static malalignments (altered length-tension relationships resulting from poor static posture, joint dysfunction, and myofascial adhesions) may lead to altered muscle recruitment patterns (altered force-couple relationships). This is caused by **altered reciprocal inhibition**. Altered reciprocal inhibition is the process by which a tight muscle (short, overactive, myofascial adhesions) causes decreased neural drive, and therefore optimal recruitment of its functional antagonist (1). This process alters the normal force-couple relationships that should be present at all segments throughout the HMS. Furthermore, altered reciprocal

Altered reciprocal inhibition: the process whereby a tight muscle (short, overactive, myofascial adhesions) causes decreased neural drive, and therefore optimal recruitment of its functional antagonist.

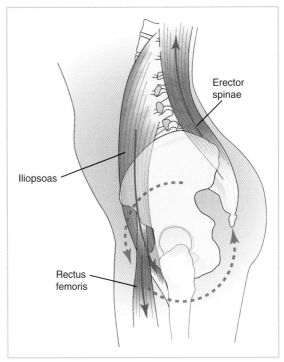

Figure 3.5 Altered reciprocal inhibition and synergistic dominance.

inhibition can lead to **synergistic dominance**, which is the process in which a synergist compensates for a prime mover to maintain force production (1,13). For example, a tight psoas decreases the neural drive and therefore optimal recruitment of the gluteus maximus. This altered recruitment and force production of the gluteus maximus (prime mover for hip extension), leads to compensation and substitution by the synergists (hamstrings) and stabilizers (erector spinae) (Figure 3-5). This can potentially lead to hamstring strains and low back pain. In another example, if a client has a weak gluteus medius, then synergists (tensor fascia latae, adductor complex, and quadratus lumborum) become synergistically dominant to compensate for the weakness (6). This altered muscle recruitment pattern further alters static alignment (alters normal joint alignment and normal length-tension relationships around the joint to which the muscles attach) and leads to injury.

DYNAMIC MALALIGNMENTS

Several authors have described common movement impairment syndromes (dynamic malalignment) that are caused by static malalignments and altered muscle recruitment patterns (1,10,14). The most common movement impairment syndromes include the **lower extremity movement impairment syndrome** and the **upper extremity movement impairment syndrome**.

Individuals with a lower extremity movement impairment syndrome are usually characterized by excessive foot pronation (flat feet), increased knee valgus (tibia internally rotated and femur internally rotated and adducted or knock-kneed), and increased movement at the LPHC (extension or flexion) during functional movements (Figure 3-6; Table 3-1). Potentially *tightened* or *overactive* muscles may include the peroneals, lateral gastrocnemius, soleus, iliotibial band, lateral hamstring complex, adductor complex, and psoas. Potentially *weakened* or *inhibited* muscles may include the posterior tibialis, flexor digitorum longus, flexor hallucis longus, anterior tibialis, vastus medialis, pes anserine complex (sartorius, gracilis, semitendinosus), gluteus medius, hip external rotators, gluteus maximus, and local stabilizers of the LPHC. Potential joint dysfunctions may include the first metatarsophalangeal joint, subtalar joint, talocrural joint, proximal tibiofibular joint, sacroiliac joint, and lumbar facet joints. Individuals who present with the lower extremity movement impairment syndrome typically exhibit predictable patterns of injury including plantar fasciitis, posterior tibialis tendinitis (shin splints), anterior knee pain, and low-back pain (1,10,14).

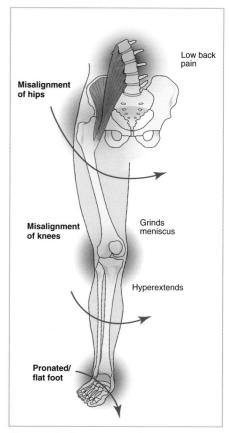

Figure 3.6 Lower extremity movement impairment syndrome.

Table 3.1   LOWER EXTREMITY MOVEMENT IMPAIRMENT SYNDROME

Tight or Overactive Muscles	Weak or Underactive Muscles	Common Joint Dysfunction	Possible Injuries
Peroneals	Posterior tibialis	First metatarsopha-langeal joint	Plantar fasciitis
Lateral gastrocnemius	Flexor digitorum longus	Subtalar joint	Posterior tibialis tendinitis
Soleus	Flexor hallucis longus	Talocrural joint	Anterior knee pain
Iliotibial band	Anterior tibialis	Proximal tibiofibular joint	Low-back pain
Lateral hamstring complex	Vastus medialis	Sacroiliac joint	
Adductor complex	Pes anserine complex	Lumbar facet joints	
Psoas	Gracilis		
	Sartorius		
	Semitendinosus		
	Gluteus medius		
	Hip external rotators		
	Gluteus maximus		
	Local stabilizers of the LPHC		

Individuals with the upper extremity movement impairment syndrome are usually characterized as having rounded shoulders and a forward head posture or improper scapulothoracic or glenohumeral kinematics during functional movements (Figure 3-7; Table 3-2). This pattern is common in individuals who sit for extended periods of time or who develop pattern overload (e.g., throwing, continual bench pressing, and swimming). Potentially *tightened* or *overactive* muscles include the pectoralis major, pectoralis minor, anterior deltoid, subscapularis, latissimus dorsi, levator scapulae, upper trapezius, teres major, sternocleidomastoid, scalenes, and rectus capitis. Potentially *weakened* or *inhibited* muscles usually include the rhomboids, lower trapezius, posterior deltoid, teres minor, infraspinatus, serratus anterior, longus coli, and longus capitis. Potential joint dysfunctions may include the sternoclavicular joint, acromioclavicular joint, and thoracic and cervical facet joints.

Individuals who present with the upper extremity movement impairment syndrome typically exhibit predictable patterns of injury including rotator cuff impingement, shoulder instability, biceps tendinitis, thoracic outlet syndrome, and headaches (1,10).

Assessing an individual for these impairment syndromes will be covered in further detail in later chapters.

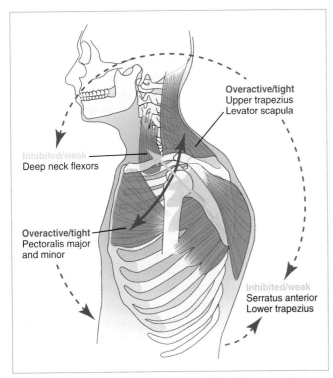

Figure 3.7   Upper extremity movement impairment syndrome.

Table 3.2 UPPER EXTREMITY MOVEMENT IMPAIRMENT SYNDROME

Tight/Overactive Muscles	Weak/Underactive Muscles	Common Joint Dysfunction	Possible Injuries
Pectoralis major	Rhomboids	Sternoclavicular joint	Rotator cuff impingement
Pectoralis minor	Lower trapezius	Acromioclavicular joint	Shoulder instability
Anterior deltoid	Posterior deltoid	Thoracic and cervical facet joints	Biceps tendinitis
Subscapularis	Teres minor		Thoracic outlet syndrome
Latissimus dorsi	Infraspinatus		Headaches
Levator scapulae	Serratus anterior		
Upper trapezius	Longus coli and longus capitis		
Teres major			
Sternocleidomastoid			
Scalenes			
Rectus capitis			

EVIDENCE-BASED REVIEW OF COMMON SEGMENTAL MOVEMENT SYSTEM IMPAIRMENTS

Foot and Ankle

SCIENTIFIC REVIEW

The ankle is the most commonly injured joint in both sports and daily life (15). Several authors have found that control at the hip is vital for maintaining control at the ankle (16–19). It has also been demonstrated that proximal factors such as LPHC muscle weakness, in particular in the frontal and transverse planes, contribute to altered lower extremity alignment, leading to increased foot pronation (9,20,21) (Figure 3-8). If the hip lacks dynamic stability in the frontal and transverse planes during functional weight-bearing activities, the femur may adduct and internally rotate, whereas the tibia may externally rotate and the foot goes into excessive pronation (9,20). These static malalignments (altered length-tension relationships and joint arthrokinematics), abnormal muscle activation patterns, and dynamic malalignments can alter neuromuscular control and can lead to plantar fasciitis (22,23), patellofemoral pain (9,24–34), ITB tendonitis (35), and increased risk of anterior cruciate ligament (ACL) tears (36–50).

STATIC MALALIGNMENTS (ALTERED LENGTH-TENSION RELATIONSHIPS OR ALTERED JOINT ARTHROKINEMATICS)

Common static malalignments of the foot and ankle include hyperpronation of the foot (9,20,51,52), which may result from overactivity of the peroneals and lateral gastrocnemius, underactivity of the anterior and posterior tibialis, and decreased joint motion of the first metatarsophalangeal (MTP) joint and talus (decreased posterior glide). It has been reported that there is decreased ankle

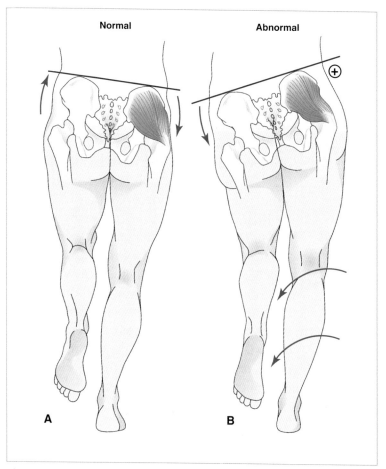

Figure 3.8   Effects of weak LPHC on lower extremity.

dorsiflexion after an ankle sprain (53,54). It is hypothesized that decreased posterior glide of the talus can decrease dorsiflexion at the ankle (55). Denegar et al. (56) found decreased posterior glide of the talus in subjects with a history of lateral ankle sprains. Green et al. (57) found a more rapid restoration of dorsiflexion and normalization of gait in patients with ankle sprains who were treated with manual posterior glide of the talus.

ABNORMAL MUSCLE ACTIVATION PATTERNS (ALTERED FORCE-COUPLE RELATIONSHIPS)

It has been demonstrated that subjects with unilateral chronic ankle sprains had weaker ipsilateral hip abduction strength (17,19) and increased postural sway (58,59). It has also been demonstrated that subjects with increased postural sway had up to seven times more ankle sprains than those subjects with better postural sway scores (60,61). Furthermore, fatigue in the knee and hip musculature (sagittal and frontal planes) creates even greater postural sway (62,63). Cerny (64) found that weakness and decreased postural stability in the stabilizing muscles of the LPHC, such as the gluteus medius, may produce deviations in subtalar joint motion during gait (Figure 3-8). Foot placement depends on hip abduction and adduction moments generated during the swing phase of gait, and subsequent subtalar joint inversion moments occur in response to medial foot placement errors secondary to overactivity of the hip adductors (16). This has led to the determination through research that proximal stability and strength deficits at the hip can lead to ankle injuries (65).

DYNAMIC MALALIGNMENT

It has been shown that excessive pronation of the foot during weight-bearing causes altered alignment of the tibia, femur, and pelvic girdle (Figure 3-5) and can lead to internal rotation stresses at the lower extremity and pelvis, which may lead to increased strain on soft tissues (Achilles' tendon, plantar fascia, patella tendon, ITB, etc.) and compressive forces on the joints (subtalar joint, patellofemoral joint, tibiofemoral joint, iliofemoral joint, and sacroiliac joint), which can become symptomatic (9,51). The LPHC alignment has been shown by Khamis and Yizhar (66) to be directly affected by bilateral hyperpronation of the feet. Hyperpronation of the feet induced an anterior pelvic tilt of the LPHC. The addition of two to three degrees of foot pronation led to a 20 to 30% increase in pelvic alignment while standing and a 50 to 75% increase in anterior pelvic tilting during walking (66). Because an anterior pelvic tilt has been correlated with increased lumbar curvature, the change in foot alignment might also influence lumbar spine position (67). Furthermore, an asymmetric change in foot alignment (as might occur from a unilateral ankle sprain) may cause asymmetric lower extremity, pelvic, and lumbar alignment, which might enhance symptoms or dysfunction.

Hip and Knee

SCIENTIFIC REVIEW

Knee injuries account for greater than 50% of injuries in college and high school (25,26) athletes, and among lower extremity injuries, the knee is one of the most commonly injured segments of the HMS. Two of the more common diagnoses resulting from physical activity are patellofemoral pain (PFP) and ACL sprains or tears. Both PFP and ACL injuries are public health concerns costing $2.5 billion annually for ACL injuries (38). Most knee injuries occur during noncontact deceleration in the frontal and transverse planes (43,68). It has also been shown that static malalignments, abnormal muscle activation patterns, and dynamic malalignments alter neuromuscular control and can lead to PFP (14,24), ACL injury (47,69–74), and ITB tendonitis (35).

STATIC MALALIGNMENTS (ALTERED LENGTH-TENSION RELATIONSHIPS AND JOINT ARTHROKINEMATICS)

Static malalignments can lead to increased PFP and knee injury. Common static malalignments include hyperpronation of the foot (9,20,51,52), increased Q angle (a 10-degree shift in Q-angle increased patellofemoral contact forces by 45%) (75) (Figure 3-9), anterior pelvic tilt (66), and decreased flexibility of the quadriceps, hamstring complex, and iliotibial band (21,22,27).

ABNORMAL MUSCLE ACTIVATION PATTERNS (ALTERED FORCE-COUPLE RELATIONSHIPS)

Abnormal muscle activation patterns can lead to PFP, ACL injury, and other knee injuries. Abnormal contraction intensity and onset timing of the vastus medialis obliquus (VMO) and vastus lateralis have been demonstrated in subjects with PFP (76). Ireland et al. have demonstrated 26% less hip abduction strength and 36% decreased strength of the hip external rotators in subjects with PFP, leading to increased femoral adduction and internal rotation (24). Other researchers have also demonstrated decreased hip abduction strength in subjects with PFP (77–79). Fredericson et al. (35) found that long-distance runners with ITB syndrome had weaker hip abduction strength on the affected leg, and also demonstrated that their symptoms were alleviated with a successful return to running after undergoing a hip abductor strengthening program. Heinert et al. (80) found that hip abductor weakness influenced knee abduction (femoral adduction or internal rotation and tibial external rotation) during the stance phase of running. Lawrence et al. (81) demonstrated that individuals with decreased hip external rotation strength had increased vertical ground reaction forces during landing, which is a potential predictor of PFP and ACL injury. Research has also demonstrated increased adductor activity and decreased dorsiflexion in subjects demonstrating increased dynamic knee valgus (82) and decreased neuromuscular control of core musculature (83,84).

DYNAMIC MALALIGNMENTS

Dynamic malalignments may occur during movement as a result of poor neuromuscular control and dynamic stability of the trunk and lower extremities (14,70,84,85). Static malalignments (altered length-tension relationships and altered joint arthrokinematics) and abnormal muscle activation patterns

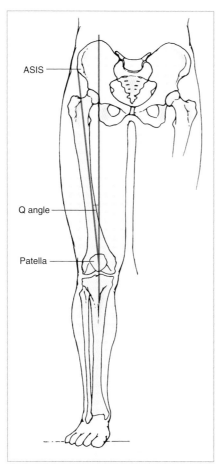

Figure 3.9   Q-Angle.

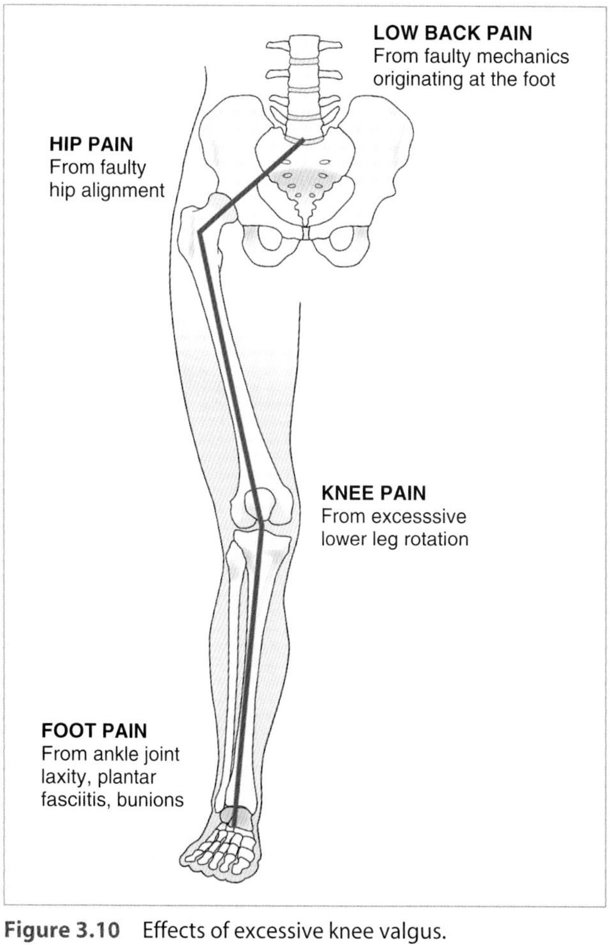

Figure 3.10   Effects of excessive knee valgus.

(altered force-couple relationships) of the LPHC compromise dynamic stability of the lower extremity and result in dynamic malalignments in the lower extremity (83,84). There is a consistent description of this dynamic malalignment (multisegmental HMS impairment) as a combination of contralateral pelvic drop, femoral adduction and internal rotation, tibia external rotation, and hyperpronation (9,14,70,73,85–92) (Figure 3-6). McLean et al. (93) have shown that an increase in knee valgus angle could increase ACL loading by approximately 100% (Figure 3-10). This multisegmental dynamic malalignment (movement impairment syndrome) has been shown to alter force production (94), proprioception (95), coordination (96), and landing mechanics (97). Deficits in neuromuscular control of the LPHC may lead to uncontrolled trunk displacement during functional movements, which in turn may place the lower extremity in a valgus position, increase knee abduction motion and torque (femoral adduction or internal rotation and tibial external rotation occurring during knee flexion), and result in increased patellofemoral contact pressure (75,98), knee ligament strain, and ACL injury (70,85).

Low Back

SCIENTIFIC REVIEW

Back injuries can be costly to both the individual and the health-care system. Previous studies have found a high incidence of low-back pain (LBP) in sports (99–101). For example, 85% of male gymnasts, 80% of weightlifters, 69% of wrestlers, 58% of soccer players, 50% of tennis players, 30% of golfers, and 60 to 80% of the general population were reported to have LBP (102–104). It is estimated that the annual costs attributable to LBP in the United States is greater than $26 billion per year (105). Individuals who have LBP are significantly more likely to have additional low-back injuries, which can predispose the individual to future osteoarthritis and long-term disability (106). It has been demonstrated that static malalignments (altered length-tension relationships or altered joint arthrokinematics), abnormal muscle activation patterns (altered force-couple relationships), and dynamic malalignments (movement system impairments) can lead to LBP.

STATIC MALALIGNMENTS (ALTERED LENGTH-TENSION RELATIONSHIPS OR ALTERED JOINT ARTHROKINEMATICS)

Optimal muscle performance is determined by the posture (length-tension) of the LPHC during functional activities (107–110). If the neutral lordotic curve of the lumbar spine is not maintained (i.e., low-back arches, low-back rounds, or excessive lean forward), the activation (107) and the relative moment arm of the muscle fibers decreases (109,110). Vertebral disk injuries occur when the outer fibrous structure of the disk (annulus fibrosis) fails,

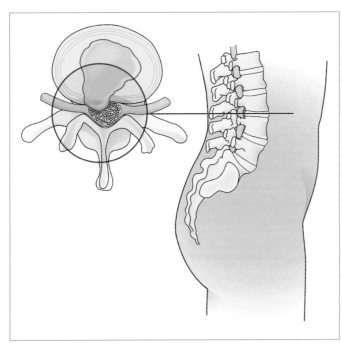

Figure 3.11   Intervertebral disk injury.

allowing the internal contents of the disk (nucleus pulposus) to be extruded and irritate nerves exiting the intervertebral foramen (Figure 3-11).

The exact mechanism underlying injury to the intervertebral disk is unclear, but it is generally proposed that it is caused by a combination of motion with compressive loading. Increases in disk pressures and stresses are influenced by the kinematics of the lumbar spine (13,111,112). Disk pressure increases with lumbar flexion (13,111,112) and a decrease in lordosis (e.g., low-back rounding) during the performance of activities (161,163). In addition, a combination of motions about the lumbar spine have been demonstrated to increase the strain placed on the disks, and include flexion with lateral bending (112). This combination of motions may generate an axial torque that Drake et al. (113) demonstrated to increase the initiation of disk herniation. Lu et al. (114) combined all of these factors and were able to demonstrate that compression combined with bending and twisting moments about the disk contributed to earlier degeneration in saturated intervertebral disks. Pelvic asymmetry (iliac rotation asymmetry or sacroiliac joint asymmetry) (Figure 3-12) has been shown to alter movement of the HMS in standing (115) and sitting (116). Pelvic asymmetry alters static posture of the entire LPHC, which alters normal arthrokinematics (coupling movement of the spine) (117–119). These changes in trunk kinematics were linked to nonspecific LBP (120). It has also been demonstrated that hip rotation asymmetry, in particular decreased hip internal rotation range of motion, is present in clients with sacroiliac joint dysfunction (121).

ABNORMAL MUSCLE ACTIVATION PATTERNS (ALTERED FORCE-COUPLE RELATIONSHIPS)

Because the LPHC musculature plays a critical role in stabilizing this complex, insufficiency of any of the musculature may induce biomechanical dysfunction and altered force-couple relationships (122). Subjects with LBP have been reported to demonstrate impaired postural control (123–125), delayed muscle relaxation (126,127), and abnormal muscle recruitment patterns (128), notably the transverse abdominus and multifidus activation is diminished in patients with LBP (129,130). A similar delay in activation of the internal oblique, multifidus, and gluteus maximus was observed on the symptomatic side of individuals with sacroiliac joint pain (131). Hides et al. (132) demonstrated that multifidus atrophy was present in clients even in the absence of continued LBP. Further, Iwai et al. (133) demonstrated that trunk extensor strength was correlated with LBP in collegiate wrestlers. Nadler et al. (134) demonstrated that a bilateral imbalance in isometric strength of the hip extensors was related to the development of LBP. The loads, forces, and movements that occur about the lumbar spine are controlled by a considerable

Figure 3.12   Pelvic asymmetry.

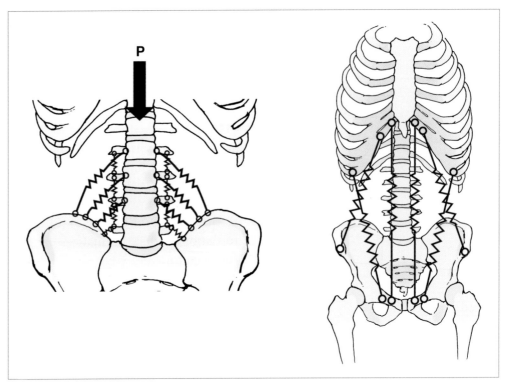

Figure 3.13   Local and global stabilizers.

number of ligaments and muscles. The ligaments that surround the spine limit intersegmental motion, maintaining the integrity of the lumbar spine. These ligaments may fail when proper motion cannot be created, proper posture cannot be maintained, or excessive motion cannot be resisted by the surrounding musculature (107–110). Therefore, decreasing the ability of local and global stabilizing muscles to produce adequate force can lead to ligamentous injury (Figure 3-13).

DYNAMIC MALALIGNMENTS

Decreased core neuromuscular control may contribute to increased valgus positioning of the lower extremity, which can lead to increased risk of knee injuries (84,135). Several studies have demonstrated that training of the trunk musculature may increase the control of hip adduction and internal rotation during functional activities and prevent dynamic malalignments and the potential injuries that arise from this impaired movement pattern (136–138).

Shoulder

SCIENTIFIC REVIEW

Shoulder pain is reported to occur in up to 21% of the general population (139,140) with 40% persisting for at least one year (141) at an estimated annual cost of $39 billion (142). Shoulder impingement is the most prevalent diagnosis, accounting for 40 to 65% of reported shoulder pain (143), while traumatic shoulder dislocations account for an additional 15 to 25% of shoulder pain (144–146). The persistent nature of shoulder pain may be the result of degenerative changes to the shoulder's capsuloligamentous structures, articular cartilage, and tendons as the result of altered shoulder mechanics. As many as 70% of individuals with shoulder dislocations experience recurrent instability within two years (146) and are at risk of developing glenohumeral osteoarthritis secondary to the increased motion at the glenohumeral joint (147,148). Degenerative changes may also affect the rotator cuff by weakening the tendons with time through intrinsic and extrinsic risk factors (142,149–151), such as repetitive overhead use (>60° of shoulder elevation), increased loads raised above shoulder height (152), and forward head and rounded shoulder posture (153), as well as altered scapular kinematics and muscle activity (154,155). Those factors are theorized to overload the shoulder muscles, especially the rotator cuff, which can lead to shoulder pain and dysfunction. Given the cost, rate of occurrence, and difficult resolution of shoulder pain, preventive exercise solutions that address these factors are essential in preventing shoulder injuries. It has been demonstrated that static malalignments (altered length-tension relationships or altered joint arthrokinematics), abnormal muscle activation patterns (altered force-couple relationships), and dynamic malalignments (movement system impairments) can lead to shoulder impairments (154–158).

STATIC MALALIGNMENTS (ALTERED LENGTH-TENSION RELATIONSHIPS OR ALTERED JOINT ARTHROKINEMATICS)

It has been demonstrated that posterior glenohumeral capsular contracture can alter normal glenohumeral kinematics, resulting in increased anterior and superior migration of the humeral head during shoulder flexion and significantly limiting shoulder internal rotation (159,160). It is also theorized that rounded shoulders (forward shoulder posture) (Figure 3-7) alters the normal length-tension relationship and joint kinematic balance of the shoulder complex (161). Any kinematic mechanism that reduces the subacromial space during humeral elevation will likely predispose an individual to impingement of the rotator cuff (162–164).

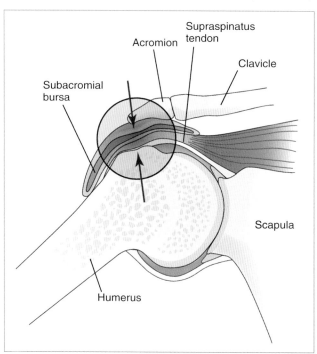

Figure 3.14 Shoulder impingement.

ABNORMAL MUSCLE ACTIVATION PATTERNS (ALTERED FORCE-COUPLE RELATIONSHIPS)

Rounded shoulder posture lengthens the rhomboids and lower trapezius musculature and shortens the serratus anterior, which alters the normal scapulothoracic force-couple relationship. This altered posture and muscle recruitment pattern would cause the scapula to remain forward-tipped and internally rotated relative to the elevating humerus, forcing the acromion and humerus to approximate and narrow the subacromial space (161,165,166) (Figure 3-14). Furthermore, a rounded shoulder posture may lead to decreased rotator cuff activation, which would decrease stabilization and lead to compression of the humeral head in the glenoid fossa (155,166).

DYNAMIC MALALIGNMENTS

There is a sequential muscle activation and force development pattern that is initiated from the ground to the core and through the extremities that has been demonstrated during kicking, running, and throwing and with a tennis serve (167–169). It has been demonstrated that approximately 85% of the muscle activation required to slow the forward-moving arm while throwing comes from the core and the scapulothoracic stabilizers (170). It has also been shown that maximal rotator cuff activation can be increased by 23 to 24% if the scapula is stabilized by the core musculature and the scapulothoracic stabilizers (trapezius, rhomboids, serratus anterior) (171). A recent study demonstrated a significant decrease in shoulder internal rotation (9.5 degrees), total shoulder motion (10.7 degrees), and elbow extension (3.2 degrees) immediately after pitching a baseball in the dominant shoulder. These changes continued to exist 24 hours after pitching (172). Altered static posture, muscle imbalances, and muscle weakness in the lower extremity, LPHC, or upper extremity can lead to dynamic malalignments.

SUMMARY • The HMS consists of the myofascial system, articular system, and neural system. Each system functions synergistically. Dysfunction in any system alters length-tension relationships, force-couple relationships, and joint kinematics, leading to movement impairment syndromes. The health and fitness professional must understand these concepts and the importance of maintaining proper structural and functional efficiency during training, reconditioning, and rehabilitation. The health and fitness professional must also be capable of performing a comprehensive HMS assessment before initiating a training program.

References

1. Sahrmann SA. Diagnosis and Treatment of Movement Impairment Syndromes. St. Louis, MO: Mosby; 2002.
2. Panjabi MM. The stabilizing system of the spine. Part I. Function, dysfunction, adaptation, and enhancement. *J Spinal Disord* 1992;5:383–9; discussion 97.
3. Panjabi MM. The stabilizing system of the spine. Part II. Neutral zone and instability hypothesis. *J Spinal Disord* 1992;5:390–6; discussion 97.
4. Neumann D. Kinesiology of the Musculoskeletal System: Foundations for Physical Rehabilitation. St. Louis, MO: Mosby; 2002.
5. Chaitow L. Muscle Energy Techniques. New York, NY: Churchill Livingstone; 1997.
6. Fredericson M, Powers CM. Practical management of patellofemoral pain. *Clin J Sport Med* 2002;12:36–8.
7. Fredericson M, White JJ, Macmahon JM, Andriacchi TP. Quantitative analysis of the relative effectiveness of 3 iliotibial band stretches. *Arch Phys Med Rehabil* 2002;83:589–92.
8. Powers CM, Ward SR, Fredericson M, Guillet M, Shellock FG. Patellofemoral kinematics during weight-bearing and non-weight-bearing knee extension in persons with lateral subluxation of the patella: a preliminary study. *J Orthop Sports Phys Ther* 2003;33: 677–85.
9. Powers CM. The influence of altered lower-extremity kinematics on patellofemoral joint dysfunction: a theoretical perspective. *J Orthop Sports Phys Ther* 2003;33:639–46.
10. Janda V. Muscles and Motor Control in Cervicogenic Disorders. In: Grant G, ed. Physical Therapy of the Cervical and Thoracic Spine. New York, NY: Churchill Livingstone; 2002:182–99.
11. Lewit K. Muscular and articular factors in movement restriction. *Man Med* 1985;1:83–5.
12. Sahrmann SA. Does postural assessment contribute to patient care? *J Orthop Sports Phys Ther* 2002;32:376–9.
13. Edgerton VR, Wolf SL, Levendowski DJ, Roy RR. Theoretical basis for patterning EMG amplitudes to assess muscle dysfunction. *Med Sci Sports Exerc* 1996;28:744–51.
14. Earl JE, Hertel J, Denegar CR. Patterns of dynamic malalignment, muscle activation, joint motion, and patellofemoral-pain syndrome. *J Sport Rehabil* 2005;14:215–33.
15. Wolfe MW, Uhl TL, Mattacola CG, McCluskey LC. Management of ankle sprains. *Am Fam Physician* 2001;63:93–104.
16. MacKinnon CD, Winter DA. Control of whole body balance in the frontal plane during human walking. *J Biomech* 1993;26:633–44.
17. Beckman SM, Buchanan TS. Ankle inversion injury and hypermobility: effect on hip and ankle muscle electromyography onset latency. *Arch Phys Med Rehabil* 1995;76:1138–43.

18. Sadeghi H, Sadeghi S, Prince F, Allard P, Labelle H, Vaughan CL. Functional roles of ankle and hip sagittal muscle moments in able-bodied gait. *Clin Biomech (Bristol, Avon)* 2001;16:688–95.

19. Friel K, McLean N, Myers C, Caceres M. Ipsilateral hip abductor weakness after inversion ankle sprain. *J Athl Train* 2006;41:74–8.

20. Hollman JH, Kolbeck KE, Hitchcock JL, Koverman JW, Krause DA. Correlations between hip strength and static foot and knee posture. *J Sport Rehabil* 2006;15:12–23.

21. Fulkerson JP. Diagnosis and treatment of patients with patellofemoral pain. *Am J Sports Med* 2002;30 447–56.

22. Riddle DL, Pulisic M, Pidcoe P, Johnson RE. Risk factors for plantar fasciitis: a matched case-control study. *J Bone Joint Surg Am* 2003;85-A:872–7.

23. Irving DB, Cook JL, Young MA, Menz HB. Obesity and pronated foot type may increase the risk of chronic plantar heel pain: a matched case-control study. *BMC Musculoskelet Disord* 2007;8:41.

24. Ireland ML, Willson JD, Ballantyne BT, Davis IM. Hip strength in females with and without patellofemoral pain. *J Orthop Sports Phys Ther* 2003;33:671–6.

25. Hootman JM, Dick R, Agel J. Epidemiology of collegiate injuries for 15 sports: summary and recommendations for injury prevention initiatives. *J Athl Train* 2007;42:311–19.

26. Fernandez WG, Yard EE, Comstock RD. Epidemiology of lower extremity injuries among U.S. high school athletes. *Acad Emerg Med* 2007;14:641–5.

27. Witvrouw E, Bellemans J, Lysens R, Danneels L, Cambier D. Intrinsic risk factors for the development of patellar tendinitis in an athletic population. A two-year prospective study. *Am J Sports Med* 2001;29: 190–5.

28. Mascal CL, Landel R, Powers C. Management of patellofemoral pain targeting hip, pelvis, and trunk muscle function: 2 case reports. *J Orthop Sports Phys Ther* 2003;33:647–60.

29. Thomee R, Renstrom P, Karlsson J, Grimby G. Patellofemoral pain syndrome in young women: a clinical analysis of alignment, pain parameters, common symptoms, functional activity level. *Scand J Med Sci Sports* 1995;5:237–44.

30. Bizzini M, Childs JD, Piva SR, Delitto A. Systematic review of the quality of randomized controlled trials for patellofemoral pain syndrome. *J Orthop Sports Phys Ther* 2003;33:4–20.

31. Crossley K, Bennell K, Green S, McConnell J. A systematic review of physical interventions for patellofemoral pain syndrome. *Clin J Sport Med* 2001;11:103–10.

32. Boling MC, Bolgla LA, Mattacola CG, Uhl TL, Hosey RG. Outcomes of a weight-bearing rehabilitation program for patients diagnosed with patellofemoral pain syndrome. *Arch Phys Med Rehabil* 2006;87: 1428–35.

33. Tyler TF, Nicholas SJ, Mullaney MJ, McHugh MP. The role of hip muscle function in the treatment of patellofemoral pain syndrome. *Am J Sports Med* 2006;34:630–6.

34. Powers CM. Rehabilitation of patellofemoral joint disorders: a critical review. *J Orthop Sports Phys Ther* 1998;28 345–54.

35. Fredericson M, Cookingham CL, Chaudhari AM, Dowdell BC, Oestreicher N, Sahrmann SA. Hip abductor weakness in distance runners with iliotibial band syndrome. *Clin J Sport Med* 2000;10:169–75.

36. Mountcastle SB, Posner M, Kragh JF, Taylor DC. Gender differences in anterior cruciate ligament injury vary with activity: epidemiology of anterior cruciate ligament injuries in a young, athletic population. *Am J Sports Med* 2007;35:1635–42.

37. Agel J, Arendt E, Bershadsky B. Anterior cruciate ligament injury in national collegiate athletic association basketball and soccer: a 13-year review. *Am J Sports Med* 2005;33:524–30.

38. Garrick JG, Requa RK. ACL Injuries in Men and Women—How Common Are They? In: Griffin LY, ed. Prevention of Noncontact ACL Injuries. Rosemont, IL: American Academy of Orthopaedic Surgeons; 2001.

39. Wilder FV, Hall BJ, Barrett JPJ, Lemrow NB. History of acute knee injury and osteoarthritis of the knee: a prospective epidemiological assessment. The Clearwater Osteoarthritis Study. *Osteoarthritis Cartilage* 2002;10:611–6.

40. Prodromos CC, Han Y, Rogowski J, Joyce B, Shi K. A meta-analysis of the incidence of anterior cruciate ligament tears as a function of gender, sport, and a knee injury-reduction regimen. *Arthroscopy* 2007;23:1320–5.

41. Arendt E, Dick R. Knee injury patterns among men and women in collegiate basketball and soccer. NCAA data and review of literature. *Am J Sports Med* 1995;23:694–701.

42. Arendt EA, Agel J, Dick R. Anterior cruciate ligament injury patterns among collegiate men and women. *J Athl Train* 1999;34:86–92.

43. Boden BP, Dean GS, Feagin JA, Garrett WE. Mechanisms of anterior cruciate ligament injury. *Orthopedics* 2000;23:573–8.

44. Ireland ML, Wall C. Epidemiology and comparison of knee injuries in elite male and female United States basketball athletes. *Med Sci Sports Exerc* 1990;22(Suppl):S82.

45. Arendt E. Anterior cruciate ligament injuries in women; review. *Sport Med Arthroscop* 1997;5:149–55.

46. Ireland ML. Anterior cruciate ligament injury in female athletes: epidemiology. *J Athl Train* 1999;34:150–4.

47. Hewett TE, Myer GD, Ford KR. Decrease in neuromuscular control about the knee with maturation in female athletes. *J Bone Joint Surg Am* 2004; 86-A:1601–8.

48. Uhorchak JM, Scoville CR, Williams GN, Arciero RA, St. Pierre P, Taylor DC. Risk factors associated with noncontact injury of the anterior cruciate ligament: a prospective four-year evaluation of 859 West Point cadets. *Am J Sports Med* 2003;31:831–42.

49. Junge A, Rosch D, Peterson L, Graf-Baumann T, Dvorak J. Prevention of soccer injuries: a prospective intervention study in youth amateur players. *Am J Sports Med* 2002;30:652–9.

50. Mandelbaum BR, Silvers HJ, Watanabe DS, et al. Effectiveness of a neuromuscular and proprioceptive training program in preventing anterior cruciate ligament injuries in female athletes: 2 year follow-up. *Am J Sports Med* 2005;33:1003–10.

51. Powers CM, Chen PY, Reischl SF, Perry J. Comparison of foot pronation and lower extremity rotation in persons with and without patellofemoral pain. *Foot Ankle Int* 2002;23:634–40.

52. Reischl SF, Powers CM, Rao S, Perry J. Relationship between foot pronation and rotation of the tibia and femur during walking. *Foot Ankle Int* 1999;20:513–20.

53. Payne KA, Berg K, Latin RW. Ankle injuries and ankle strength, flexibility, and proprioception in college basketball players. *J Athl Train* 1997;32:221–5.

54. Wiesler ER, Hunter DM, Martin DF, Curl WW, Hoen H. Ankle flexibility and injury patterns in dancers. *Am J Sports Med* 1996;24:754–7.

55. Greenman PE. Principles of Manual Medicine. Baltimore, MD: Lippincott Williams &Wilkins; 1996.

56. Denegar CR, Hertel J, Fonseca J. The effect of lateral ankle sprain on dorsiflexion range of motion, posterior talar glide, and joint laxity. *J Orthop Sports Phys Ther* 2002;32:166–73.

57. Green T, Refshauge K, Crosbie J, Adams R. A randomized controlled trial of a passive accessory joint mobilization on acute ankle inversion sprains. *Phys Ther* 2001;81:984–94.

58. Lentell G, Baas B, Lopez D, McGuire L, Sarrels M, Snyder P. The contributions of proprioceptive deficits, muscle function, and anatomic laxity to functional instability of the ankle. *J Orthop Sports Phys Ther* 1995;21:206–15.

59. Cornwall MW, Murrell P. Postural sway following inversion sprain of the ankle. *J Am Pediatr Med Assoc* 1991;81:243–7.

60. McGuine TA, Greene JJ, Best T, Leverson G. Balance as a predictor of ankle injuries in high school basketball players. *Clin J Sports Med* 2000;10:239–44.

61. Tropp H, Askling C, Gillquist J. Prevention of ankle sprains. *Am J Sports Med* 1985;13:259–62.

62. Gribble PA, Hertel J. Effect of hip and ankle muscle fatigue on unipedal postural control. *J Electromyogr Kinesiol* 2004;14:641–6.

63. Gribble PA, Hertel J. Effect of lower-extremity muscle fatigue on postural control. *Arch Phys Med Rehabil* 2004;85:589–92.

64. Cerny K. Pathomechanics of stance. Clinical concepts for analysis. *Phys Ther* 1984;64:1851–9.

65. Nicholas JA, Strizak AM, Veras G. A study of thigh muscle weakness in different pathological states of the lower extremity. *Am J Sports Med* 1976;4:241–8.

66. Khamis S, Yizhar Z. Effect of feet hyperpronation on pelvic alignment in a standing position. *Gait Posture* 2007;25:127–34.

67. Levine D, Whittle MW. The effects of pelvic movement on lumbar lordosis in the standing position. *J Orthop Sports Phys Ther* 1996;24:130–5.

68. Olsen OE, Myklebust G, Engebretsen L, Bahr R. Injury mechanisms for anterior cruciate ligament injuries in team handball: a systematic video analysis. *Am J Sports Med* 2004;32:1002–12.

69. Hewett TE. Neuromuscular and hormonal factors associated with knee injuries in female athletes. Strategies for intervention. *Sports Med* 2000;29:313–27.

70. Hewett TE, Myer GD, Ford KR, et al. Biomechanical measures of neuromuscular control and valgus loading of the knee predict anterior cruciate ligament injury risk in female athletes: a prospective study. *Am J Sports Med* 2005;33:492–501.

71. Hewett TE, Stroupe AL, Nance TA, Noyes FR. Plyometric training in female athletes. Decreased impact forces and increased hamstring torques. *Am J Sports Med* 1996;24:765–73.

72. Hewett TE, Ford KR, Myer GD, Wanstrath K, Scheper M. Gender differences in hip adduction motion and torque during a single-leg agility maneuver. *J Orthop Res* 2006;24:416–21.

73. Hewett TE, Myer GD, Ford KR. Reducing knee and anterior cruciate ligament injuries among female athletes: a systematic review of neuromuscular training interventions. *J Knee Surg* 2005;18:82–8.

74. Hewett TE, Ford KR, Myer GD. Anterior cruciate ligament injuries in female athletes: part 2, a meta-analysis of neuromuscular interventions aimed at injury prevention. *Am J Sports Med* 2006;34:490–8.

75. Mizuno Y, Kumagai M, Mattessich SM, et al. Q-angle influences tibiofemoral and patellofemoral kinematics. *J Orthop Res* 2001;19:834–40.

76. Cowan SM, Bennell KL, Hodges PW, Crossley KM, McConnell J. Delayed onset of electromyographic activity of vastus medialis obliquus relative to vastus lateralis in subjects with patellofemoral pain syndrome. *Arch Phys Med Rehabil* 2001;82:183–9.

77. Dierks TA, Manal KT, Hamill J, Davis IS. Proximal and distal influences on hip and knee kinematics in runners with patellofemoral pain during a prolonged run. *J Orthop Sports Phys Ther* 2008;38:448–56.

78. Cichanowski HR, Schmitt JS, Johnson RJ, Niemuth PE. Hip strength in collegiate female athletes with patellofemoral pain. *Med Sci Sports Exerc* 2007;39:1227–32.

79. Robinson RL, Nee RJ. Analysis of hip strength in females seeking physical therapy treatment for unilateral patellofemoral pain syndrome. *J Orthop Sports Phys Ther* 2007;37:232–8.

80. Heinert BL, Kernozek TW, Greany JF, Fater DC. Hip abductor weakness and lower extremity kinematics during running. *J Sport Rehabil* 2008;17:243–56.

81. Lawrence RK, Kernozek TW, Miller EJ, Torry MR, Reuteman P. Influences of hip external rotation strength on knee mechanics during single-leg drop landings in females. *Clin Biomech (Bristol, Avon)* 2008;23:806–13.

82. Vesci BJ, Padua DA, Bell DR, Strickand LJ, Guskiewicz KM, Hirth CJ. Influence of hip muscle strength, flexibility of hip and ankle musculature, and hip muscle activation on dynamic knee valgus motion during a double-legged squat. *J Athl Train* 2007;42:Supplement 83.

83. Wilson JD, Ireland ML, Davis I. Core strength and lower extremity alignment during single leg squats. *Med Sci Sports Exerc* 2006;38:945–52.

84. Zazulak BT, Hewett TE, Reeves NP, Goldberg B, Cholewicki J. Deficits in neuromuscular control of the trunk predict knee injury risk: a prospective biomechanical-epidemiologic study. *Am J Sports Med* 2007;35:1123–30.
85. Hewett TE, Zazulak BT, Myer GD, Ford KR. A review of electromyographic activation levels, timing differences, and increased anterior cruciate ligament injury incidence in female athletes. *Br J Sports Med* 2005;39:347–50.
86. Chaudhari AM, Andriacchi TP. The mechanical consequences of dynamic frontal plane limb alignment for non-contact ACL injury. *J Biomech* 2006;39:330–8.
87. Ford KR, Myer GD, Smith RL, Vianello RM, Seiwert SL, Hewett TE. A comparison of dynamic coronal plane excursion between matched male and female athletes when performing single leg landings. *Clin Biomech (Bristol, Avon)* 2006;21:33–40.
88. Jacobs CA, Uhl TL, Mattacola CG, Shapiro R, Rayens WS. Hip abductor function and lower extremity landing kinematics: sex differences. *J Athl Train* 2007;42:76–83.
89. Kernozek TW, Torry MR, H VANH, Cowley H, Tanner S. Gender differences in frontal and sagittal plane biomechanics during drop landings. *Med Sci Sports Exerc* 2005;37:1003–12; discussion 13.
90. Hewett TE, Myer GD, Ford KR. Anterior cruciate ligament injuries in female athletes: part 1, mechanisms and risk factors. *Am J Sports Med* 2006;34:299–311.
91. Zazulak BT, Ponce PL, Straub SJ, Medvecky MJ, Avedisian L, Hewett TE. Gender comparison of hip muscle activity during single-leg landing. *J Orthop Sports Phys Ther* 2005;35:292–9.
92. McLean SG, Fellin RE, Suedekum N, Calabrese G, Passerallo A, Joy S. Impact of fatigue on gender-based high-risk landing strategies. *Med Sci Sports Exerc* 2007;39:502–14.
93. McLean SG, Lipfert SW, van den Bogert AJ. Effect of gender and defensive opponent on the biomechanics of sidestep cutting. *Med Sci Sports Exerc* 2004;36:1008–16.
94. Millet GY, Lepers R. Alterations of neuromuscular function after prolonged running, cycling and skiing exercises. *Sports Med* 2004;34:105–16.
95. Miura K, Ishibashi Y, Tsuda E, Okamura Y, Otsuka H, Toh S. The effect of local and general fatigue on knee proprioception. *Arthroscopy* 2004;20:414–8.
96. Rodacki AL, Fowler NE, Bennett SJ. Multi-segment coordination: fatigue effects. *Med Sci Sports Exerc* 2001;33:1157–67.
97. Carcia CR, Shultz SJ, Granata KP, Perrin DH, Martin RL. Females recruit quadriceps faster than males at multiple knee flexion angles following a weight-bearing rotary perturbation. *Clin J Sport Med* 2005;15:167–71.
98. Lee TQ, Yang BY, Sandusky MD, McMahon PJ. The effects of tibial rotation on the patellofemoral joint: assessment of the changes in in situ strain in the peripatellar retinaculum and the patellofemoral contact pressures and areas. *J Rehabil Res Dev* 2001;38:463–9.
99. Dreisinger TE, Nelson B. Management of back pain in athletes. *Sports Med* 1996;21(4):313–20.
100. Kujala UM, Taimela S, Erkintalo M, Salminen JJ, Kaprio J. Low-back pain in adolescent athletes. *Med Sci Sports Exerc* 1996;28:165–70.
101. Nadler SF, Wu KD, Galski T, Feinberg JH. Low back pain in college athletes. A prospective study correlating lower extremity overuse or acquired ligamentous laxity with low back pain. *Spine* 1998;23:828–33.
102. Ganzit GP, Chisotti L, Albertini G, Martore M, Gribaudo CG. Isokinetic testing of flexor and extensor muscles in athletes suffering from low back pain. *J Sports Med Phys Fitness* 1998;38:330–6.
103. Lundin O, Hellstrom M, Nilsson I, Sward L. Back pain and radiological changes in the thoraco-lumbar spine of athletes. A long-term follow-up. *Scand J Med Sci Sports* 2001;11:103–9.
104. Sward L, Hellstrom M, Jacobsson B, Peterson L. Back pain and radiologic changes in the thoraco-lumbar spine of athletes. *Spine* 1990;15:124–9.
105. Luo X, Pietrobon R, Sun SX, Liu GG, Hey L. Estimates and patterns of direct health care expenditures among individuals with back pain in the United States. *Spine* 2004;29:79–86.
106. Greene HS, Cholewicki J, Galloway MT, Nguyen CV, Radebold A. A history of low back injury is a risk factor for recurrent back injuries in varsity athletes. *Am J Sports Med* 2001;29:795–800.
107. Holmes JA, Damaser MS, Lehman SL. Erector spinae activation and movement dynamics about the lumbar spine in lordotic and kyphotic squat-lifting. *Spine* 1992;17:327–34.
108. Kong WZ, Goel VK, Gilbertson LG, Weinstein JN. Effects of muscle dysfunction on lumbar spine mechanics. A finite element study based on a two motion segments model. *Spine* 1996;21:2197–206; discussion 206–7.
109. Arjmand N, Shirazi-Adl A. Biomechanics of changes in lumbar posture in static lifting. *Spine* 2005;30:2637–48.
110. McGill SM, Hughson RL, Parks K. Changes in lumbar lordosis modify the role of the extensor muscles. *Clin Biomech (Bristol, Avon)* 2000;15:777–80.
111. Hammer W. Functional Soft Tissue Examination and Treatment by Manual Methods. New York, NY: Aspen Publishers; 1999.
112. Evjenth O, Hamberg J, Brady MM. The Extremities: Muscle Stretching in Manual Therapy: A Clinical Manual. 3rd ed. Alfta, Sweden: New Intherlitho, Spa; 1993.
113. Drake JD, Callaghan JP. Intervertebral neural foramina deformation due to two types of repetitive combined loading. *Clin Biomech* 2009;24(1):1–6.
114. Lu YM, Hutton WC, Gharpuray VM. Do bending, twisting, and diurnal fluid changes in the disc affect the propensity to prolapse? A viscoelastic finite element model. *Spine* 1996;21(22):2570–9.
115. Young RS, Andrew PD, Cummings GS. Effect of simulating leg length inequality on pelvic torsion and trunk mobility. *Gait Posture* 2000;11:217–23.
116. Al-Eisa E, Egan D, Deluzio K, Wassersug R. Effects of pelvic asymmetry and low back pain on trunk kinematics during sitting: a comparison with standing. *Spine* 2006;31:E135–43.

117. White AA, Panjabi MM. Clinical Biomechanics of the Spine. 2nd ed. Philadelphia, PA: Lippincott Williams & Wilkins; 1990.

118. Cholewicki J, Crisco JJ III, Oxland TR, Yamamoto I, Panjabi MM. Effects of posture and structure on three-dimensional coupled rotations in the lumbar spine. A biomechanical analysis. *Spine* 1996;21:2421–8.

119. Panjabi M, Yamamoto I, Oxland T, Crisco J. How does posture affect coupling in the lumbar spine? *Spine* 1989;14:1002–11.

120. Lund T, Nydegger T, Schlenzka D, Oxland TR. Three-dimensional motion patterns during active bending in patients with chronic low back pain. *Spine* 2002;27:1865–74.

121. Cibulka MT, Sinacore DR, Cromer GS, Delitto A. Unilateral hip rotation range of motion asymmetry in patients with sacroiliac joint regional pain. *Spine* 1998;23:1009–15.

122. Takemasa R, Yamamoto H, Tani T. Trunk muscle strength in and effect of trunk muscle exercises for patients with chronic low back pain. The differences in patients with and without organic lumbar lesions. *Spine* 1995;20:2522–30.

123. Cholewicki J, Silfies SP, Shah RA, Greene HS, Reeves NP, Alvi K, Goldberg B. Delayed trunk muscle reflex responses increase the risk of low back injuries. *Spine* 2005;30:2614–20.

124. Cholewicki J, VanVliet JJ. Relative contribution of trunk muscles to the stability of the lumbar spine during isometric exertions. *Clin Biomech (Bristol, Avon)* 2002;17:99–105.

125. Radebold A, Cholewicki J, Polzhofer GK, Greene HS. Impaired postural control of the lumbar spine is associated with delayed muscle response times in patients with chronic idiopathic low back pain. *Spine* 2001;26:724–30.

126. Radebold A, Cholewicki J, Panjabi MM, Patel TC. Muscle response pattern to sudden trunk loading in healthy individuals and in patients with chronic low back pain. *Spine* 2000;25:947–54.

127. Reeves NP, Cholewicki J, Milner TE. Muscle reflex classification of low-back pain. *J Electromyogr Kinesiol* 2005;15:53–60.

128. van Dieen JH, Cholewicki J, Radebold A. Trunk muscle recruitment patterns in patients with low back pain enhance the stability of the lumbar spine. *Spine* 2003;28:834–41.

129. Ferreira PH, Ferreira ML, Hodges PW. Changes in recruitment of the abdominal muscles in people with low back pain: ultrasound measurement of muscle activity. *Spine* 2004;29:2560–6.

130. Hodges PW, Richardson CA. Inefficient muscular stabilization of the lumbar spine associated with low back pain. A motor control evaluation of transversus abdominis. *Spine* 1996;21:2640–50.

131. Hungerford BP, Gilleard WP, Hodges, PP. Evidence of altered lumbopelvic muscle recruitment in the presence of sacroiliac joint pain. *Spine* 2003;28: 1593–600.

132. Hides JA, Richardson CA, Jull GA. Multifidus muscle recovery is not automatic after resolution of acute, first-episode low back pain. *Spine* 1996;21:2763–9.

133. Iwai K, Nakazato K, Irie K, Fujimoto H, Nakajima H. Trunk muscle strength and disability level of low back pain in collegiate wrestlers. *Med Sci Sports Exerc* 2004;36:1296–300.

134. Nadler SF, Malanga GA, Feinberg JH, Prybicien M, Stitik TP, DePrince M. Relationship between hip muscle imbalance and occurrence of low back pain in collegiate athletes: a prospective study. *Am J Phys Med Rehabil* 2001;80:572–7.

135. Leetun DT, Ireland ML, Willson JD, Ballantyne BT, Davis IM. Core stability measures as risk factors for lower extremity injury in athletes. *Med Sci Sports Exerc* 2004;36:926–34.

136. Myer GD, Ford KR, Brent JL, Hewett TE. The effects of plyometric vs. dynamic stabilization and balance training on power, balance, and landing force in female athletes. *J Strength Cond Res* 2006;20:345–53.

137. Myer GD, Ford KR, Palumbo JP, Hewett TE. Neuromuscular training improves performance and lower-extremity biomechanics in female athletes. *J Strength Cond Res* 2005;19:51–60.

138. Paterno MV, Myer GD, Ford KR, Hewett TE. Neuromuscular training improves single-limb stability in young female athletes. *J Orthop Sports Phys Ther* 2004;34:305–16.

139. Bongers PM. The cost of shoulder pain at work. *BMJ* 2001;322:64–5.

140. Urwin M, Symmons D, Allison T, et al. Estimating the burden of musculoskeletal disorders in the community: the comparative prevalence of symptoms at different anatomical sites, and the relation to social deprivation. *Ann Rheum Dis* 1998;57:649–55.

141. Van der Heijden G. Shoulder disorders: a state of the art review. *Baillieres Best Pract Res Clin Rheumatol* 1999;13:287–309.

142. Johnson M, Crosley K, O'Neil M, Al Zakwani I. Estimates of direct health care expenditures among individuals with shoulder dysfunction in the United States. *J Orthop Sports Phys Ther* 2005;35:A4–PL8.

143. van der Windt DA, Koes BW, Boeke AJ, Deville W, De Jong BA, Bouter LM. Shoulder disorders in general practice: prognostic indicators of outcome. *Br J Gen Pract* 1996;46:519–23.

144. Matsen FA III, Thomas SC, Rockwood CA Jr. Anterior Glenohumeral Instability. In: Rockwood CA Jr, Matsen FA III, eds. The Shoulder, Vol 1. Philadelphia, PA: WB Saunders; 1990. p 526–622.

145. Dobson CC, Cordasco FA. Anterior glenohumeral joint dislocations. *Orthop Clin North Am* 2008;39(4):507–18, vii.

146. Blasier RB, Guldberg RE, Rothman ED. Anterior shoulder instability: contributions of rotator cuff forces and the capsular ligaments in a cadaver model. *J Shoulder Elbow Surg* 1992;1:140–50.

147. Buscayret F, Edwards TB, Szabo I, Adeleine P, Coudane H, Walch G. Glenohumeral arthrosis in anterior instability before and after surgical intervention. *Am J Sports Med* 2004;32:1165–72.

148. Cameron ML, Kocher MS, Briggs KK, Horan MP, Hawkins RJ. The prevalence of glenohumeral osteoarthrosis in unstable shoulders. *Am J Sports Med* 2003;31:53–5.

149. Bigliani LU, Levine WN. Subacromial impingement syndrome. *J Bone Joint Surg Am* 1997;79:1854–68.

150. Yamaguchi K, Ditsios K, Middleton WD, Hildebolt CF, Galatz LM, Teefey SA. The demographic and morphological features of rotator cuff disease. A comparison of asymptomatic and symptomatic shoulders. *J Bone Joint Surg Am* 2006;88:1699–704.

151. Yamaguchi K, Sher JS, Andersen WK, et al. Glenohumeral motion in patients with rotator cuff tears: a comparison of asymptomatic and symptomatic shoulders. *J Shoulder Elbow Surg* 2000;9:6–11.

152. NIOSH. Shoulder Musculoskeletal Disorders: Evidance for Work Readiness. In: Bernard, ed. Musculoskeletal disorders (MSD's) and workplace factors: a Critical Review of Epidemiologic Evidence for Work-related Musculoskeletal Disorders of the Neck, Upper Extremity, and Low Back. Cincinnati, OH: Centers for Disease Control and Prevention, 1997:122–95.

153. Szeto GPY, Straker L, Raine S. A field comparison of neck and shoulder postures in symptomatic and asymptomatic office workers. *Appl Ergon* 2002;33:75–84.

154. Thigpen CA, Padua DA, Karas SG. Comparison of scapular kinematics between individuals with and without multidirectional shoulder instability. *J Athl Train* 2005;40.

155. Thigpen CA, Padua DA, Xu N, Karas SG. Comparison of serratus anterior and upper trapezius muscle activation between subjects with and without multidirectional shoulder instability. *J Orthop Sports Phys Ther* 2005;35:A80–PL22.

156. Yamaguchi T, Ishii K, Yamanaka M, Yasuda K. Acute effect of static stretching on power output during concentric dynamic constant external resistance leg extension. *J Strength Cond Res* 2006;20:804–10.

157. Schmitt L, Snyder-Mackler L. Role of scapular stabilizers in etiology and treatment of impingement syndrome. *J Orthop Sports Phys Ther* 1999;29:31–8.

158. Meister K. Injuries to the shoulder in the throwing athlete. Part 1: biomechanics/pathophysiology/classification of injury. *Am J Sports Med* 2000;28:265–75.

159. Tyler TF, Nicholas SJ, Roy T, Gleim GW. Quantification of posterior capsule tightness and motion loss in patients with shoulder impingement. *Am J Sports Med* 2000;28:668–73.

160. Harryman DT, Sidles JA, Clark JM, McQuade KJ, Gibb TD, Matsen FA. Translation of the humeral head on the glenoid with passive glenohumeral motion. *J Bone Joint Surg Am* 1990;72:1334–43.

161. Hebert LJ, Moffet H, McFadyen BJ, Dionne CE. Scapular behavior in shoulder impingement syndrome. *Arch Phys Med Rehabil* 2002;83:60–9.

162. Fu FH, Harner CD, Klein AH. Shoulder impingement syndrome. A critical review. *Clin Orthop Relat Res* 1991:162–73.

163. Michener LA, McClure PW, Karduna AR. Anatomical and biomechanical mechanisms of subacromial impingement syndrome. *Clin Biomech (Bristol, Avon)* 2003;18:369–79.

164. Gohlke F, Barthel T, Gandorfer A. The influence of variations of the coracoacromial arch on the development of rotator cuff tears. *Arch Orthop Trauma Surg* 1993;113:28–32.

165. Cools AM, Witvrouw EE, Declercq GA, Vanderstraeten GG, Cambier DC. Scapular muscle recruitment patterns: trapezius muscle latency with and without impingement symptoms. *Am J Sports Med* 2003;31:542–9.

166. Halder AM, Halder CG, Zhao KD, O'Driscoll SW, Morrey BF, An KN. Dynamic inferior stabilizers of the shoulder joint. *Clin Biomech (Bristol, Avon)* 2001;16:138–43.

167. Putnam C. Sequential motions of body segments in striking and throwing skills: descriptions and explanations. *J Biomech* 1993;26(Suppl 1):125–35.

168. Kibler W, Chandler T, Livingston B, Roetert E. Shoulder range of motion in elite tennis players. Effect of age and years of tournament play. *Am J Sports Med* 1996;24:279–85.

169. Hirashima M, Kadota H, Sakurai S, Kudo K, Ohtsuki T. Sequential muscle activity and its functional role in the upper extremity and trunk during overarm throwing. *J Sports Sci* 2002;20:301–10.

170. Happee R, Van der Helm FC. The control of shoulder muscles during goal directed movements, an inverse dynamic analysis. *J Biomech* 1995;28:1179–91.

171. Kebaetse M, McClure P, Pratt NA. Thoracic position effect on shoulder range of motion, strength, and three-dimensional scapular kinematics. *Arch Phys Med Rehabil* 1999;80:945–50.

172. Reinold MM, Wilk KE, Macrina LC, et al. Changes in shoulder and elbow passive range of motion after pitching in professional baseball players. *Am J Sports Med* 2008;36:523–7.

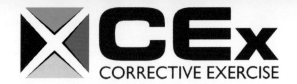

SECTION 2 | ASSESSING FOR HUMAN MOVEMENT DYSFUNCTION

CHAPTER 4

Health Risk Appraisal

OBJECTIVES

Upon completion of this chapter, you will be able to:

➤ Explain the components and function of a health appraisal.

➤ Ask appropriate general and medical questions to gather subjective information from clients.

➤ Recognize potential "red flags" that may need to be considered when designing a corrective exercise program.

INTRODUCTION

ASSESSMENTS are crucial in the design of a safe, individualized corrective exercise program. The first step in the assessment process is to perform a health risk appraisal on your client. The subjective information obtained in the health risk appraisal can offer insight into the individual's past, present, and, perhaps, future. The assessment will also provide the health and fitness professional any potential "red flags" that may need to be taken into account before starting a program. Some of the key pieces of information to obtain from a health risk appraisal include one's physical readiness for activity, general lifestyle information, and medical history.

READINESS FOR ACTIVITY

Gathering personal background information about an individual can be very valuable in gaining an understanding of the individual's physical condition and can also provide insights into what types of imbalances they may exhibit. One of the easiest methods of gathering this information is through the Physical Activity Readiness Questionnaire (PAR-Q) (Figure 4-1), which was designed to help determine whether a person is ready to undertake low-to-moderate-to-high activity levels (1). Furthermore, it aids in identifying people for whom

	Questions	Yes	No
1	Has your doctor ever said that you have a heart condition and that you should only perform physical activity recommended by a doctor?	☐	☐
2	Do you feel pain in your chest when you perform physical activity?	☐	☐
3	In the past month, have you had chest pain when you were not performing any physical activity?	☐	☐
4	Do you lose your balance because of dizziness or do you ever lose consciousness?	☐	☐
5	Do you have a bone or joint problem that could be made worse by a change in your physical activity?	☐	☐
6	Is your doctor currently prescribing any medication for your blood pressure or for a heart condition?	☐	☐
7	Do you know of <u>any</u> other reason why you should not engage in physical activity?	☐	☐

If you have answered "Yes" to one or more of the above questions, consult your physician <u>before</u> engaging in physical activity. Tell your physician which questions you answered "Yes" to. After a medical evaluation, seek advice from your physician on what type of activity is suitable for your current condition.

Figure 4.1 Sample physical activity readiness questionnaire (PAR-Q).

certain activities may not be appropriate or who may need further medical attention.

The PAR-Q is directed toward detecting any possible cardiorespiratory dysfunction, such as coronary heart disease, and is a good beginning point for gathering personal background information concerning one's cardiorespiratory function. However, it is only one component of a thorough corrective exercise assessment. Although this information is extremely important, asking other questions can provide additional information about an individual. This includes questions about an individual's general lifestyle and medical history.

GENERAL LIFESTYLE INFORMATION

Asking some very basic questions concerning an individual's history or personal background can provide a wealth of information. Two important areas to understand include one's occupation and lifestyle.

Occupation

Knowing a client's occupation can provide the health and fitness professional with insight into what his or her movement capacity is and what kinds of movement patterns are performed throughout the day. Examples of typical questions are shown in Figure 4-2.

By obtaining this information, a health and fitness professional can begin to recognize important clues about the structure and, ultimately, the function of a client. Each question provides relevant information about one's structure.

	Questions	Yes	No
1	What is your current occupation?		
2	Does your occupation require extended periods of sitting?	☐	☐
3	Does your occupation require extended periods of repetative movements? (If yes, please explain.)	☐	☐
4	Does your occupation require you to wear shoes with a heel (dress shoes)?	☐	☐
5	Does your occupation cause you anxiety (mental stress)?	☐	☐

Figure 4.2 Sample questions: client occupation.

EXTENDED PERIODS OF SITTING

This is a very important question that provides a lot of information. First, if an individual is sitting a large portion of the day, his or her hips are flexed for prolonged periods of time. This, in turn, can lead to tight hip flexors that can cause postural imbalances within the kinetic chain. Second, if an individual is sitting for prolonged periods of time, especially at a computer, there is a tendency for the shoulders and cervical spine to fatigue under the constant influence of gravity. This often leads to a postural imbalance of rounding of the shoulders and a forward head.

REPETITIVE MOVEMENTS

Repetitive movements can create a pattern overload to muscles and joints that may lead to tissue trauma and eventually kinetic chain dysfunction (2). This can be seen in jobs that require a lot of overhead work such as construction and painting. Working with the arms overhead for long periods may lead to shoulder soreness that could be the result of tightness in the latissimus dorsi and pectorals and weakness in the rotator cuff. This imbalance does not allow for proper shoulder motion or stabilization during activity which can lead to shoulder and neck pain.

DRESS SHOES

Wearing shoes with a heel puts the ankle complex in a plantarflexed position for extended periods. This can lead to tightness in the gastrocnemius and soleus, causing postural imbalance, such as overpronation at the foot and ankle complex (flattening of the arch of the foot) which can lead to foot and ankle injury.

MENTAL STRESS

Mental stress or anxiety can lead to a dysfunctional breathing pattern that can further lead to postural distortion and kinetic chain dysfunction (3,4).

Lifestyle

Questions pertaining to an individual's lifestyle will reflect what an individual does in his or her free time. This is generally known as their recreation or hobbies. Examples of typical questions are shown in Figure 4-3.

	Questions	Yes	No
1	Do you partake in any recreational activities (golf, tennis, skiing, etc.)? (If yes, please explain.)	☐	☐
2	Do you have any hobbies (reading, gardening, working on cars, etc.)? (If yes, please explain.)	☐	☐

Figure 4.3   Sample questions: client's lifestyle.

RECREATION

Recreation, in the context of an assessment, refers to an individual's physical activities outside of the work environment. By finding out what recreational activities an individual performs, a health and fitness professional can better design a program to fit these needs. This information also provides insight on the types of stresses being placed on one's structure that can lead to muscle imbalances. For example, many people like to golf, ski, play tennis, or engage in a variety of other sporting activities in their spare time. Proper program strategies must be incorporated to ensure that individuals are trained in a manner that optimizes the efficiency of the human movement system while addressing potential muscles imbalances that may be a result of their activity.

HOBBIES

Hobbies, in the context of an assessment, refer to activities that an individual may partake in regularly, but are not necessarily athletic in nature. Examples include gardening, working on cars, reading, watching television, and playing video games. In many of these cases, the individual must maintain a particular posture for an extended period of time, leading to potential muscle imbalances.

MEDICAL HISTORY

The medical history (Figure 4-4) is absolutely crucial. Not only does it provide information about any life-threatening chronic diseases (such as coronary heart disease, high blood pressure, and diabetes), it also provides information about the structure and function of the individual by uncovering important information such as past injuries, surgeries, imbalances, and chronic conditions.

	Questions	Yes	No
1	Have you ever had any pain or injuries (ankle, knee, hip, back, shoulder, etc.)? (If yes, please explain.)	☐	☐
	_____		
	_____		
2	Have you ever had any surgeries? (If yes, please explain.)	☐	☐
	_____		
	_____		
3	Has a medical doctor ever diagnosed you with a chronic disease, such as coronary heart disease, coronary artery disease, hypertension (high blood pressure), high cholesterol or diabetes? (If yes, please explain.)	☐	☐
	_____		
	_____		
4	Are you currently taking any medication? (If yes, please explain.)	☐	☐
	_____		
	_____		

Figure 4.4   Sample questions: client's medical history.

Past Injuries

Inquiring about an individual's past injuries can illuminate possible dysfunctions. One of the best predictors of future injuries is past injury. There is a vast array of research that has demonstrated past injuries affect the functioning of the human movement system (5–46). Beyond the risk of suffering the same injury again or compensating for an incompletely rehabilitated injury leading to another (possibly more serious) injury, a prior injury can also have effects up and down the kinetic chain:

1. Ankle Sprains

   Ankle sprains have been shown to decrease the neural control to the gluteus medius and gluteus maximus muscles. This, in turn, can lead to poor control of the lower extremities during many functional activities, which can eventually lead to injury (5–8).

2. Knee Injuries Involving Ligaments

   Knee injury can cause a decrease in the neural control to muscles that stabilize the patellofemoral and tibiofemoral joints and lead to further injury. Noncontact knee injuries are often the result of ankle or hip dysfunctions. The knee is caught between the ankle and the hip. If the ankle or hip joint begins to function improperly this results in altered movement and force distribution of the knee. Over time, this can lead to further injury (9–25).

3. Low-Back Injuries

   Low-back injuries can cause decreased neural control to stabilizing muscles of the core, resulting in poor stabilization of the spine. This can further lead to dysfunction in upper and lower extremities (26–33).

4. Shoulder Injuries
   Shoulder injuries cause altered neural control of the rotator cuff muscles, which can lead to instability of the shoulder joint during functional activities (34–42).
5. Other Injuries
   Injuries that result from human movement system imbalances include repetitive hamstring complex strains, groin strains, patellar tendonitis (jumper's knee), plantar fasciitis (pain in the arch of the foot), posterior tibialis tendonitis (shin splints), biceps tendonitis (shoulder pain), and headaches.

All of the aforementioned past injuries should be taken into consideration while assessing individuals, as the mentioned imbalances will manifest over time, unless proper care has been given. However, at best, individuals can recall only half their injury history, mostly the severe injuries. So a close examination of imbalances through further assessments performed by the health and fitness professional can turn up areas of potential risks.

Past Surgeries

Surgical procedures create trauma for the body and may have similar effects to those of an injury. They can create dysfunction, unless properly rehabilitated. Some common surgical procedures include the following:

- Foot and ankle surgery
- Knee surgery
- Back surgery
- Shoulder surgery
- Cesarean section for birth (cutting through the abdominal wall to deliver a baby)
- Appendectomy (cutting through the abdominal wall to remove the appendix)

In each case, surgery will cause pain and inflammation that can alter neural control to the affected muscles and joints if not rehabilitated properly (43,44).

Chronic Conditions

Numerous governmental, health-care organizations, professional medical societies, social organizations, and even special interest groups point out that chronic medical conditions will cost ever-increasing amounts of public and private money for ongoing, and sometimes lifetime, treatment. Routine care and care of complications from chronic conditions such as hypertension, hyperlipidemia, obesity, osteoarthritis, cardiopulmonary diseases, and diabetes may well become the greatest expense a nation can endure. It should not be surprising that many of these conditions have a lifestyle component that has some influence on the development of the disease, and in many cases the condition begins with the sedentary child, meaning the focus on prevention of chronic diseases needs to start maybe even as early as elementary school.

The American College of Sports Medicine has begun an *Exercise Is Medicine* initiative in an attempt to raise awareness in the medical community of the physician's obligation to prescribe and encourage an active lifestyle in all his or her patients. It is estimated that more than 75% of the American adult population does not partake, on a daily basis, in 30 minutes of low-to-moderate physical activity (45). The risk of chronic disease goes up significantly in individuals who are not as physically active as this minimal standard (45,46). In all likelihood, the health and fitness professional will work not only with relatively healthy clients, but also with clients with any number of chronic diseases such as:

- Cardiovascular disease, coronary artery disease, congenital heart disease, valvular disorders, or congestive heart failure
- Hypertension (high blood pressure)
- High cholesterol or other blood lipid disorders
- Stroke or peripheral artery disease
- Lung or breathing problems from smoking, asthma, obstructive pulmonary diseases, or exposure to inflammatory stimuli
- Obesity in children or adults
- Type 1 or type 2 diabetes mellitus
- Cancer

Medications

Some individuals may be under the care of a medical professional and may be required to use any one of a variety of medications. It is *not* the role of a health and fitness professional to administer, prescribe, or educate on the usage and effects of any of these medications.

The purpose of this section is to briefly outline some of the primary classes of drugs and their proposed physiologic effects (Tables 4-1 and 4-2). The tables are merely intended to present a simplistic overview of medications. They are *not* intended to serve as conclusive evidence regarding the medications

Table 4.1   COMMON MEDICATIONS BY CLASSIFICATION

Medication	Basic Function
Beta-Blockers (ß-Blockers)	Generally used as antihypertensive (high blood pressure); may also be prescribed for arrhythmias (irregular heart rate)
Calcium Channel Blockers	Generally prescribed for hypertension and angina (chest pain)
Nitrates	Generally prescribed for hypertension, congestive heart failure
Diuretics	Generally prescribed for hypertension, congestive heart failure, and peripheral edema
Bronchodilators	Generally prescribed to correct or prevent bronchial smooth muscle constrictor in individuals with asthma or other pulmonary diseases
Vasodilators	Used in the treatment of hypertension and congestive heart failure
Antidepressants	Use in the treatment of various psychiatric and emotional disorders

Table 4.2 EFFECTS OF MEDICATION ON HEART RATE AND BLOOD PRESSURE		
Medication	**Heart Rate**	**Blood Pressure**
Beta-Blockers (ß-Blockers)	↓	↓
Calcium Channel Blockers	↑ ↔ or ↓	↓
Nitrates	↑ ↔	↔ ↓
Diuretics	↔	↔ ↓
Bronchodilators	↔	↔
Vasodilators	↑ ↔ or ↓	↓
Antidepressants	↑ or ↔	↔ or ↓

↓, decrease; ↑, increase; ↔, no effect.

or their effects. For more complete information about medications, contact a health-care provider or refer to the *Physician's Desk Reference*.

SUMMARY • A health and fitness professional's primary responsibility is to safely and effectively guide clients to successful attainment of their goals. To do so requires a comprehensive understanding of an individual's background as well as his or her physical capabilities and desires. A health risk appraisal is the first step in gathering this information about clients to design an individualized corrective exercise program. A corrective exercise program is only as good as the assessment process, making all aspects of the assessment process crucial to ensure the program is safe and specific to meet the client's needs.

References

1. Thomas S, Reading J, Shephard R. Revision of the Physical Activity Readiness Questionnaire (PAR-Q). *Can J Sport Sci* 1992;17:338–45.
2. Bachrach RM. The relationship of low back pain to psoas insufficiency. *J Orthop Med* 1991;13:34–40.
3. Janda V. Muscles and Motor Control in Cervicogenic Disorders In: Grant R, ed. Physical Therapy of the Cervical and Thoracic Spine. Edinburgh: Churchill Livingstone; 1988:182–99.
4. Leahy PM. Active Release Techniques: Logical Soft Tissue Treatment. In: Hammer WI, ed. Functional Soft Tissue Examination and Treatment by Manual Methods. Gaithersburg, MD: Aspen Publishers, Inc; 1999: 549–60.
5. Bullock-Saxton JE. Local sensation changes and altered hip muscle function following severe ankle sprain. *Phys Ther* 1994;74:17–28; discussion 28–31.
6. Guskiewicz K, Perrin D. Effect of orthotics on postural sway following inversion ankle sprain. *J Orthop Sports Phys Ther* 1996;23:326–31.
7. Nitz A, Dobner J, Kersey D. Nerve injury and grades II and III ankle sprains. *Am J Sports Med* 1985;13: 177–82.
8. Wilkerson G, Nitz A. Dynamic ankle stability: mechanical and neuromuscular interrelationships. *J Sport Rehab* 1994;3:43–57.
9. Barrack R, Lund P, Skinner H. Knee proprioception revisited. *J Sport Rehab* 1994;3:18–42.
10. Beard D, Kyberd P, O'Connor J, Fergusson C. Reflex hamstring contraction latency in ACL deficiency. *J Orthop Res* 1994;12:219–28.
11. Boyd I. The histological structure of the receptors in the knee joint of the cat correlated with their physiological response. *J Physiol* 1954;124:476–88.
12. Corrigan J, Cashman W, Brady M. Proprioception in the cruciate deficient knee. *J Bone Joint Surg Br* 1992;74B:247–50.
13. DeCarlo M, Klootwyk T, Shelbourne D. ACL surgery and accelerated rehabilitation. *J Sport Rehab* 1997;6:144–56.

14. Ekholm J, Eklund G, Skoglund S. On the reflex effects from knee joint of the cat. *Acta Physiol Scand* 1960;50:167–74.
15. Feagin J. The syndrome of the torn ACL. *Orthop Clin North Am* 1979;10:81–90.
16. Fredericson M, Cookingham CL, Chaudhari AM, Dowdell BC, Oestreicher N, Sahrmann SA. Hip abductor weakness in distance runners with iliotibial band syndrome. *Clin J Sport Med* 2000;10:169–75.
17. Hewett TE, Lindenfeld TN, Riccobene JV, Noyes FR. The effect of neuromuscular training on the incidence of knee injury in female athletes. A prospective study. *Am J Sports Med* 1999;27:699–706.
18. Ireland ML, Willson JD, Ballantyne BT, Davis IM. Hip strength in females with and without patellofemoral pain. *J Orthop Sports Phys Ther* 2003;33:671–6.
19. Irrgang J, Harner C. Recent advances in ACL rehabilitation: clinical factors. *J Sport Rehab* 1997;6:111–24.
20. Irrgang J, Whitney S, Cox E. Balance and proprioceptive training for rehabilitation of the lower extremity. *J Sport Rehab* 1994;3:68–83.
21. Johansson H. Role of knee ligaments in proprioception and regulation of muscle stiffness. *J Electromyogr Kinesiol* 1991;1:158–79.
22. Johansson H, Sjolander P, Sojka P. A sensory role for the cruciate ligaments. *Clin Orthop Relat Res* 1991;268:161–78.
23. Johansson H, Sjölander P, Sojka P. Receptors in the knee joint ligaments and their role in the biomechanics of the joint. *Crit Rev Biomed Eng* 1991;18:341–68.
24. Nyland J, Smith S, Beickman K, Armsey T, Caborn D. Frontal plane knee angle affects dynamic postural control strategy during unilateral stance. *Med Sci Sports Exerc* 2002;34:1150–7.
25. Powers C. The influence of altered lower-extremity kinematics on patellofemoral joint dysfunction: a theoretical perspective. *J Orthop Sports Phys Ther* 2003;33:639–46.
26. Bullock-Saxton JE, Janda V, Bullock MI. Reflex activation of gluteal muscles in walking. An approach to restoration of muscle function for patients with low-back pain. *Spine* 1993;18:704–8.
27. Hodges P, Richardson C, Jull G. Evaluation of the relationship between laboratory and clinical tests of transversus abdominis function. *Physiother Res Int* 1996;1:30–40.
28. Hodges PW, Richardson CA. Inefficient muscular stabilization of the lumbar spine associated with low back pain. A motor control evaluation of transversus abdominis. *Spine* 1996;21:2640–50.
29. Hodges PW, Richardson CA. Contraction of the abdominal muscles associated with movement of the lower limb. *Phys Ther* 1997;77:132–42; discussion 142–4.
30. Janda V. Muscles and Motor Control in Low Back Pain: Assessment and Management. In: Twomey L, ed. Physical Therapy of the Low Back. New York, NY: Churchill Livingstone;1987.
31. Lewit K. Muscular and articular factors in movement restriction. *Manual Med* 1985;1:83–5.
32. O'Sullivan P, Twomey L, Allison G, Sinclair J, Miller K, Knox J. Altered patterns of abdominal muscle activation in patients with chronic low back pain. *Aust J Physiother* 1997;43:91–8.
33. Richardson C, Jull G, Toppenberg R, Comerford M. Techniques for active lumbar stabilization for spinal protection. *Aust J Physiother* 1992;38:105–12.
34. Broström L-Å, Kronberg M, Nemeth G. Muscle activity during shoulder dislocation. *Acta Orthop Scand* 1989;60:639–41.
35. Glousman R. Electromyographic analysis and its role in the athletic shoulder. *Clin Orthop Relat Res* 1993;288:27–34.
36. Glousman R, Jobe F, Tibone J, Moynes D, Antonelli D, Perry J. Dynamic electromyographic analysis of the throwing shoulder with glenohumeral instability. *J Bone Joint Surg Am* 1988;70A:220–6.
37. Hanson ED, Leigh S, Mynark RG. Acute effects of heavy- and light-load squat exercise on the kinetic measures of vertical jumping. *J Strength Cond Res* 2007;21:1012–7.
38. Howell S, Kraft T. The role of the supraspinatus and infraspinatus muscles in glenohumeral kinematics of anterior shoulder instability. *Clin Orthop Relat Res* 1991;263:128–34.
39. Kedgley A, Mackenzie G, Ferreira L, Johnson J, Faber K. In vitro kinematics of the shoulder following rotator cuff injury. *Clin Biomech (Bristol, Avon)* 2007;22:1068–73.
40. Kronberg M, Broström L-Å, Nemeth G. Differences in shoulder muscle activity between patients with generalized joint laxity and normal controls. *Clin Orthop Relat Res* 1991;269:181–92.
41. Yanagawa T, Goodwin C, Shelburne K, Giphart J, Torry M, Pandy M. Contributions of the individual muscles of the shoulder to glenohumeral joint stability during abduction. *J Biomech Eng* 2008;130:21–4.
42. Yasojima T, Kizuka T, Noguchi H, Shiraki H, Mukai N, Miyanaga Y. Differences in EMG activity in scapular plane abduction under variable arm positions and loading conditions. *Med Sci Sports Exerc* 2008;40:716–21.
43. Graven-Nielsen T, Mense S. The peripheral apparatus of muscle pain: evidence from animal and human studies. *Clin J Pain* 2001;17:2–10.
44. Mense S, Simons D. Muscle Pain. Understanding its Nature, Diagnosis, and Treatment. Philadelphia, PA: Williams & Wilkins;2001.
45. Lambert E, Bohlmann I, Cowling K. Physical activity for health: understanding the epidemiological evidence for risk benefits. *Int J Sports Med* 2001;1:1–15.
46. Pate R, Pratt M, Blair S, et al. Physical activity and public health: a recommendation from the Centers for Disease Control and Prevention and the American College of Sports Medicine. *JAMA* 1995;273:402–7.

CHAPTER 5

Static Postural Assessments

OBJECTIVES *Upon completion of this chapter, you will be able to:*

➤ Define the function of a static postural assessment.

➤ Describe the kinetic chain implications for static postural alignment.

➤ Discuss the avenues through which static postural alignment may alter over time.

➤ Discuss the implications for existing postural distortions.

➤ Perform a static postural assessment.

INTRODUCTION

POSTURAL assessments have been a tool available to clinicians across the ages. Before the availability of data-driven technologies, postural assessments were a critical component of any evaluation. As the limitations of some of these data-driven technologies to provide kinetic chain–related information are being realized, postural assessments and functional movement assessments are being given greater credence (1–3). The renaissance of these qualitative assessments has then posed the difficulty of quantifying qualitative information in an attempt to provide objective and measurable baselines. In this new age of evidence-based medicine, there has been little time to allow for the applied clinical research to objectively evaluate these qualitative techniques. Therefore, there is limited clinical research and subsequently limited evidence-based research on the efficacy of postural assessments.

Static posture: how individuals physically present themselves in stance. It is reflected in the alignment of the body.

POSTURE

Posture can be thought of as static or dynamic. **Static posture**, or how individuals physically present themselves in stance, could be considered the base from which an individual moves. It is reflected in the alignment of the body (Figure 5-1). It provides the foundation or the platform from which

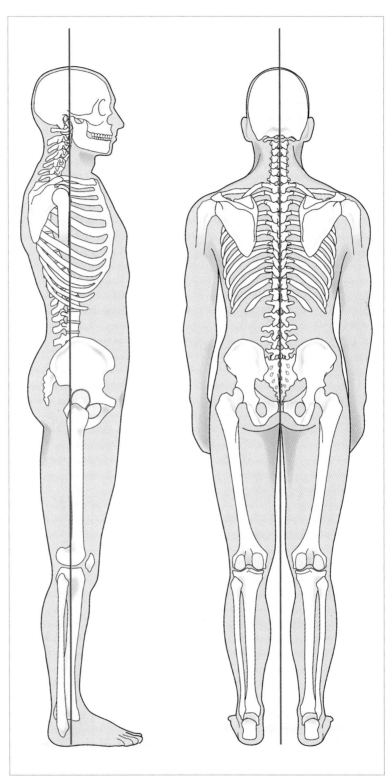

Figure 5.1 Static posture.

Dynamic posture: how an individual is able to maintain posture while performing functional tasks.

the extremities function. As with any structure, a weak foundation leads to secondary problems elsewhere in the system. For instance, the shifting foundation of a house may not be noticed until the cracks appear in the walls or problems occur at the roof.

Dynamic posture is reflective of how an individual is able to maintain posture while performing functional tasks. This will be covered in further detail in chapter six. For the sake of this chapter, we will be focusing on static postural assessments.

IMPORTANCE OF POSTURE AS IT RELATES TO INJURY

The use of a static postural assessment has been the basis for identifying muscle imbalances. The assessment may not be able to specifically identify whether a problem is structural (or biomechanical) in nature or whether it is derived from the development of poor muscular recruitment patterns with resultant muscle imbalances. However, a static postural assessment provides excellent indicators of problem areas that must be further evaluated to clarify the problems at hand. This allows for intervention at the level of the causative factor rather than simply treating the symptomatic complaints. For instance, it is easy to add a bit more plaster to a crack in the wall, sand it out, and paint over it. However, if the weakened and shifted foundation of the house is left as is, the visible cracks in the wall will return, accompanied by perhaps larger cracks in the wall and problems with the ceiling. At some point, the "patch and go" approach no longer works, forcing a larger intervention, perhaps a renovation or reconstruction. The same is true within the body. We can continue to treat the symptomatic complaints using anti-inflammatory medications, modification of activities, or simply pushing through the pain, all leading to further dysfunction adding layer upon layer of structural and neuromuscular adaptations. However, if we return to looking for the causative factors of the inflammation, discomfort, or poor performance, we will more likely be successful in selecting the most effective intervention to alleviate the dysfunction and provide the pain-free functional outcomes we seek for our clients. Beginning with a static postural assessment is a fundamental step to achieve this goal-oriented outcome.

MUSCLE IMBALANCE

Myofascial: the connective tissue in and around muscles and tendons.

There may be several causative factors for changes in joint alignment, including quality and function of **myofascial** tissue, and alterations in muscle-tendon function. Whatever the reason, the body will continually adapt in an attempt to produce the functional outcome that is requested by the system. Unfortunately, this adaptability will lead to imbalances and eventually to imbalances that move beyond a dysfunction and into tissue damage and pathology. Along the continuum of the adaptation, the muscle-tendon units will shorten or lengthen as the stressors demand. This can result in the stabilizing muscles being less efficient to stabilize joints as they are pulled out of optimal alignment (4–7).

Muscle imbalance: alteration in the functional relationship between pairs or groups of muscles.

Muscle imbalance is a condition in which there is a lack of balance between certain types of muscles. This tendency appears to be fairly systematic. It seems that certain muscles are prone to shortening (tightness), whereas other muscles are susceptible to lengthening and weakness (inhibition) (8, 9). The combination of tight and weak muscles can alter normal movement patterns (10, 11). This results in an alteration of the biomechanics of joints leading to degeneration. Table 5-1 lists the muscles prone to shortening and lengthening.

Table 5.1 MUSCLES PRONE TO SHORTENING AND LENGTHENING	
Typically Shortened Muscles	**Typically Lengthened Muscles**
Gastrocnemius	Anterior tibialis
Soleus	Posterior tibialis
Adductors	Vastus medialis oblique (VMO)
Hamstring complex	Gluteus maximus/medius
Psoas	Transverse abdominus
Tensor fascia latae	Internal oblique
Rectus femoris	Multifidus
Piriformis	Serratus anterior
Quadratus lumborum	Middle/lower trapezius
Erector spinae	Rhomboids
Pectoralis major/minor	Teres minor
Latissimus dorsi	Infraspinatus
Teres major	Posterior deltoid
Upper trapezius	Deep cervical flexors
Levator scapulae	
Sternocleidomastoid	
Scalenes	

Adapted from Janda V. Muscles and Motor Control in Low Back Pain: Assessment and Management. In: Twomey LT, ed. Physical Therapy of the Low Back. Edinburgh: Churchill Livingstone; 1987:253–78.

HOW DO ALTERATIONS IN STATIC POSTURE OCCUR?

The main factors that cause postural imbalance include the following:

1. Habitual movement patterns
2. Altered movement patterns from repetitive movement
3. Altered movement patterns from injury
4. Altered movement patterns from surgery
5. Altered movement patterns from incompletely rehabilitated injuries

Habitual Movement Patterns

It is essential for the health and fitness professional to have an understanding of posture and the importance it has in our daily lives. It is even more important to realize what effects posture has on a daily basis. Individuals may have developed some poor postural habits without even realizing it. Many individuals carry overstuffed briefcases on just one side of their body, which chronically overloads it. Frequently the body does not readjust itself to neutral positioning and continues to move in this imbalanced position, even when not loaded. The same may be true for those who do a lot of driving. Chronic use of the right lower extremity without awareness of trying to maintain symmetry causes the body to shift to the right and promote external rotation of the left lower extremity. Workstations both at home and at the office frequently contribute to neck and arm dysfunction. Positioning of the computer monitor, the keyboard, and the chair may all create an environment for the development of postural deviations (Figure 5-2).

Altered Movement Patterns from Repetitive Movement

Repetition of movement as in chronic overuse or injury can lead to a change in the elasticity of the muscle (12). Poor posture and a lack of daily movement are also considered a contributing factor (13). Muscle that is repeatedly placed in a shortened position, such as the iliopsoas complex during sitting, will eventually adapt and tend to remain short (10,14). Stress and chronic fatigue may also result in muscle imbalances (15,16).

Repetitive movements can cause imbalances by placing demands on certain muscle groups more predominantly. This is evident when looking at many athletes such as swimmers, runners, and tennis players. Swimmers often exhibit overemphasized pectoral muscles in relation to the scapular retractors, giving them a rounded shoulder posture (17) (Figure 5-3).

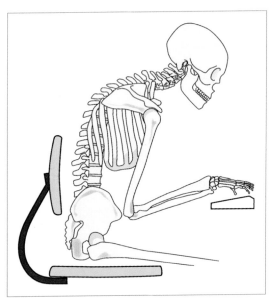

Figure 5.2   Habitual patterns.

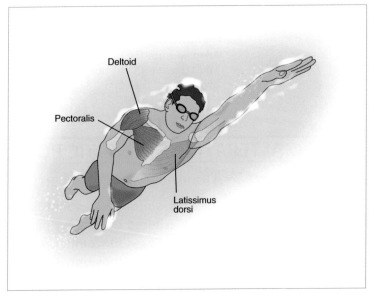

Figure 5.3   Overused muscles on swimmers.

Repetitive movement also affects everyday people such as a construction worker who is hammering with the same hand day in and day out (Figure 5-4). Waiters and waitresses often carry large trays with the same arm, much the same as a mother carries her child on the same hip.

Postural imbalances are also seen in the gym with people who focus on certain muscle groups more so than others. This is evident in individuals who overemphasize chest, shoulder, and biceps work (Figure 5-5). This often results in rounded shoulders, a forward head, and internal rotation at the shoulder joint.

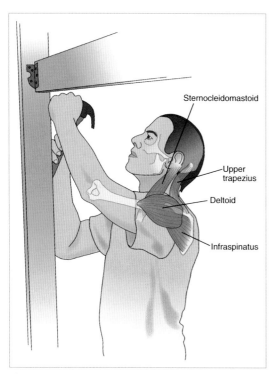

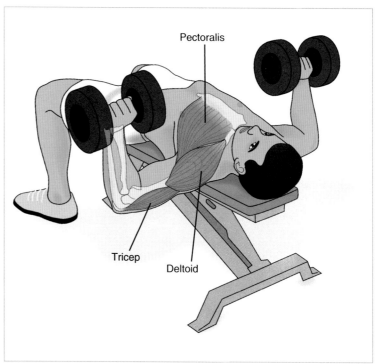

Figure 5.4 Overused muscles on construction workers.

Figure 5.5 Overused muscles on gym members.

Altered Movement Patterns from Injury

Acute injury may result in chronic muscle imbalances. An individual may assume adaptive postures to avoid pain or to create function. Oftentimes, even after the pain has subsided and motion restrictions or strength has returned, the individual may not change his or her adaptive movement strategies unless reminded to return to a more normal motor pattern. It is those mild yet repetitive ankle sprains, or the occasional sore back, that continues to promote modified motion. The changing movement patterns alter loads across the joints and alter recruitment strategies of muscles, all leading to muscular imbalances reflected in postural changes.

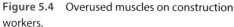

Hypomobility: restricted motion.

Injury may also result in tissue that becomes restricted (**hypomobility**). Immobilizations through splinting or self-immobilization as a result of pain may allow tissue to shorten. Without restoring mobility, the reciprocal muscles are lengthened, creating weakness. Muscles that are too short and tight are then functionally paired with muscles that are lengthened and weak, disrupting the neuromuscular balance in the interdependent relationship. Postural changes caused by the muscle imbalances become evident.

Altered Movement Patterns from Surgery

Even the best of surgeries results in scar tissue. Scar mobility is often an overlooked aspect of the rehabilitation paradigm. Lack of mobility alters the tissue alignment and pulls on the fascia, affecting joints and muscle function. There may have been some compensatory altered movement patterns used for functional mobility before the surgery or shortly after the surgical intervention. Balanced movement must be actively restored, or resultant muscle imbalances and postural changes will develop.

Altered Movement Patterns from Incompletely Rehabilitated Injuries

In these days of a limited number of visits for insurance-covered rehabilitation, many clients may have initiated a rehabilitative intervention after an injury, but have been discharged before return to their required functional level. They then continue on their own well-intended programs that may be overlooking the imbalances that were never resolved. Or they may simply discontinue rehabilitation and be willing to live within their current limitations. In either case, the body will adapt to the available mobility and stability, creating compensatory movement patterns that are eventually reflective in postural imbalance.

By knowing what can cause improper postural habits, the health and fitness professional can begin to properly address the client's needs. As a common denominator, improper posture usually results from or leads to muscle imbalances (4, 5, 10, 14, 15, 18–22). The health and fitness professional's job is to identify those muscle imbalances, identify the causative agents, and institute a comprehensive corrective exercise program. A postural assessment is the first step in assessing the client's status.

COMMON DISTORTIONAL PATTERNS

How an individual presents himself or herself in static stance is, in a sense, a road map of how the body has been used over time. Twists and turns in what should otherwise be a fairly erect and cylindrical structure are evidence of compensatory movement patterns. Something is not working as well as the body requires it to work; therefore, it has called on other structures or muscle groups to "jump in and help" (synergistic dominance). Most structures and muscle groups in the body have very defined functional roles. Although they may be appropriately used to create more than one movement, for instance the quadriceps may flex the hip (rectus femoris) or extend the knee; however, when asked to provide rotational stability at the knee, the quadriceps may be hypertrophied from the overtaxing use and result in symptomatic complaints of infrapatellar tendonitis, anterior knee pain, or patellofemoral dysfunction. Hips shifted off of midline may indicate load-bearing habits to one side and may be reflective of imbalances in the pelvis as a result of carrying a heavy briefcase. Or those driving may develop fatigue and tightness in the right leg.

What is interesting is that the body has a tendency to compensate in particular patterns or by particular relationships between muscles. These patterns were studied and described by Janda (19) in the early 1970s. Florence and Henry Kendall similarly studied these patterns and took an alternative approach of addressing these postural deviations through the relationship of agonist–antagonist muscle groups. Their work was continued by one of Florence Kendall's students, Shirley Sahrmann (23).

JANDA'S POSTURAL DISTORTION SYNDROMES

Lower crossed syndrome: a postural distortion syndrome characterized by an anterior tilt to the pelvis and lower-extremity muscle imbalances.

Upper crossed syndrome: a postural distortion syndrome characterized by a forward head and rounded shoulders with upper-extremity muscle imbalances.

Pronation distortion syndrome: a postural distortion syndrome characterized by foot pronation and lower-extremity muscle imbalances.

Janda identified three basic compensatory patterns (19). This is not to say that other compensations do not occur. He simply suggested that there was a cascading effect of alterations or deviations in static posture that would more likely than not present themselves in a particular pattern. The three postural distortion patterns to be assessed during a static postural assessment include the **lower crossed syndrome**, **upper crossed syndrome**, and **pronation distortion syndrome**. These three static postural distortion syndromes can translate into the lower and upper extremity movement impairment syndromes discussed in chapter three during functional movement. Assessments for the movement impairment syndromes will be done through the use of movement assessments discussed in the next chapter.

Lower Crossed Syndrome

An individual with lower crossed syndrome is characterized by increased lumbar lordosis and an anterior pelvic tilt (Figure 5-6). There are common muscles that are too tight and others that are too weak. The muscles that may be tight include the gastrocnemius, soleus, adductor complex, hip flexor complex (psoas, rectus femoris, tensor fascia latae), latissimus dorsi, and the erector spinae (Table 5-2). The muscles that are commonly weak or lengthened include the posterior tibialis, anterior tibialis, gluteus maximus, gluteus medius, transverse abdominus, and internal oblique (Table 5-2). The pattern of tightness and weakness indicative of lower crossed syndrome causes predictable patterns of joint dysfunctions, movement imbalances, and injury patterns. Associated joint dysfunctions include the subtalar joint, tibiofemoral joint, iliofemoral joint, sacroiliac joint, and lumbar facet joints. Common movement dysfunctions include decreased stabilization of the lumbar spine during functional movements. This is characterized by excessive lumbar lordosis with squatting, lunging, or overhead pressing.

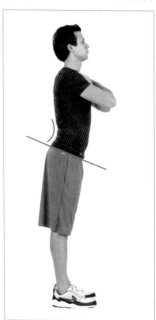

Figure 5.6   Lower crossed syndrome.

Table 5.2	LOWER CROSSED SYNDROME SUMMARY		
Short Muscles	**Lengthened Muscles**	**Altered Joint Mechanics**	**Possible Injuries**
Gastrocnemius	Anterior tibialis	**Increased:**	Hamstring complex strain
Soleus	Posterior tibialis	Lumbar extension	Anterior knee pain
Hip flexor complex	Gluteus maximus		Low-back pain
Adductors	Gluteus medius	**Decreased:**	
Latissimus dorsi	Transversus abdominis	Hip extension	
Erector spinae	Internal oblique		

Common injury patterns include hamstring complex strains, anterior knee pain, and low-back pain (5,10,14).

Upper Crossed Syndrome

Individuals with upper crossed syndrome are characterized by rounded shoulders and a forward head posture (Figure 5-7). This pattern is common in individuals who sit a lot or who develop pattern overload from one-dimensional training protocols. Functionally tightened muscles include the pectoralis major, pectoralis minor, subscapularis, latissimus dorsi, levator scapulae, upper trapezius, teres major, sternocleidomastoid, and scalenes (Table 5-3). Functionally weakened or lengthened muscles include the rhomboids, lower trapezius, teres minor, infraspinatus, serratus anterior, and deep cervical flexors (Table 5-3). Potential joint dysfunctions include the sternoclavicular joint, acromioclavicular joint, and thoracic and cervical facet joints. Potential injury patterns include rotator cuff impingement, shoulder instability, biceps tendinitis, thoracic outlet syndrome, and headaches (5,10,14).

Pronation Distortion Syndrome

Individuals with pronation distortion syndrome are characterized by excessive foot pronation (flat feet), knee flexion, internal rotation, and adduction ("knock-kneed") (Figure 5-8). Functionally tightened muscles include the peroneals, gastrocnemius, soleus, iliotibial band, hamstring complex, adductor complex, and psoas (Table 5-4). Functionally weakened or inhibited areas include the posterior tibialis, anterior tibialis, vastus medialis, gluteus medius, gluteus maximus, and hip external rotators (Table 5-4). Potential joint dysfunctions include the first metatarsophalangeal joint, subtalar joint, talocrural joint, sacroiliac joint, and lumbar facet joints. Individuals with pronation distortion syndrome develop predictable patterns of injury, including plantar fasciitis, posterior tibialis tendinitis (shin splints), patellar tendonitis, and low-back pain (24–26).

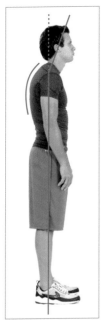

Figure 5.7 Upper crossed syndrome.

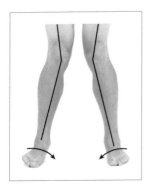

Figure 5.8 Pronation distortion syndrome.

Table 5.3	UPPER CROSS SYNDROME SUMMARY		
Short Muscles	**Lengthened Muscles**	**Altered Joint Mechanics**	**Possible Injuries**
Upper trapezius	Deep cervical flexors	**Increased:**	Headaches
Levator scapulae	Serratus anterior	Cervical extension	Biceps tendonitis
Sternocleidomastoid	Rhomboids	Scapular protraction/elevation	Rotator cuff impingement
Scalenes	Mid-trapezius		Thoracic outlet syndrome
Latissimus dorsi	Lower trapezius	**Decreased:**	
Teres major	Teres minor	Shoulder extension	
Subscapularis	Infraspinatus	Shoulder external rotation	
Pectoralis major/minor			

Table 5.4   PRONATION DISTORTION SYNDROME SUMMARY

Short Muscles	Lengthened Muscles	Altered Joint Mechanics	Possible Injuries
Gastrocnemius	Anterior tibialis	**Increased:**	Plantar fascitis
Soleus	Posterior tibialis	Knee adduction	Posterior tibialis tendonitis (shin splints)
Peroneals	Vastus medialis	Knee internal rotation	Patellar tendonitis
Adductors	Gluteus medius/maximus	Foot pronation	Low-back pain
Iliotibial band	Hip external rotators	Foot external rotation	
Hip flexor complex		**Decreased:**	
Biceps femoris (short head)		Ankle dorsiflexion	
		Ankle inversion	

(*Text continues on page 103*)

SYSTEMATIC APPROACH TO ASSESS STATIC POSTURE

Static postural assessments require a strong visual observation skill from the practitioner. This can be developed with time and practice. It requires a systematic approach. Commonly, static postural assessments begin at the feet and travel upward toward the head. We are bipedal in nature, and our feet interact with the external environment with every step we take. Often, alterations or deviations observed in the lower part of the body are then reflected in compensatory alterations or deviations farther up the kinetic chain. Many of these compensations can be identified through a comprehensive static postural assessment.

➤ KINETIC CHAIN CHECKPOINTS

Postural assessments require observation of the kinetic chain (human movement system). To structure this observation, NASM has devised the use of kinetic chain checkpoints to allow the health and fitness professional to systematically view the body statically and during motion (which will be reviewed in the next chapter). The kinetic chain checkpoints refer to major joint regions of the body including the following:

1. Foot and ankle
2. Knee
3. Lumbo-pelvic-hip complex (LPHC)
4. Shoulders
5. Head/cervical spine

ANTERIOR VIEW

- Foot/ankles: straight and parallel, not flattened or externally rotated
- Knees: in line with toes, not adducted or abducted
- LPHC: pelvis level with both anterior superior iliac spines in same transverse plane
- Shoulders: level, not elevated or rounded
- Head: neutral position, not tilted or rotated

Note: An imaginary line should begin midway between the heels, extending upward between the lower extremities, through the midline of the pelvis and through the trunk and skull.

Continued on page 102

Kinetic Chain Checkpoints, Anterior View

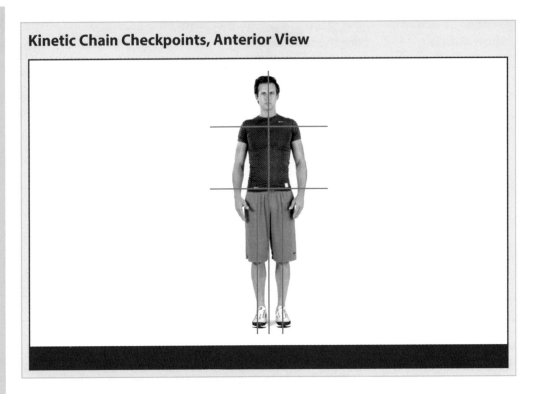

LATERAL VIEW

- Foot/ankle: neutral position, leg vertical at right angle to sole of foot
- Knees: neutral position, not flexed or hyperextended
- LPHC: pelvis in neutral position, not anteriorly (lumbar extension) or posteriorly rotated (lumbar flexion)
- Shoulders: normal kyphotic curve, not excessively rounded
- Head: neutral position, not in excessive extension ("jutting" forward)

Note: An imaginary line should run slightly anterior to the lateral malleolus, through the middle of the femur, center of the shoulder, and middle of the ear.

Kinetic Chain Checkpoints, Lateral View

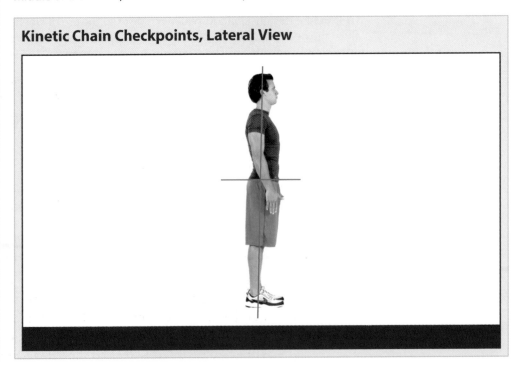

POSTERIOR VIEW

- Foot/ankle: heels are straight and parallel, not overly pronated
- Knees: neutral position, not adducted or abducted
- LPHC: pelvis level with both posterior superior iliac spines in same transverse plane
- Shoulders/scapulae: level, not elevated or protracted (medial borders essentially parallel and approximately 3 to 4 inches apart)
- Head: neutral position neither tilted nor rotated

Note: An imaginary line should begin midway between the heels, extending upward between the lower extremities, through the midline of the pelvis and through the spine and skull.

Kinetic Chain Checkpoints, Posterior View

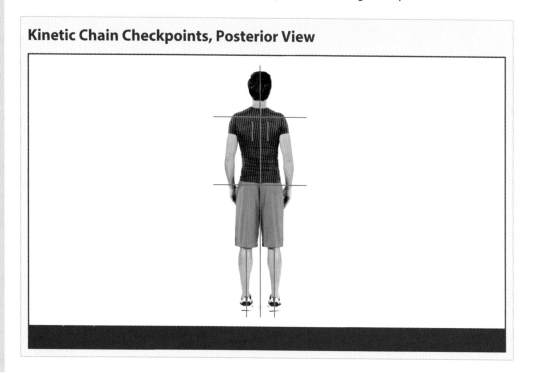

SUMMARY • A static postural assessment is a simple yet effective tool to quickly "size up" your client. Consider yourself a detective looking for structural deviations within a kinetic chain as well as for symmetry from the right to left side of the body. Alterations in structure will lead to or could be caused by muscle imbalances. Many muscle imbalances can be inferred simply from the deviations noted in the static postural assessment. Using a static postural assessment on an initial evaluation of your client will give you a "big picture" view of how that individual uses his or her body day in and day out. Consider the body as a road map. Movement patterns commonly used will be expressed in the alignment the body naturally assumes. Identifying these static deviations and asymmetries in conjunction with those identified in the dynamic postural assessment (see chapter six, Movement Assessments) will provide the clues as to how an individual uses his or her body biomechanically. Knowing that and understanding how interconnected all the body systems are, the health and fitness professional can begin to identify what other components have been affected by the altered alignment. How have these alterations distorted the feedback from the proprioceptors? How has the altered alignment affected the function of the soft tissue? Has the fascia been overloaded? Have compensatory muscle imbalances been generated creating altered length-tension relationships, altered force production, synergistic dominance, and altered reciprocal inhibition relationships? How have these changes affected the entire kinetic chain and overall coordination of movement within the limbs and between the limbs and the trunk? What further questions will you need to ask your clients about their day-to-day postural habits (how they stand, sit, and carry packages, briefcases, or babies)? Do you need to dig further into prior injuries, surgeries, or "minor" aches and pains that with time may have altered their freedom of movement? Do they appear to fall neatly into one of the more common postural disorders or do they have combined compensations leading to further complexities in biomechanical and neuromuscular loading? The static postural assessment is the first step in assessing the biomechanical and neuromuscular pieces of the puzzle necessary to create a program for functional rebalancing for your client.

References

1. Bell DR, Padua DA. Influence of ankle dorsiflexion range of motion and lower leg muscle activation on knee valgus during a double legged squat. *J Athl Train* 2007;42:S-84.
2. Padua DA, Marshall SW, Boling MC, Thigpen CA, Garrett WE, Beutler AI. The landing error scoring system (LESS) is a valid and reliable clinical assessment tool of jump-landing biomechanics: the JUMP-ACL study. *Am J Sports Med* 2009;37(10):1996–2002.
3. Vesci BJ, Padua DA, Bell DR, Strickland LJ, Guskiewicz KM, Hirth CJ. Influence of hip muscle strength, flexibility of hip and ankle musculature, and hip muscle activation on dynamic knee valgus motion during a double-legged squat. *J Athl Train* 2007;42:S-83.
4. Lewit K. Muscular and articular factors in movement restriction. *Manual Med* 1985;1:83–5.
5. Janda V. Muscle Strength in Relation to Muscle Length, Pain and Muscle Imbalance. In: Harms-Rindahl K, ed. Muscle Strength. New York, NY: Churchill Livingstone; 1993:83–91.
6. Beimborn DS, Morrissey MC. A review of literature related to trunk muscle performance. *Spine* 1988;13:655–70.
7. Liebenson C. Active muscular relaxation techniques. Part II: clinical application. *J Manipulative Physiol Ther* 1990;13(1):2–6.
8. Janda V. On the concept of postural muscles and posture in man. *Aust J Physiother* 1983;29(3):83–4.
9. Janda V. Muscle Function Testing. London: Butterworths; 1983.
10. Liebenson C. Integrating Rehabilitation into Chiropractic Practice (Blending Active and Passive Care). In: Liebenson C, ed. *Rehabilitation of the Spine*. Baltimore, MD: Williams & Wilkins;1996:13–44.
11. Edgerton VR, Wolf S, Roy RR. Theoretical basis for patterning EMG amplitudes to assess muscle dysfunction. *Med Sci Sports Exerc* 1996;28(6):744–51.
12. Leahy PM. Improved treatments for carpal tunnel syndrome. *Chiro Sports Med* 1995;9:6–9.
13. Guyer B, Ellers B. Childhood injuries in the United States: mortality, morbidity, and cost. *Am J Dis Child* 1990;144:649–52.
14. Hammer WI. Muscle Imbalance and Post-facilitation Stretch. In: Hammer WI, ed. Functional Soft Tissue Examination and Treatment by Manual Methods. 2nd ed. Gaithersburg, MD: Aspen Publishers, Inc; 1999:415–46.
15. Chaitow L. Cranial Manipulation Theory and Practice: Osseous and Soft Tissue Approaches. London: Churchill Livingstone; 1999.
16. Timmons B. Behavioral and Psychological Approaches to Breathing Disorders. New York, NY: Plenum Press; 1994.
17. Hammer WI. The shoulder. In: Hammer WI, ed. Functional Soft Tissue Examination and Treatment by Manual Methods. 2nd ed. Gaithersburg, MD: Aspen Publishers, Inc; 1999:35–136.
18. Lewitt K. Manipulation in Rehabilitation of the Locomotor System. London: Butterworths; 1993.
19. Janda V. Muscles and Motor Control in Cervicogenic Disorders. In: Grant R, ed. Physical Therapy of the Cervical and Thoracic Spine. St. Louis, MO: Churchill Livingstone; 2002:182–99.
20. Hodges PW. Motor control of the trunk. In: Grieve GP, ed. Modern Manual Therapy of the Vertebral Column. 3rd ed. New York, NY: Churchill Livingstone; 2004:119–40.
21. Spring H, Illi U, Kunz H, Rothlin K, Schneider W, Tritschler T. Stretching and Strengthening Exercises. New York, NY: Theime Medicals Publishers, Inc; 1991.
22. Sarhmann S. Posture and muscle imbalance: faulty lumbopelvic alignment and associated musculoskeletal pain syndromes. *Orthop Div Rev Can Phys Ther* 1992;12:13–20.
23. Sahrmann S. Diagnosis and Treatment of Movement Impairment Syndromes. St. Louis, MO: Mosby; 2002.
24. Irving DB, Cook JL, Young MA, Menz HB. Obesity and pronated foot type may increase the risk of chronic plantar heel pain: a matched case-control study. *BMC Musculoskelet Disord* 2007;8:41.
25. Kaufman KR, Brodine SK, Shaffer RA, Johnson CW, Cullison TR. The effect of foot structure and range of motion on musculoskeletal overuse injuries. *Am J Sports Med* 1999;27:585–93.
26. Moen MH, Tol JL, Weir A, Steunebrink M, De Winter TC. Medial tibial stress syndrome: a critical review. *Sports Med* 2009;39:523–46.

CHAPTER 6

Movement Assessments

OBJECTIVES *Upon completion of this chapter, you will be able to:*

➤ Explain the rationale for performing movement assessments.

➤ Understand the difference between transitional and dynamic movement assessments.

➤ Determine potential muscle imbalances based on certain movement compensations.

➤ Design a corrective exercise strategy to improve movement impairments.

INTRODUCTION

MOVEMENT is the means by which we are able to perform all activities, ranging from those necessary for daily living to job tasks and recreational enjoyment. Our ability to move is one of the most important aspects of our existence. Recognizing optimal movement requires a thorough understanding and application of human movement science, specifically functional anatomy, kinesiology, biomechanics, physiology, and motor control. Understanding normal movement allows identification of abnormal movement, which can indicate possible muscle imbalances and corrective strategies. This chapter will review the rationale for movement assessments, present how to perform movement assessments, and discuss how to correlate the findings of these assessments to possible muscle imbalances.

THE SCIENTIFIC RATIONALE FOR MOVEMENT ASSESSMENTS

Movement assessments, based on sound human movement science, are the cornerstone of a comprehensive and integrated assessment process (1,2). Other assessments in this integrated approach include those for both muscle length (goniometric assessment) and muscle strength (manual muscle testing), which will be reviewed in later chapters (1,2).

Movement represents the integrated functioning of many systems within the human body, primarily the muscular, skeletal, and nervous systems (1–3). These

105

systems form an interdependent triad that, when operating correctly, allows for optimal structural alignment, neuromuscular control (coordination), and movement (4). Each of these outcomes is important to establishing normal length-tension relationships, which ensure proper length and strength of each muscle around a joint (1,5,6). This is known as **muscle balance** (Figures 6-1, 6-2).

As mentioned in previous chapters, muscle balance is essential for optimal recruitment of force-couples to maintain precise joint motion and ultimately decrease excessive stress placed on the body (1–3,6). All of this translates into the efficient transfer of forces to accelerate, decelerate, and stabilize the interconnected joints of the body, and is the source from which the term

> Muscle balance: establishing normal length-tension relationships, which ensure proper length and strength of each muscle around a joint.

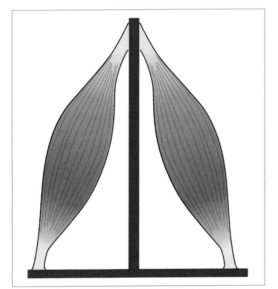

Figure 6.1   Muscle balance.

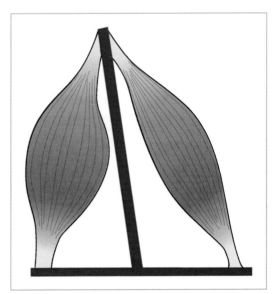

Figure 6.2   Muscle imbalance.

> Kinetic chain: "kinetic" denotes the force transference from the nervous system to the muscular and skeletal systems as well as from joint to joint, and "chain" refers to the interconnected linkage of all joints in the body.

kinetic chain is derived. "Kinetic" denotes the force transference from the nervous system to the muscular and skeletal systems as well as from joint to joint, and "chain" refers to the interconnected linkage of all joints in the body. Essentially, the kinetic chain can be considered the human movement system (HMS).

However, as mentioned in chapter three, for many reasons such as repetitive stress, impact trauma, disease, and sedentary lifestyle, dysfunction can occur in one or more of these systems (1,2,6,7). When this occurs, muscle balance, muscle recruitment, and joint motion are altered, leading to changes in structural alignment, neuromuscular control (coordination), and movement patterns of the HMS (1–4, 8–10). The result is a HMS impairment and, ultimately, injury (1–6, 8–11). When HMS impairments exist, there are muscles that are overactive and muscles that are underactive around a joint (Table 6-1) (1–3,6,9,10). The terms "overactive" and "underactive" are used in this text to refer to the activity level of a muscle relative to *another* muscle or muscle group, not necessarily to its own normal functional capacity. Any muscle, whether in a shortened or lengthened state, can be underactive or weak because of altered length-tension relationships or altered reciprocal inhibition (chapter three) (10). This results in an altered recruitment strategy and ultimately an altered movement pattern (1,2,6,7,10,11). Alterations in muscle activity will

Table 6.1 TYPICAL OVERACTIVE AND UNDERACTIVE MUSCLES	
Typically Overactive Muscles	**Typically Underactive Muscles**
Gastrocnemius	Anterior tibialis
Soleus	Posterior tibialis
Adductors	Vastus medialis oblique (VMO)
Hamstring complex	Gluteus maximus/medius
Psoas	Transverse abdominus
Tensor fascia latae	Internal oblique
Rectus femoris	Multifidus
Piriformis	Serratus anterior
Quadratus lumborum	Middle/lower trapezius
Erector spinae	Rhomboids
Pectoralis major/minor	Teres minor
Latissimus dorsi	Infraspinatus
Teres major	Posterior deltoid
Upper trapezius	Deep cervical flexors
Levator scapulae	
Sternocleidomastoid	
Scalenes	

change the biomechanical motion of the joint and lead to increased stress on the tissues of the joint, and eventual injury (1–4,6,9,10).

A movement assessment allows a health and fitness professional to observe for HMS impairments including muscle imbalances (length and strength deficits) and altered recruitment strategies (2). This information can then be correlated to subjective findings and isolated assessments such as goniometric and manual muscle testing. Collectively, this data will produce a more comprehensive representation of the client or patient and thus a more individualized corrective exercise strategy.

TYPES OF MOVEMENT ASSESSMENTS

Transitional movement assessments: assessments that involve movement without a change in one's base of support.

Dynamic movement assessments: assessments that involve movement with a change in one's base of support.

Movement assessments can be categorized into two types: **transitional assessments** and **dynamic assessments**. Transitional movement assessments are assessments that involve movement without a change in one's base of support. This would include movements such as squatting, pressing, pushing, pulling, and balancing. Dynamic movement assessments are assessments that involve movement with a change in one's base of support. This would include movements such as walking and jumping.

Because posture is a dynamic quality, these observations can show postural distortions and potential overactive and underactive muscles in a naturally dynamic setting. Both types of assessments place a different demand on the HMS, so performing both transitional and dynamic assessments can help provide a better observation of one's functional status.

KINETIC CHAIN CHECKPOINTS

Movement assessments require observation of the kinetic chain (HMS). To structure this observation, NASM has devised the use of kinetic chain checkpoints to allow the health and fitness professional to systematically view the body during motion. The kinetic chain checkpoints refer to major joint regions of the body including the:

1. Foot and ankle
2. Knee
3. Lumbo-pelvic-hip complex (LPHC)
4. Shoulders and head/cervical spine (upper body)

Each joint region has a specific biomechanical motion that it produces based on its structure and function (12) as well as the joints above and below it (8). When that specific motion deviates from its normal path, it is considered a compensation and can be used to presume possible HMS impairments (muscle imbalance) (1,6,7,9–11).

(*Text continues on page 139*)

TRANSITIONAL MOVEMENT ASSESSMENTS

As stated earlier, transitional movement assessments are assessments in which movement is occurring without a change in one's base of support. The transitional movement assessments that will be covered in this chapter include the:

1. Overhead squat
2. Single-leg squat
3. Push-up
4. Standing cable row
5. Standing overhead dumbbell press
6. Star balance excursion
7. Upper extremity assessments

➤ OVERHEAD SQUAT ASSESSMENT

PURPOSE

This is designed to assess dynamic flexibility, core strength, balance, and overall neuromuscular control. There is evidence to support the use of transitional movement assessments such as the overhead squat assessment (13–17). This assessment appears to be a reliable and valid measure of lower extremity movement patterns when standard protocols are applied. The overhead squat assessment has also been shown to reflect lower extremity movement patterns during jump landing tasks (14). Knee valgus during the overhead squat test is influenced by decreased hip abductor and hip external rotation strength (15), increased hip adductor activity (16), and restricted ankle dorsiflexion (16,17). These results suggest that the movement impairments observed during this transitional movement assessment may be the result of alterations in available joint motion, muscle activation, and overall neuromuscular control that can point toward people with an elevated injury risk (16,17).

PROCEDURE

Position

1. The individual stands with the feet shoulder-width apart and pointed straight ahead. The foot and ankle complex should be in a neutral position. It is suggested that the assessment is performed with the shoes off to better view the foot and ankle complex.

2. Have individual raise his or her arms overhead, with elbows fully extended. The upper arm should bisect the torso.

Overhead Squat Position

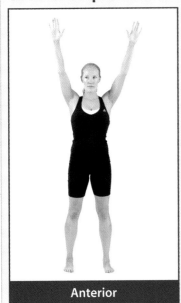

Anterior

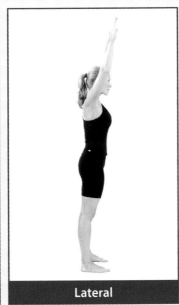

Lateral

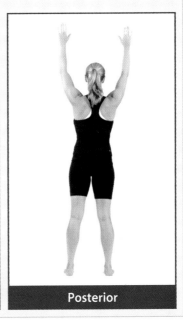

Posterior

Movement

1. Instruct the individual to squat to roughly the height of a chair seat and return to the starting position.

2. Repeat the movement for 5 repetitions, observing from each position (anterior, lateral, and posterior).

Overhead Squat Movement

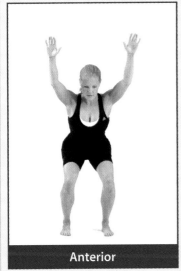

Anterior

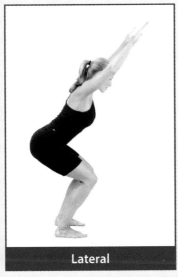

Lateral

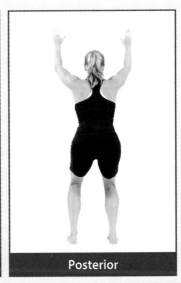

Posterior

Continued on page 110

Views

1. View feet, ankles, and knees from the front. The feet should remain straight with the knees tracking in line with the foot (second and third toes).
2. View the LPHC, shoulder, and cervical complex from the side. The tibia should remain in line with the torso while the arms also stay in line with the torso.
3. View the foot and ankle complex and the LPHC from behind. The foot and ankle complex will demonstrate slight pronation, but the arch of the foot will remain visible. The feet should also remain straight while the heels stay in contact with the ground. The LPHC should not shift from side to side.

Overhead Squat Views

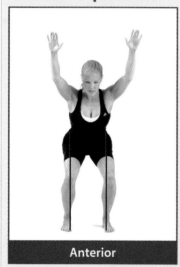
Anterior

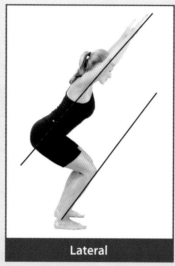
Lateral

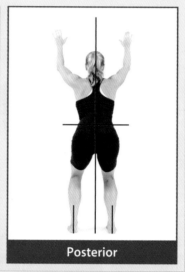
Posterior

Compensations: Anterior View

1. Feet:
   a. Do the feet flatten and/or turn out?
2. Knees:
   a. Do the knees move inward (adduct and internally rotate)?
   b. Do the knees move outward (abduct and externally rotate)?

Overhead Squat Compensations, Anterior View

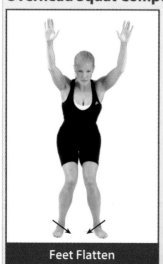
Feet Flatten

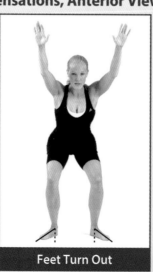
Feet Turn Out

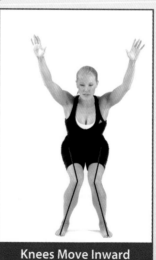
Knees Move Inward

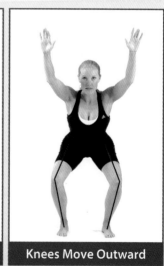
Knees Move Outward

Compensations: Lateral View

1. LPHC:
   a. Does the low back arch (excessive spinal extension)?
   b. Does the low back round (excessive spinal flexion)?
   c. Does the torso lean forward excessively?
2. Shoulder:
   a. Do the arms fall forward?

Overhead Squat Compensations, Lateral View

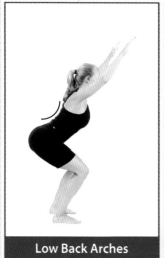 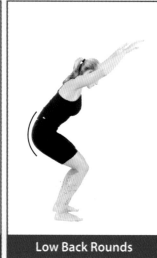 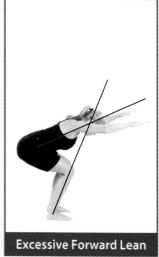 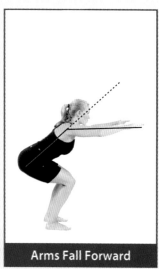

| Low Back Arches | Low Back Rounds | Excessive Forward Lean | Arms Fall Forward |

Compensations: Posterior View

1. Feet:
   a. Do the feet flatten (excessive pronation)?
   b. Do the heels rise off the floor?
2. LPHC:
   a. Is there an asymmetric weight shift?

Overhead Squat Compensations, Posterior View

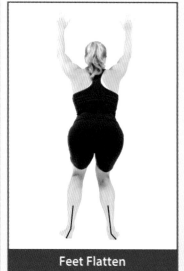 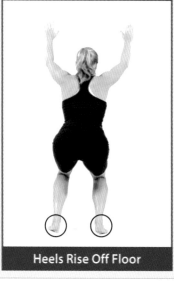 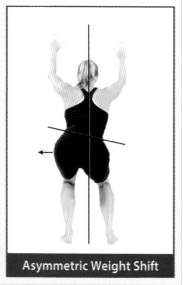

| Feet Flatten | Heels Rise Off Floor | Asymmetric Weight Shift |

Continued on page 112

When performing the assessment, record all of your findings. You can then refer to the table below to determine potential overactive and underactive muscles that will need to be addressed through corrective flexibility and strengthening techniques to improve the individual's quality of movement, decreasing the risk for injury and improving overall performance.

OVERHEAD SQUAT OBSERVATIONAL FINDINGS				
View	**Checkpoints**	**Movement Observation**	**Right - Y**	**Left - Y**
Anterior	Feet	Turn out		
		Flatten		
	Knees	Move inward		
Lateral	LPHC	Excessive forward lean		
		Low back arches		
	Shoulder complex	Arms fall forward		
Posterior	Feet	Flatten		
	LPHC	Asymmetric weight shift		

MOVEMENT COMPENSATIONS FOR THE OVERHEAD SQUAT ASSESSMENT					
View	**Checkpoint**	**Compensation**	**Probable Overactive Muscles**	**Probable Underactive Muscles**	**Possible Injuries**
Anterior	Feet	Turns Out	Soleus Lat. Gastroc-nemius Biceps Femoris (short head) Tensor Fascia Latae (TFL)	Med. Gastrocnemius Med. Hamstring Gluteus Medius/Maximus Gracilis Popliteus Sartorius	Plantar fasciitis Achilles tendinopathy Medial tibial stress syndrome Ankle sprains Patellar Tedinopathy (jumper's knee)
		Flatten	Peroneal Complex Lat. Gastrocnemius Biceps Femoris TFL	Anterior Tibialis Posterior Tibialis Med. Gastrocnemius Gluteus Medius	
	Knees	Move Inward (Valgus)	Adductor Complex Biceps Femoris (short head) TFL Lat Gastroc-nemius Vastus Lateralis	Med. Hamstring Med. Gastrocnemius Gluteus Medius/ Maximus Vastus Medialis Oblique (VMO) Anterior Tibialis Posterior Tibialis	Patellar tendinopathy (jumpers knee) Patellofemoral Syndrome ACL Injury IT band tendonitis
		Move Outward	Piriformis Biceps Femoris TFL/Gluteus Minimus	Adductors Complex Med. Hamstring Gluteus Maximus	

MOVEMENT COMPENSATIONS FOR THE OVERHEAD SQUAT ASSESSMENT (*CONTINUED*)

View	Checkpoint	Compensation	Probable Overactive Muscles	Probable Underactive Muscles	Possible Injuries
Lateral	LPHC	Excessive Forward Lean	Soleus Gastrocnemius Hip Flexor Complex Piriformis Abdominal Complex (rectus abdominus, external oblique)	Anterior Tibialis Gluteus Maximus Erector Spinae Intrinsic Core Stabilizers (transverse abdominis, multifidus, transversospinalis, internal oblique, pelvic floor muscles)	Hamstring, quad & groin strain Low back pain
		Low Back Arches	Hip Flexor Complex Erector Spinae Latissimus Dorsi	Gluteus Maximus Hamstrings Intrinsic Core Stabilizers	
		Low Back Rounds	Hamstrings Adductor Magnus Rectus Abdominis External Obliques	Gluteus Maximus Erector Spinae Intrinsic Core Stabilizers Hip Flexor Complex Latissimus Dorsi	
	Shoulders	Arms Fall Forward	Latissimus Dorsi Pectoralis Major/Minor Coracobrachialis Teres Major	Mid/Lower Trapezius Rhomboids Posterior Deltoid Rotator Cuff	Headaches Biceps tendonitis Shoulder injuries
Posterior	Foot	Foot Flattens	Peroneal Complex Lat. Gastrocnemius Biceps Femoris (short head) TFL	Anterior Tibialis Posterior Tibialis Med. Gastrocnemius Gluteus Medius	Plantar fascitis Achilles tendinopathy Medial tibial stress syndrome Ankle sprains Patellar Tedinopathy (jumper's knee)
		Heel of Foot Rises	Soleus	Anterior Tibialis	
	LPHC	Asymmetrical Weight Shift	Adductor Complex TFL (same side of shift) Gastrocnemius/soleus Piriformis Bicep Femoris Gluteus Medius (opposite side of shift)	Gluteus Medius, (same side of shift) Anterior Tibialis Adductor Complex (opposite side of shift)	Hamstring, Quad & Groin strain Low back pain SI joint pain

Continued on page 114

MODIFICATIONS TO THE OVERHEAD SQUAT ASSESSMENT

There are a couple of modifications to the overhead squat assessment that the health and fitness professional can make to gain a clearer picture of the possible overactive and underactive muscles. These include elevating the individual's heels or performing the overhead squat assessment with the hands on the hips.

Elevating Heels

Elevating the heels does two primary things. First, it places the foot and ankle complex in plantarflexion, which decreases the stretch (or extensibility) required from the plantarflexor muscles (gastrocnemius and soleus). This is important because deviation through the foot and ankle complex can cause many of the deviations to the kinetic chain, especially the feet, knees, and LPHC. Second, it alters the client's center of gravity (CoG) by decreasing the base of support (less or shorter contact surface of the foot on the ground) and shifting the CoG forward. When the CoG is moved forward, it allows the individual to sit more upright or lean back more. This is also important because with less forward lean there will be less hip flexion needed and less emphasis placed on the LPHC. In all, this modification allows the health and fitness professional to see the influence the foot and ankle has on the individual's deviations. For example, if an individual's knees move inward during the overhead squat assessment, but the compensation is then corrected after elevating the heels, then the primary region that mostly likely needs to be addressed is the foot and ankle complex. If the knees still move inward after the heels are elevated, then the primary region that most likely needs to be addressed is the hip.

Overhead Squat Assessment Modifications

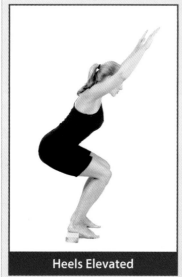

Heels Elevated

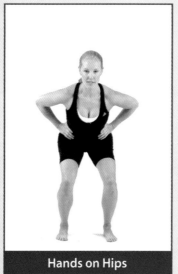

Hands on Hips

Hands on Hips

Placing the hands on the hips directly removes the stretch placed on the latissimus dorsi, pectoralis major and minor, and coracobrachialis and requires less demand from the intrinsic core stabilizers. This allows the health and fitness professional to see the influence the upper body has on the individual's compensations. For example, if an individual's low back arches during the overhead squat assessment, but the compensation is then corrected when performing the squat with the hands on the hips, then the primary regions that most likely need to be addressed are the latissimus dorsi and pectoral muscles. If the compensation still exists with the hands on the hips, then the primary regions that most likely need to be stretched include the hip flexors and the regions that need to be strengthened are the hips and intrinsic core stabilizers.

➤ SINGLE-LEG SQUAT ASSESSMENT

PURPOSE

This transitional movement assessment also assesses dynamic flexibility, core strength, balance, and overall neuromuscular control. There is evidence to support the use of the single-leg squat as a transitional movement assessment (13). This assessment also appears to be a reliable and valid measure of lower extremity movement patterns when standard application protocols are applied. Knee valgus has been shown to be influenced by decreased hip abductor and hip external rotation strength (15), increased hip adductor activity (16), and restricted ankle dorsiflexion (16,17). These results suggest that the movement impairments observed during this transitional movement assessment may be the result of alterations in available joint motion, muscle activation, and overall neuromuscular control.

PROCEDURE

Position
1. The individual should stand with hands on the hips and eyes focused on an object straight ahead.
2. Foot should be pointed straight ahead and the foot, ankle, knee, and the LPHC should be in a neutral position.

Single-Leg Squat Assessment, Position

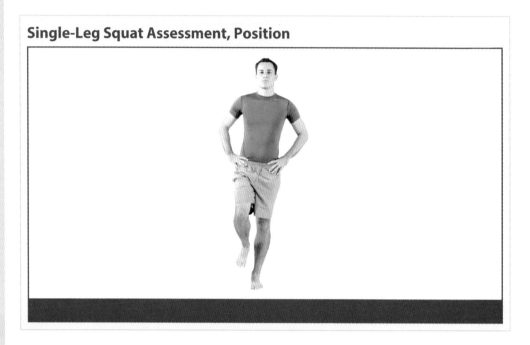

Movement
1. Have the individual squat to a comfortable level and return to the starting position.
2. Perform up to 5 repetitions before switching sides.

Views
1. View the knee, LPHC, and shoulders from the front. The knee should track in line with the foot (second and third toes). The LPHC and shoulders should remain level and face straight ahead.

Single-Leg Squat Assessment, Movement

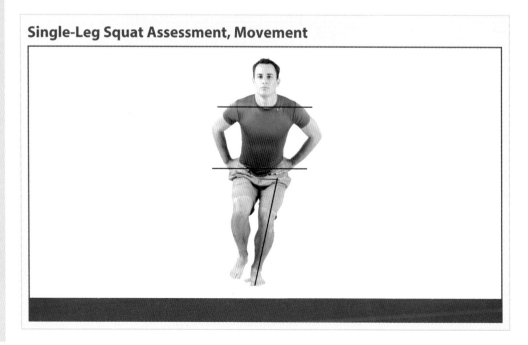

Continued on page 116

Compensations

1. Knee:
   a. Does the knee move inward (adduct and internally rotate)?
2. LPHC:
   a. Does the hip hike?
   b. Does the hip drop?
   c. Does the torso rotate inward?
   d. Does the torso rotate outward?

Single-Leg Squat Assessment, Compensations

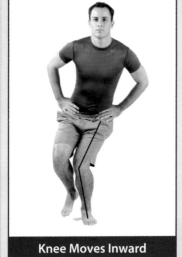

Knee Moves Inward

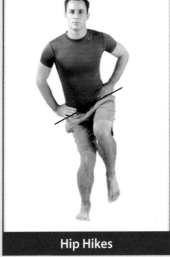

Hip Hikes

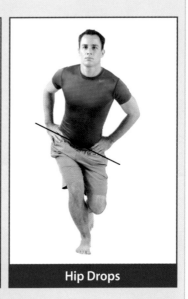

Hip Drops

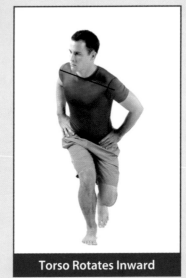

Torso Rotates Inward

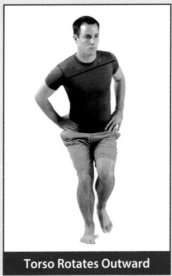

Torso Rotates Outward

Like the overhead squat assessment, record your findings. You can then refer to the table to determine potential overactive and underactive muscles that will need to be addressed through corrective flexibility and strengthening techniques to improve the individual's quality of movement, decreasing the risk for injury and improving overall performance.

SINGLE-LEG SQUAT OBSERVATIONAL FINDINGS

View	Checkpoints	Movement Observation	Right - Y	Left - Y
Anterior	Knees	Move inward		
	LPHC	Hip hikes		
		Hip drops		
		Inward rotation		
		Outward rotation		

MOVEMENT COMPENSATIONS FOR THE SINGLE-LEG SQUAT ASSESSMENT

View	Checkpoint	Compensation	Probable Overactive Muscles	Probable Underactive Muscles
Anterior	Knee	Move Inward (Valgus)	Adductor Complex Bicep Femoris (short head) TFL Lat. Gastrocnemius Vastus Lateralis	Med. Hamstring Med. Gastrocnemius Gluteus Medius/ Maximus VMO
	LPHC	Hip Hike	Quadratus Lumborum (opposite side of stance leg) TFL/ Gluteus Minimus (same side as stance leg)	Adductor Complex (same side as stance leg) Gluteus Medius (same side)
		Hip Drop	Adductor Complex (same side as stance leg)	Gluteus Medius (same side as stance leg) Quadratrus Lumborum (same side as stance leg)
	Upper Body	Inward Trunk Rotation	Internal Oblique (same side as stance leg) External Oblique (opposite side of stance leg) TFL (same side) Adductor complex (same side as stance leg)	Internal Oblique (opposite side of stance leg) External Oblique (same side as stance leg) Gluteus Medius/ Maximus
		Outward Trunk Rotation	Internal Oblique (opposite side of stance leg) External Oblique (same side as stance leg) Piriformis (same side as stance leg)	Internal Oblique (same side) External Oblique (opposite side of stance leg) Adductor Complex (opposite side of stance leg) Gluteus Medius/ Maximus

Continued on page 118

➤ **PUSHING ASSESSMENT: PUSH-UPS**

PURPOSE

The push-up assessment is related to pushing activities and evaluates the function of the LPHC and the scapular and cervical spine stabilizers.

PROCEDURE

Position
1. Instruct the individual to assume a prone position with hands roughly shoulder-width apart and knees fully extended. A modified version of the push-up can also be used depending on the capabilities of the individual.

Push-Ups Assessment, Position

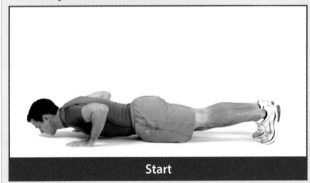
Start

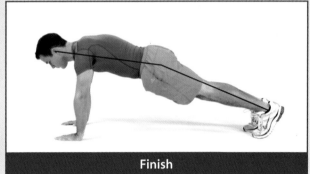
Finish

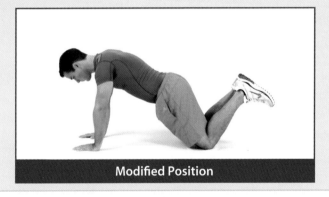
Modified Position

Movement
1. Instruct the individual to push against the floor, displacing the thorax backward until the scapulae are in a position of protraction.
2. The individual should move slowly and consistently as most faults will not be exhibited until the individual is fatigued. A 2-0-2 speed per repetition is recommended (two seconds up, zero-second hold, two seconds down).
3. Perform 10 repetitions.

Views
1. View the knees, LPHC, shoulders, and cervical spine from the side. The body should lift as one functional unit.

Compensations

1. LPHC:
   a. Does the low back sag?
   b. Does the low back round?
2. Shoulders:
   a. Do the shoulders elevate?
   b. Does the scapulae wing (lift away from the rib cage)?
3. Head/cervical spine:
   a. Does the cervical spine hyperextend?

Push-Ups Assessment, Compensations

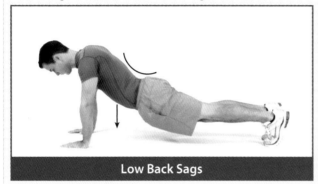

Low Back Sags

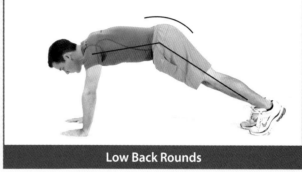

Low Back Rounds

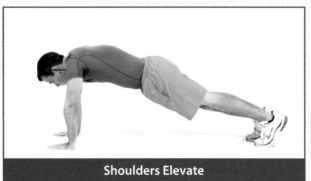

Shoulders Elevate

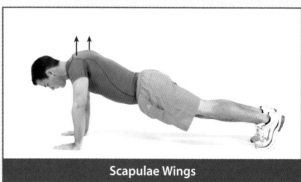

Scapulae Wings

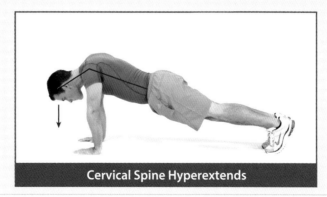

Cervical Spine Hyperextends

Record your findings. You can then refer to the table on the following page to determine potential overactive and underactive muscles that will need to be addressed through corrective flexibility and strengthening techniques to improve the individual's quality of movement, decreasing the risk for injury and improving overall performance.

Continued on page 120

PUSH-UP OBSERVATIONAL FINDINGS		
Checkpoints	**Movement Observation**	**Yes**
LPHC	Low back sags	
	Low back rounds	
Shoulders	Shoulders elevate	
	Scapular winging	
Head/Cervical Spine	Hyperextension	

MOVEMENT COMPENSATIONS FOR THE PUSH-UP ASSESSMENT			
Checkpoint	**Compensation**	**Probable Overactive Muscles**	**Probable Underactive Muscles**
LPHC	Low Back Sags	Erector Spinae Hip Flexors	Instrinsic Core Stabilizers Gluteus Maximus
	Low Back Rounds	Rectus Abdominus External Obliques	Instrinsic Core Stabilizers
Shoulders	Shoulders Elevate	Upper Trapezius Levator Scapulae Sternocleidomastoid	Mid and Lower Trapezius
	Scapular Winging	Pectoralis Minor	Serratus Anterior Mid and Lower Trapezius
Cervical Spine	Hyperextension	Upper Trapezius Sternocliedomastoid Levator Scapulae	Deep Cervical Flexors

PUSHING ASSESSMENT OPTION

If a standard or modified push-up is too difficult for the individual, pushing assessments can also be done in a standing position using cables or tubing or seated using a machine.

➤ PULLING ASSESSMENT: STANDING ROWS

PURPOSE

The standing row assessment is related to pulling activities and evaluates the function of the LPHC and the scapular and cervical spine stabilizers.

PROCEDURE

Position 1. Instruct the individual to stand in a staggered stance with the toes pointing forward.

Movement 1. Viewing from the side, instruct the individual to pull handles toward the body and return to the starting position. Like the pushing assessment, the lumbar and cervical spines should remain neutral while the shoulders stay level.

2. Perform 10 repetitions in a controlled fashion using a 2-0-2 tempo.

Standing Row Assessment, Position

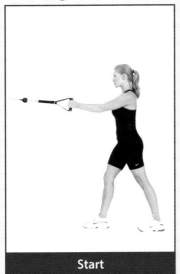

Start

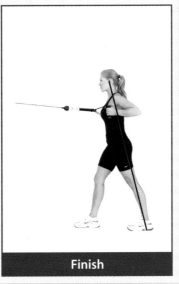

Finish

Compensations

1. Low back:
   a. Does the low back arch?
2. Shoulders:
   a. Do the shoulders elevate?
3. Head:
   a. Does the head migrate forward?

Standing Row Assessment, Compensations

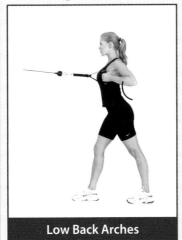

Low Back Arches

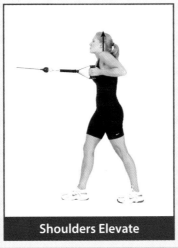

Shoulders Elevate

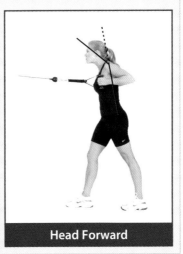

Head Forward

Record your findings. You can then refer to the table on the following page to determine potential overactive and underactive muscles that will need to be addressed through corrective flexibility and strengthening techniques to improve the individual's quality of movement, decreasing the risk for injury and improving overall performance.

Continued on page 122

STANDING ROW OBSERVATIONAL FINDINGS		
Checkpoints	**Movement Observation**	**Yes**
LPHC	Low back arches	
Shoulders	Shoulders elevates	
Head	Head migrates forward	

MOVEMENT COMPENSATIONS FOR THE STANDING ROW ASSESSMENT			
Checkpoint	**Compensation**	**Probable Overactive Muscles**	**Probable Underactive Muscles**
LPHC	Low Back Arches	Hip Flexors, Erector Spinae	Intrinsic Core Stabilizers
Shoulders	Shoulder Elevation	Upper Trapezius, Sternocleido-mastoid, Levator Scapulae	Mid and Lower Trapezius
Head	Head Migrates Forward	Upper Trapezius, Sternocleido-mastoid, Levator Scapulae	Deep Cervical Flexors

PULLING ASSESSMENT OPTION

Like the pushing assessment, the pulling assessment can also be performed on a machine, depending on the individual's physical capabilities.

➤ PRESSING ASSESSMENT: STANDING OVERHEAD DUMBBELL PRESS

PURPOSE

The pressing assessment is related to everyday pressing activities and evaluates the function of the LPHC, scapular stabilizers, and cervical spine stabilizers as well as shoulder range of motion.

PROCEDURE

Position
1. Instruct the individual to stand with feet shoulder-width apart and toes pointing forward.
2. Choose a dumbbell weight at which the individual can perform 10 repetitions comfortably.

Standing Overhead Dumbbell Press Assessment, Position

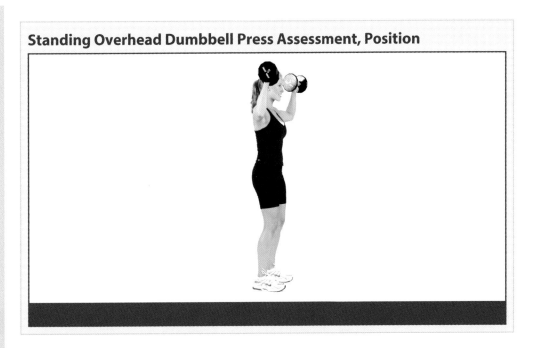

Movement

1. Viewing from the anterior and lateral positions, instruct the individual to press the dumbbells overhead and return to the starting position. The lumbar and cervical spines should remain neutral while the shoulders stay level and the arms bisect the ears.
2. Perform 10 repetitions in a controlled fashion using a 2-0-2 tempo.

Standing Overhead Dumbbell Press Assessment, Movement

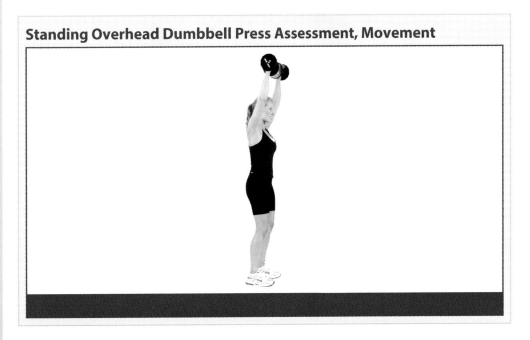

Compensations

1. Low back:
   a. Does the low back arch?
2. Shoulders:
   a. Do the shoulders elevate?
   b. Do the arms migrate forward?
   c. Do the elbows flex?
3. Head:
   a. Does the head migrate forward?

Continued on page 124

Standing Overhead Dumbbell Press Assessment, Compensations

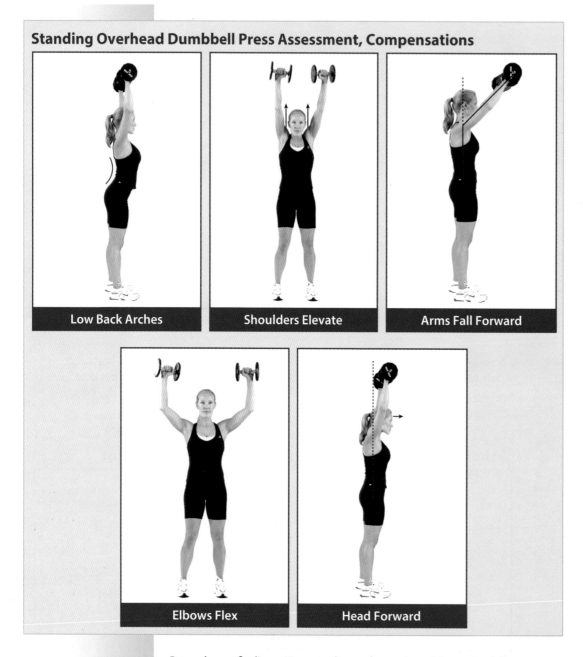

Low Back Arches　　Shoulders Elevate　　Arms Fall Forward

Elbows Flex　　Head Forward

Record your findings. You can then refer to the table on the following page to determine potential overactive and underactive muscles that will need to be addressed through corrective flexibility and strengthening techniques to improve the individual's quality of movement, decreasing the risk for injury and overall improving performance.

OVERHEAD PRESS OBSERVATIONAL FINDINGS		
Checkpoints	**Movement Observation**	**Yes**
LPHC	Low back arches	
Shoulders	Shoulders elevates	
	Arms migrate forward	
	Elbows flex	
Head	Head migrates forward	

MOVEMENT COMPENSATIONS FOR THE OVERHEAD PRESS ASSESSMENT

Checkpoint	Compensation	Probable Overactive Muscles	Probable Underactive Muscles
LPHC	Low Back Arches	Hip Flexors Erector Spinae Latissimus Dorsi	Intrinsic Core Stabilizers Gluteus Maximus
Shoulders	Shoulder Elevation	Upper Trapezius, Sternocleido-Mastoid, Levator Scapulae	Mid and Lower Trapezius
	Arms Migrate Forward	Latissimus Dorsi Pectorals	Rotator Cuff Mid and Lower Trapezius
	Elbows Flex	Latissimus Dorsi Pectorals Biceps Brachii	Rotator Cuff Mid and Lower Trapezius
Head	Head Migrates Forward	Upper Trapezius, Sternocleidomastoid, Levator Scapulae	Deep Cervical Flexors

➤ STAR BALANCE EXCURSION TEST

PURPOSE

This assessment measures multiplanar balance and neuromuscular efficiency of the testing leg during closed-chain functional movements (18–20).

PROCEDURE

Position
1. The individual is instructed to stand on the testing leg.
2. This individual is instructed to squat down as far as he or she can control with the knee aligned in a neutral position (**balance threshold**).

Star Balance Excursion Test, Position

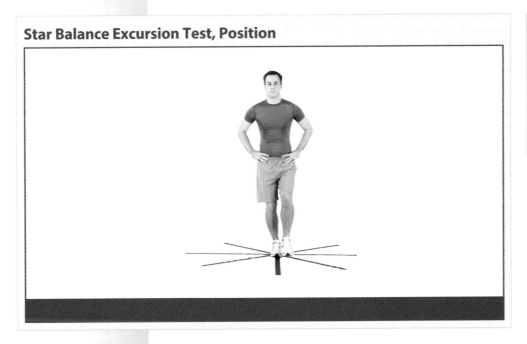

Balance threshold: the distance one can squat down on one leg while keeping the knee aligned in a neutral position (in line with the second and third toes).

Continued on page 126

Movement

1. The individual is then to reach with the opposite leg in the sagittal, frontal, and transverse planes while trying to maintain balance and keeping the knee in line with the second and third toes of the balance foot. The health and fitness professional assesses in which plane of motion the individual has the least amount of control (i.e., cannot maintain balance or knee moves inward). This can help in determining which plane(s) of motion may need to be emphasized in the individual's corrective exercise strategy.

Star Balance Excursion Test, Movement

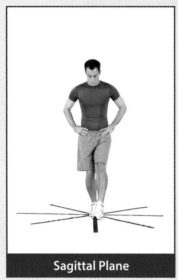

Sagittal Plane

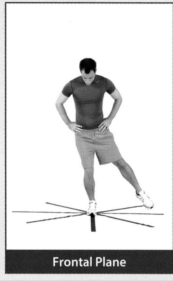

Frontal Plane

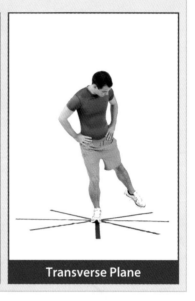

Transverse Plane

➤ UPPER EXTREMITY TRANSITIONAL ASSESSMENTS

PURPOSE

The upper extremity transitional assessments are used to determine any specific movement deficits in the shoulder complex. These assessments include the:

- Horizontal abduction test
- Rotation test
- Shoulder flexion test

PROCEDURE

Position

All three tests are performed with the client standing with heels, buttocks, shoulders, and head against a wall (the low back should be held in a neutral lumbar position).

Movement

1. For the horizontal abduction test, raise both arms straight out in front to 90 degrees of flexion with the thumbs up. Keeping the elbows extended, horizontally abduct the arms back toward the wall. Properly performed, the back of the hands will touch the wall with no movement compensations.

2. For the rotation test, abduct the shoulders to 90 degrees and bend the elbows to 90 degrees. With each humerus parallel to the floor, internally rotate the palms toward the floor then externally rotate the arms back toward the wall. The goal is to internally rotate the humerus until the palms of the hands and the forearms are within 20 degrees of the wall, then to externally rotate the humerus to touch the back of the hands against the wall with no movement compensations in either direction.

3. The shoulder flexion test begins as described above. The elbows are extended with thumbs up, then the straight arms are extended straight up toward the wall. The goal is to touch the thumbs against the wall with no compensatory movements such as shrugging or increasing lumbar lordosis.

Upper Extremity Transitional Assessments, Movement

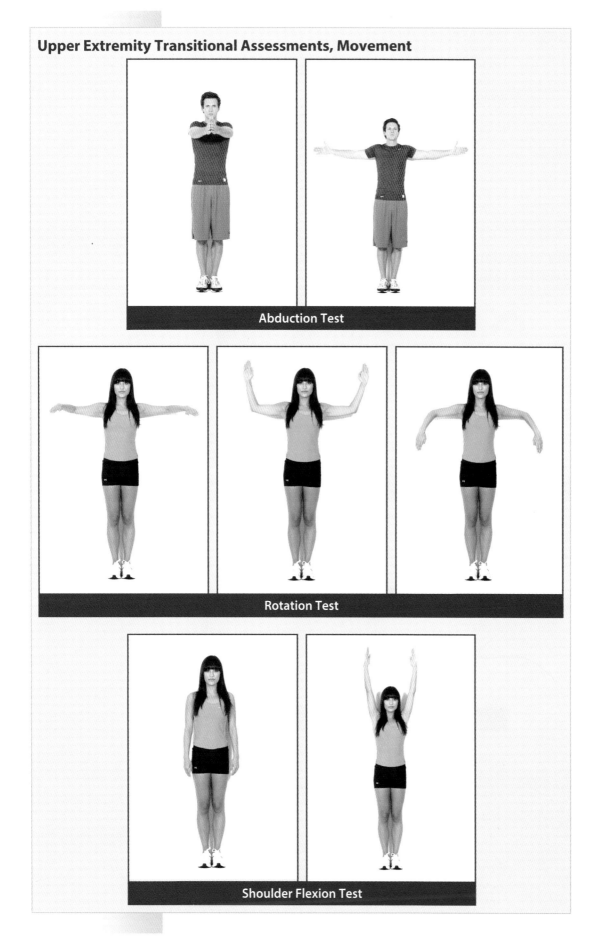

Abduction Test

Rotation Test

Shoulder Flexion Test

Continued on page 128

Compensations

1. Horizontal abduction test:
   a. Do the shoulders elevate?
   b. Do the shoulders protract?
   c. Do the elbows flex?
2. Rotation test:
   a. Do the shoulders elevate (internal rotation)?
   b. Do the shoulders protract (internal rotation)?
   c. Are the hands far from the wall (internal and external rotation)?
3. Shoulder flexion test:
   a. Do the shoulders elevate?
   b. Does the low back arch?
   c. Do the elbows flex?

Upper Extremity Transitional Assessments, Compensations
Horizontal Abduction Test Compensations

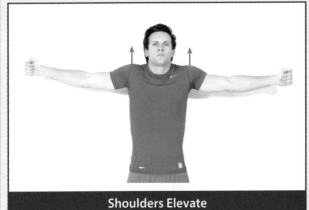

Shoulders Elevate

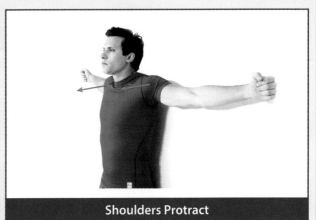

Shoulders Protract

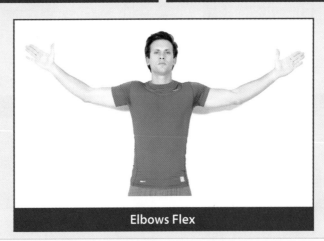

Elbows Flex

Rotation Test Compensations

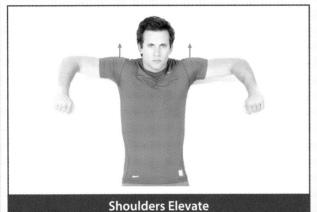

Shoulders Elevate

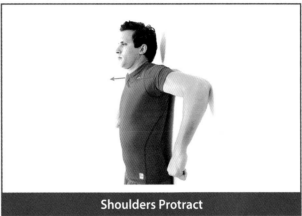

Shoulders Protract

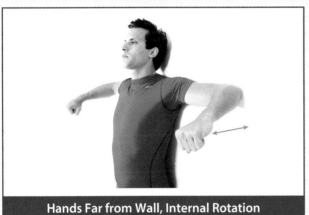

Hands Far from Wall, Internal Rotation

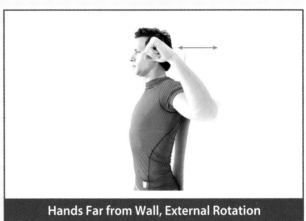

Hands Far from Wall, External Rotation

Shoulder Flexion Test Compensations

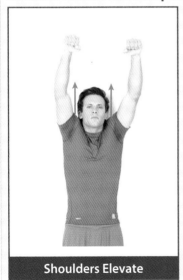

Shoulders Elevate

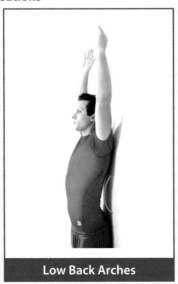

Low Back Arches

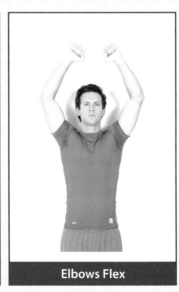

Elbows Flex

You can then refer to the table on the following page to determine potential overactive and underactive muscles that will need to be addressed through corrective flexibility and strengthening techniques to improve the individual's quality of movement, decreasing the risk for injury and overall improving performance.

Continued on page 130

UPPER EXTREMITY TRANSITIONAL ASSESSMENT SOLUTIONS TABLE

Probable Compensations for the Horizontal Abduction Test

Compensation	Potential Meaning
Elbows consistently flex even when properly shown or told not to	Overactive biceps brachii (long head) Underactive triceps brachii (long head) and rotator cuff
Shoulder protracts (humeral head moves forward and upward)	Overactive pectoralis major/minor and hypomobile posterior capsule Underactive rotator cuff, rhomboids, and middle/lower trapezius
Shoulders elevate	Overactive upper trapezius and levator scapulae Underactive rotator cuff, rhomboids, and middle/lower trapezius

Probable Compensations for the Rotation Test

Compensation	Potential Meaning
Internal Rotation	
Hands are far from wall	Overactive teres minor and infraspinatus and hypomobile posterior capsule Underactive subscapularis and teres major
Shoulder protracts (humeral head moves forward and upward)	Overactive pectoralis major/minor and hypomobile posterior capsule Underactive rotator cuff, rhomboids, and middle/lower trapezius
Shoulders elevate	Overactive upper trapezius and levator scapulae Underactive rotator cuff, rhomboids, and middle/lower trapezius
External Rotation	
Hands are far from wall	Overactive subscapularis, pectoralis major, teres major, and latissimus dorsi Underactive teres minor and infraspinatus

Probable Compensations for the Standing Shoulder Flexion Test

Compensation	Potential Meaning
Elbows flex	Overactive biceps brachii (long head), latissimus dorsi, teres major, and pectoralis major Underactive triceps brachii (long head) and rotator cuff
Shoulders elevate	Overactive upper trapezius and levator scapulae Underactive rotator cuff, rhomboids, and middle/lower trapezius
Low back arches off the wall	Overactive erector spinae, latissimus dorsi and pectoralis major/minor Underactive rotator cuff, rhomboids, and middle/lower trapezius

➤ DYNAMIC POSTURAL ASSESSMENTS

As stated earlier in the chapter, dynamic movement assessments are assessments in which movement is occurring with a change in one's base of support. The dynamic movement assessments that will be covered in this chapter include:

1. Gait
2. Landing error scoring system (LESS) test
3. Tuck jump test
4. Davies test

➤ GAIT: TREADMILL WALKING

PURPOSE

To assess one's dynamic posture during ambulation.

PROCEDURE

Movement

1. Have the individual walk on a treadmill at a comfortable pace at a 0-degree incline.

Views

1. From an anterior view, observe the feet and knees. The feet should remain straight with the knees in line with the toes. From a lateral view, observe the low back, shoulders, and head. The low back should maintain a neutral lordotic curve. The shoulders and head should also be in neutral alignment. From a posterior view, observe the feet and LPHC. The feet should remain straight and the LPHC should remain level.

Gait: Treadmill Walking Assessment, Views

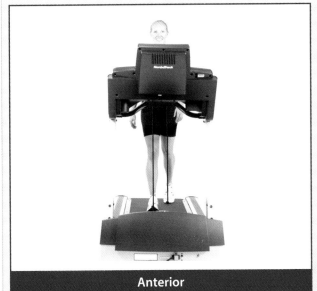

Anterior

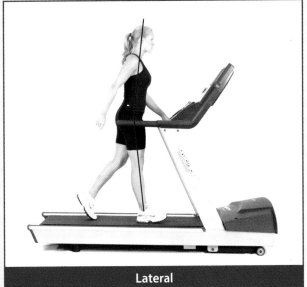

Lateral

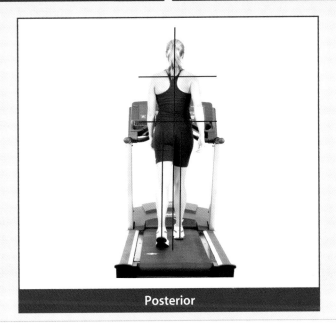

Posterior

Continued on page 132

Compensations:
Anterior View

1. Feet:
   a. Do the feet flatten and/or turn out
2. Knees:
   a. Do the knees move inward?

Gait: Treadmill Walking Assessment Compensations, Anterior View

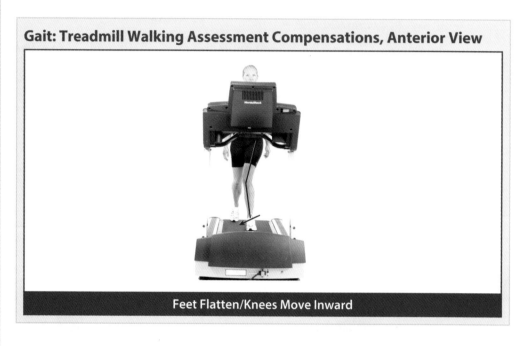

Feet Flatten/Knees Move Inward

Compensations:
Lateral View

1. LPHC:
   a. Does the low back arch?
2. Shoulders and head:
   a. Do the shoulders round?
   b. Does the head migrate forward?

Gait: Treadmill Walking Assessment Compensations, Lateral View

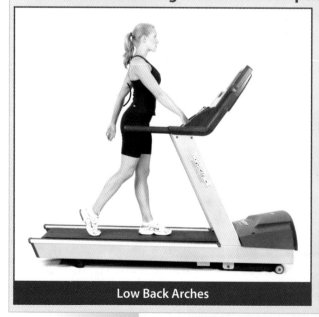

Low Back Arches

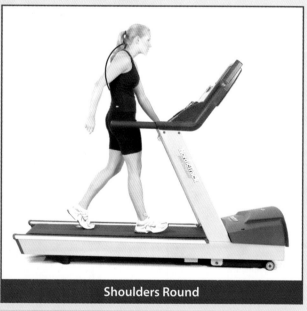

Shoulders Round

Gait: Treadmill Walking Assessment Compensations, Lateral View

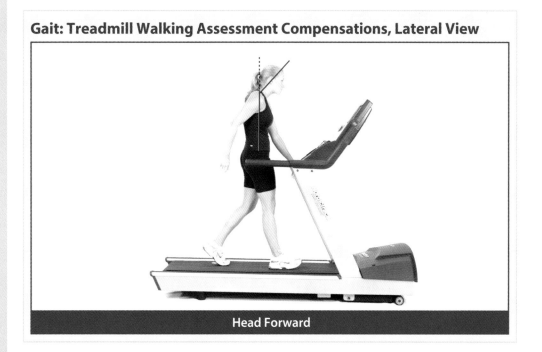

Head Forward

Compensations:
Posterior View

1. Feet:
   a. Do the feet flatten and/or turn out?
2. LPHC:
   a. Is there excessive pelvic rotation?
   b. Do the hips hike?

Gait: Treadmill Walking Assessment Compensations, Posterior View

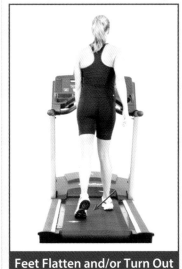

Feet Flatten and/or Turn Out

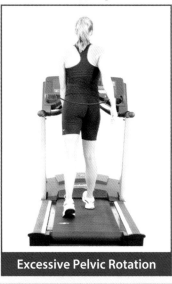

Excessive Pelvic Rotation

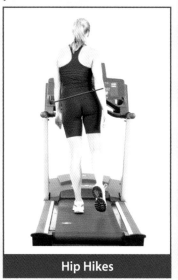

Hip Hikes

When performing the assessment, record all of your findings. You can then refer to the table on the following page to determine potential overactive and underactive muscles that will need to be addressed through corrective flexibility and strengthening techniques to improve the individual's quality of movement, decreasing the risk for injury and improving overall performance.

Continued on page 134

GAIT OBSERVATIONAL FINDINGS		
Checkpoints	**Movement Observation**	**Yes**
Feet	Flatten	
	Turn out	
Knees	Move inward	
LPHC	Low back arches	
	Excessive rotation	
	Hip hikes	
Shoulders	Rounded	
Head	Forward	

MOVEMENT COMPENSATIONS FOR THE GAIT ASSESSMENT			
Checkpoint	**Compensation**	**Probable Overactive Muscles**	**Probable Underactive Muscles**
Feet	Flatten	Peroneal Complex Lat. Gastrocnemius Biceps Femoris (short head) TFL	Anterior Tibialis Posterior Tibialis Med. Gastrocnemius Gluteus Medius
	Turn Out	Soleus Lat. Gastrocnemius Biceps Femoris (short head) TFL	Med. Gastrocnemius Med. Hamstring Gluteus Medius/Maximus Gracilis Sartorius Popliteus
Knees	Move Inward (Valgus)	Adductor Complex Biceps Femoris (short head) TFL Lat Gastrocnemius Vastus Lateralis	Med. Hamstring Med. Gastrocnemius Gluteus Medius/Maximus Vastus Medialis Oblique Anterior Tibialis Posterior Tibialis
LPHC	Low Back Arches	Hip Flexor Complex Erector Spinae Latissimus Dorsi	Gluteus Maximus Intrinsic Core Stabilizers Hamstrings
	Excessive Rotation	External Obliques Adductor Complex Hamstrings	Gluteus Maximus and Medius Intrinsic Core Stabilizers
	Hip Hike	Quadratus Lumborum (opposite side of stance leg) TFL/Gluteus Minimus (same side as stance leg)	Adductor Complex (same side as stance leg) Gluteus Medius (same side as stance leg)
Shoulders	Rounded	Pectorals Latissimus Dorsi	Mid and Lower Trapezius Rotator Cuff
Head	Forward	Upper Trapezius Levator Scapulae Sternocliedomastoid	Deep Cervical Flexors

➤ **LANDING ERROR SCORING SYSTEM (LESS) TEST**

PURPOSE

The LESS test is a clinical dynamic movement assessment tool for identifying improper movement patterns during the jump landing tasks (21,22). This test evaluates landing technique based on nine jump landing concepts using 13 different yes or no questions.

PROCEDURE

Position

1. The individual stands on a 30-cm (12-inch) box. A target line is drawn on the floor at a distance of half the individual's height.

Movement

1. The individual is instructed to "jump forward from the box with both feet so that you land with both feet just after the line" and "as soon as you land, jump up for maximum height and land back down."

Landing Error Scoring System (LESS) Test

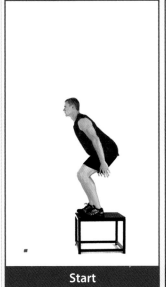

Start

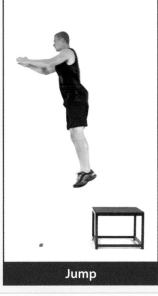

Jump

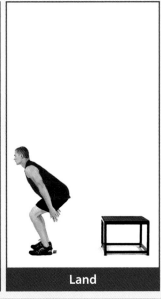

Land

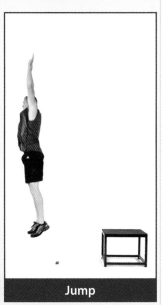

Jump

2. The individual views a demonstration performed by the health and fitness professional, then gets the opportunity to practice.
3. Ideally, video cameras are place 10 feet in front and to the right of the landing area.
4. Three trials are performed.
5. The videos are evaluated as follows:
   a. Knee flexion angle at initial contact >30 degrees; 0 = yes, 1 = no
   b. Knee valgus at initial contact, knees over midfoot; 0 = yes, 1 = no
   c. Trunk flexion angle at contact; 0 = trunk is flexed, 1 = not flexed
   d. Lateral trunk flexion at contact; 0 = trunk is vertical, 1 = not vertical
   e. Ankle plantar flexion at contact; 0 = toe to heel, 1 = no
   f. Foot position at initial contact, toes > 30 degrees external rotation; 0 = no, 1 = yes
   g. Foot position at initial contact, toes > 30 degrees internal rotation; 0 = no, 1 = yes
   h. Stance width at initial contact < shoulder width; 0 = no, 1 = yes
   i. Stance width at initial contact > shoulder width; 0 = no, 1 = yes
   j. Initial foot contact symmetric; 0 = yes, 1 = no

Continued on page 136

      k. Knee flexion displacement (knee position before jumping), > 45 degrees; 0 = yes, 1 = no

      l. Knee valgus displacement (knee position before jumping), knee inside great toe;
         0 = no, 1 = yes

      m. Trunk flexion at maximal knee angle, trunk flexed more than at initial contact;
         0 = yes, 1 = no

      n. Hip flexion angle at initial contact, hips flexed; 0 = yes, 1 = no

      o. Hip flexion at maximal knee angle, hips flexed more than at initial contact; 0 = yes,
         1 = no

      p. Joint displacement, sagittal plane; 0 = soft, 1 = average, 2 = stiff

      q. Overall impression; 0 = excellent, 1 = average, 2 = poor

6. A higher LESS score indicates a greater number of landing errors committed and therefore a higher risk for injury.

Although the above process for the LESS test will provide the health and fitness professional with the most comprehensive analysis of one's functional status, this assessment may be difficult to perform in some settings in which video cameras are not an option. In this case, a modified version of this assessment can be used to assess some of the primary compensations that can be indicators of potential injury. In the modified version, the health and fitness professional would view the individual from an anterior view. The primary compensations to look for would include the:

1. Foot position:
    a. Foot position at initial contact, toes > 30 degrees external rotation; 0 = no, 1 = yes

2. Knee position:
    a. Knee valgus at initial contact, knees over midfoot; 0 = yes, 1 = no
    b. Knee valgus displacement, knee inside great toe; 0 = no, 1 = yes

If these compensations are present, the professional can use Table 6-1 to determine potential muscle imbalances that should be addressed through a corrective exercise program.

➤ TUCK JUMP TEST

PURPOSE

The tuck jump exercise may be useful to the health and fitness professional for the identification of lower extremity technical flaws during a plyometric activity (23,24). The tuck jump requires a high effort level from the individual. Initially, the individual may place most of his or her cognitive efforts solely on the performance of this difficult jump. The health and fitness professional may readily identify potential deficits especially during the first few repetitions (23,24).

PROCEDURE

Movement

1. The individual performs repeated tuck jumps for 10 seconds (see the figure on opposite page), which allows the health and fitness professional to visually grade the outlined criteria (23). To further improve the accuracy of the assessment, a standard two-dimensional camera in the frontal and sagittal planes may be used to assist the health and fitness professional.

2. The individual's techniques are subjectively rated as either having an apparent deficit (checked) or not. The movement deficits to be evaluated are listed on the following page.

3. The deficits are then tallied for the final assessment score. Indicators of flawed techniques should be noted for each individual and should be the focus of feedback during subsequent training sessions (23).

4. The individual's baseline performance can be compared with repeated assessments performed at the midpoint and conclusion of training protocols to objectively track improvement with jumping and landing technique.

Tuck Jump Test

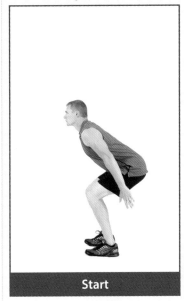 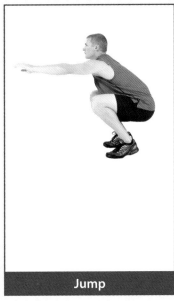 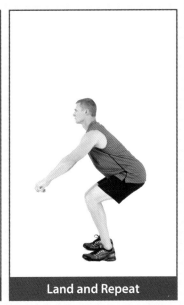

| Start | Jump | Land and Repeat |

5. Empirical laboratory evidence suggests that individuals who do not improve their scores, or who demonstrate six or more flawed techniques, should be targeted for further technique training (23).

TUCK JUMP ASSESSMENT OBSERVATIONS

Tuck Jump Assessment	Pre	Mid	Post	Comments
Knee and Thigh Motion				
1. Lower extremity valgus at landing	❑	❑	❑	
2. Thighs do not reach parallel (peak of jump)	❑	❑	❑	
3. Thighs not equal side-to-side (during flight)	❑	❑	❑	
Foot Position During Landing				
4. Foot placement not shoulder width apart	❑	❑	❑	
5. Foot placement not parallel (front to back)	❑	❑	❑	
6. Foot contact timing not equal	❑	❑	❑	
7. Excessive landing contact noise	❑	❑	❑	
Plyometric Technique				
8. Pause between jumps	❑	❑	❑	
9. Technique declines prior to 10 seconds	❑	❑	❑	
10. Does not land in same footprint (excessive in-flight motion)	❑	❑	❑	
	Total_____	Total_____	Total_____	

Continued on page 138

➤ **UPPER EXTREMITY DAVIES TEST**

PURPOSE

This assessment measures upper extremity agility and stabilization. This assessment may not be suitable for individuals who lack shoulder stability.

PROCEDURE

Position

1. Place two pieces of tape on the floor, 36 inches apart.
2. Have individual assume a push-up position, with one hand on each piece of tape.

Upper Extremity Davies Test, Position

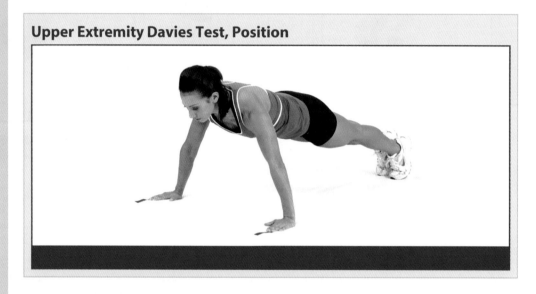

Movement

1. Instruct individual to quickly move the right hand to touch the left hand.
2. Perform alternating touching on each side for 15 seconds.
3. Repeat for three trials.
4. Record the number of lines touched by both hands.
5. Reassess in the future to measure improvement of number of touches and improvements in movement efficiency.

Upper Extremity Davies Test, Movement

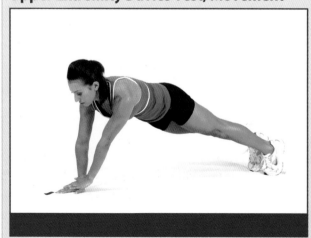
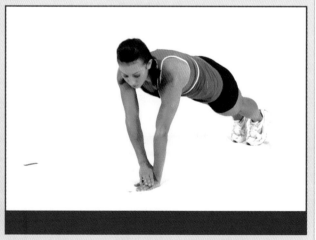

CHECKLIST FOR THE DAVIES TEST			
Distance of Points	Trial Number	Time	Repetitions Performed
36 inches	One	15 seconds	
36 inches	Two	15 seconds	
36 inches	Three	15 seconds	

WHEN NOT TO PERFORM THE LESS, TUCK JUMP, AND DAVIES TESTS

Although very helpful in uncovering movement deficiencies, these dynamic movement assessments may not be appropriate for all populations. This is one reason why subjective assessments, static posture, and transitional movement assessments are important to perform before dynamic assessments as these assessments can be used to qualify one's ability to perform these assessments.

For example, if an individual has difficulty performing the single-leg squat assessment, then the LESS and tuck jump tests may not be appropriate for that individual. Or, if an individual exhibits poor scapular stability during the push-up assessment, then the Davies test should be discouraged. In these examples, the transitional movement assessments should provide all of the answers necessary to begin developing a corrective exercise strategy.

ASSESSMENT IMPLEMENTATION OPTIONS

Movement assessments are a key component in determining movement efficiency and potential risks for injury. These assessments, along with previous and future assessments covered in this textbook, can help in designing a specific corrective exercise program to enhance one's functionality and overall performance, thus decreasing the risk for injury. We reviewed a number of example movement assessments in this chapter, and although all of them can provide valuable information about your client, time is of the essence. So it will be important to maximize your time by choosing assessments that will provide you with the most amount of information in the least amount of time. If time becomes an issue, the primary movement assessments that should be performed in the assessment process are the overhead squat and the single-leg squat. These assessments will provide you with the most information about your client's functional status in a relatively short time. The remaining assessments (push-up, standing cable row, overhead dumbbell press, star excursion, upper extremity, gait, LESS test, tuck jump, and Davies test) could be viewed as secondary assessments and performed if time allowed.

A second option to consider is that all of the assessments covered in this chapter can become one's first workout. From this first workout, the health and fitness professional can obtain the necessary information about the individual. The client will think he or she is getting a workout, but you as the health and fitness professional are obtaining valuable information about the client's structural integrity to help design and implement a corrective exercise program specific to the needs of that client. It's important to remember that depending on one's physical capabilities, not all assessments will be appropriate for all clients, so only choose assessments that the individual can perform safely.

Third, using these movement assessments could be a way to help build your client base. Offering 30- to 45-minute "assessment sessions" that take individuals through these assessments and a customized corrective exercise program based on the assessment findings can be a way to help generate revenue as well as to potentially have individuals working with you long term.

SUMMARY • Movement assessments are the cornerstone of an integrated assessment process (1,2). They allow the health and fitness professional to observe the length-tension relationships, force-couple relationships, and joint motions of the entire kinetic chain.

With a thorough understanding of human movement science and the use of the kinetic chain checkpoints to systematically detect compensation in joint motion, inferences as to HMS impairments can be made (1–3,9,10). This data can then be correlated to other assessments such as goniometric measurements and manual muscle testing so that a comprehensive corrective strategy can be developed.

References

1. Sahrmann SA. Diagnosis and Treatment of Movement Impairment Syndromes. St. Louis, MO: Mosby; 2002.
2. Liebenson C. Integrated Rehabilitation Into Chiropractic Practice (blending active and passive care). In: Liebenson C, ed. Rehabilitation of the Spine. Baltimore, MD: Williams & Wilkins; 1996:13–43.
3. Comerford MJ, Mottram SL. Movement and stability dysfunction—contemporary developments. *Man Ther* 2001;6(1):15–26.
4. Panjabi MM. The stabilizing system of the spine. Part I: function, dysfunction, adaptation, and enhancement. *J Spinal Disord* 1992;5(4):383–9.
5. Kendall FP, McCreary EK, Provance PG, Rodgers MM, Romani WA. Muscles Testing and Function with Posture and Pain. 5th ed. Baltimore, MD: Lippincott Williams & Wilkins; 2005.
6. Janda V. Evaluation of Muscle Imbalances. In: Liebenson C, ed. Rehabilitation of the Spine. Baltimore, MD: Williams & Wilkins; 1996:97–112.
7. Sahrmann SA. Posture and muscle imbalance. Faulty lumbar pelvic alignments. *Phys Ther* 1987;67:1840–4.
8. Powers CM. The influence of altered lower-extremity kinematics on patellofemoral joint dysfunction: a theoretical perspective. *J Orthop Sports Phys Ther* 2003;33(11):639–46.
9. Janda V. Muscles and Motor Control in Low Back Pain: Assessment and Management. In: Twomey LT, ed. Physical Therapy of the Low Back. Edinburgh: Churchill Livingstone; 1987:253–78.
10. Janda V. Muscle Strength in Relation to Muscle Length, Pain, and Muscle Imbalance. In: Harms-Ringdahl, ed. International Perspectives in Physical Therapy VIII. Edinburgh: Churchill Livingstone; 1993:83–91.
11. Edgerton VR, Wolf SL, Levendowski DJ, Roy RR. Theoretical basis for patterning EMG amplitudes to assess muscle dysfunction. *Med Sci Sports Exerc* 1996;28(6):744–51.
12. Neumann DA. Kinesiology of the Musculoskeletal System: Foundations for Physical Rehabilitation. St. Louis, MO: Mosby; 2002.
13. Zeller B, McCrory J, Kibler W, Uhl T. Differences in kinematics and electromyographic activity between men and women during the single-legged squat. *Am J Sports Med* 2003;31:449–56.
14. Buckley BD, Thigpen CA, Joyce CJ, Bohres SM, Padua DA. Knee and hip kinematics during a double leg squat predict knee and hip kinematics at initial contact of a jump landing task. *J Athl Train* 2007;42:S-81.
15. Ireland ML, Willson JD, Ballantyne BT, Davis IM. Hip strength in females with and without patellofemoral pain. *J Orthop Sports Phys Ther* 2003;33:671–6.
16. Vesci BJ, Padua DA, Bell DR, Strickland LJ, Guskiewicz KM, Hirth CJ. Influence of hip muscle strength, flexibility of hip and ankle musculature, and hip muscle activation on dynamic knee valgus motion during a double-legged squat. *J Athl Train* 2007;42:S-83.
17. Bell DR, Padua DA. Influence of ankle dorsiflexion range of motion and lower leg muscle activation on knee valgus during a double legged squat. *J Athl Train* 2007;42:S-84.
18. Herrington L, Hatcher J, Hatcher A, McNicholas M. A comparison of star excursion balance test reach distances between ACL deficient patients and asymptomatic controls. *Knee* 2009;16(2):149–52.
19. McKeon PO, Ingersoll CD, Kerrigan DC, Saliba E, Bennett BC, Hertel J. Balance training improves function and postural control in those with chronic ankle instability. *Med Sci Sports Exerc* 2008;40(10):1810–9.
20. Plisky PJ, Rauh MJ, Kaminski TW, Underwood FB. Star excursion balance test as a predictor of lower extremity injury in high school basketball players. *J Orthop Sports Phys Ther* 2006;36(12):911–9.
21. DiStefano LJ, Padua DA, DiStefano MJ, Marshall SW. Influence of age, sex, technique, and exercise program on movement patterns after anterior cruciate ligament

injury prevention in youth soccer players. *Am J Sports Med* 2009;37(3):495–505.

22. Padua DA, Marshall SW, Boling MC, Thigpen CA, Garrett WE, Beutler AI. The landing error scoring system (LESS) is a valid and reliable clinical assessment tool of jump-landing biomechanics: the JUMP-ACL study. *Am J Sports Med* 2009;37(10):1996-2002.

23. Myer GD, Ford KR, Hewett TE. Tuck jump assessment for reducing anterior cruciate ligament injury risk. *Athl Ther Today* 2008;13(5):39–44.

24. Myer GD, Ford KR, Hewett TE. Rationale and clinical techniques for anterior cruciate ligament injury prevention among female athletes. *J Athl Train* 2004;39(4):352–364.

Range of Motion Assessments

Upon completion of this chapter, you will be able to:

➤ Identify the importance of achieving optimal range of motion in human movement.

➤ Explain how the integrated function of the muscular, skeletal, and nervous systems collectively influences the ability to move through a full range of motion.

➤ Discuss how a goniometer and an inclinometer can be used to measure joint range of motion and why it is important for the health and fitness professional to develop skill in taking these measures.

➤ Discuss the various components of a goniometer and specifically explain how to use this instrument to measure joint range of motion.

➤ Demonstrate the ability to measure joint range of motion at the foot, knee, hip, and shoulder joints.

➤ Explain how optimal range of motion at these joints correlates to the overhead squat and single-leg squat assessments.

➤ For each joint movement identified, discuss the muscles being assessed, the antagonist muscles, positioning of the client, the execution of the goniometric measurement, common errors in measurement, and the movement compensations to look for.

INTRODUCTION

OPTIMAL human movement requires optimum range of motion (ROM) at each joint. The ability to identify proper and altered joint motion and muscle lengths, correlate them to movement dysfunctions, and develop a methodological strategy is vital for all health and fitness professionals to develop safe and effective corrective strategies for their clients. This chapter is intended to guide the health and fitness professional in the assessment of joint ROM and muscle length by using goniometric measurement.

THE SCIENTIFIC RATIONALE FOR GONIOMETRIC MEASUREMENT

Goniometric measurement is a major component of a comprehensive and integrated assessment process (1–3). Other assessments in this integrated approach include movement assessments and muscle strength (manual muscle testing) (1,2).

Range of motion: the amount of motion available at a specific joint.

The movement of a joint through its biomechanical ROM represents the integrated functioning of the HMS (1,2,4). When operating correctly, this system allows for optimal structural alignment, optimal neuromuscular control (coordination), and optimal ROM to occur at each joint (5). This is essential to help ensure proper length and strength of each muscle as well as optimal joint ROM (1,6,7).

Precise neuromuscular control of ROM at each joint will ultimately decrease excessive stress placed on the body (1,2,4,8). Herein lies the importance of assessing joint ROM. If one joint lacks proper ROM, then adjacent joints and tissues (above and/or below) must move more to compensate for the dysfunctional joint ROM. For example, if clients possess less than adequate ankle dorsiflexion, they may be at greater risk of injury to the knee (9,10), hip, or low back.

In all, each joint must exhibit proper ROM for the efficient transference of forces to accelerate, decelerate, and stabilize the interconnected joints of the body and produce optimal human movement.

The concept of human movement system impairment is important to understand because it is essentially what is being assessed with goniometric measurements. As mentioned in chapter three, human movement system impairments are an alteration in the ability of the muscular, nervous, and skeletal systems to function interdependently and effectively to perform their functional tasks (8,11). Some muscles will become overactive, shortened, and restrict joint motion whereas other muscles will become underactive, lengthened, and not promote joint motion (1,2,4,7,11,12). A noted decrease in the ROM of a joint may signify overactive muscles, underactive muscles, and/or altered arthrokinematics (3).

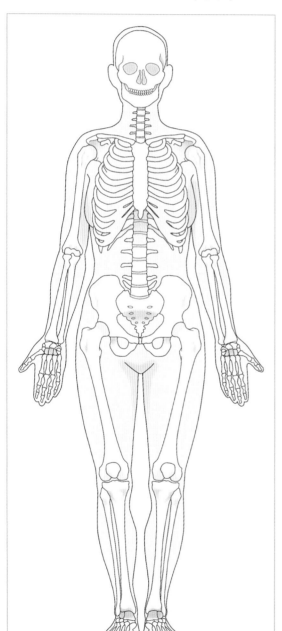

Figure 7.1 Anatomic position.

RANGE OF MOTION

Range of motion is the amount of motion available at a specific joint. To understand ROM measurement a complete understanding of the starting position is crucial. In all motions except rotations, the body is in the anatomic position (Figure 7-1). In this position, the body is at rest at 0 degrees of flexion, extension, abduction, and adduction. The ROM is affected by the type of motion applied (passive or active).

Passive range of motion: the amount obtained by the examiner without any assistance by the client.

Passive range of motion is the amount obtained by the examiner without any assistance by the client. In most normal subjects, passive ROM is slightly greater than active ROM. Passive ROM provides information regarding joint-play motion and physiologic end-feel to the movement. This helps create an objective look at the articular surfaces of the joint as well as tissue extensibility of both contractile and noncontractile tissues.

Active range of motion: the amount of motion obtained solely through voluntary contraction from the client.

Active range of motion refers to the amount of motion obtained solely through voluntary contraction from the client. Active ROM can be determined through the use of movement assessments such as the overhead squat assessment. Information provided here includes muscular strength, neuromuscular control, painful arcs, and overall functional abilities. Comparisons of passive and active ROM provide a complete objective assessment of the articulations and the soft tissue that envelops and moves it.

PHYSIOLOGIC END-FEEL

Some joints are constructed so that the joint capsule is the limiting factor in movement, whereas other joints rely solely on ligamentous structures for stability (Figure 7-2). The extent of passive ROM is limited by the uniqueness of the structure being evaluated. For example, a soft end-feel may acknowledge the presence of edema. A firm end-feel may describe increased muscular tonicity or a normal ligamentous structure. This information is important because it describes the integrity of the structures being evaluated. Initiating a training program that fails to correct mechanical movement flaws and

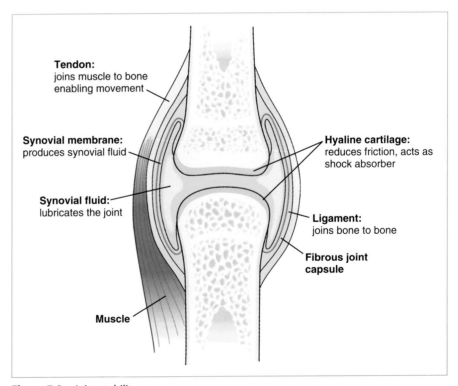

Tendon: joins muscle to bone enabling movement

Synovial membrane: produces synovial fluid

Synovial fluid: lubricates the joint

Hyaline cartilage: reduces friction, acts as shock absorber

Ligament: joins bone to bone

Fibrous joint capsule

Muscle

Figure 7.2 Joint stability.

Table 7.1	PATHOLOGIC (ABNORMAL) END-FEEL	
End-Feel	**Description**	**Examples**
Soft	Occurs later or earlier in the motion than is normal, or in a joint which usually has a firm or hard end-feel	Soft tissue edema Synovitis
Firm	Occurs later or earlier in the motion than is normal, or in a joint that usually has a hard or soft end-feel	Increased muscle tone Capsular, ligamentous, or muscular shortening
Hard	Occurs later or earlier in the motion than is normal, or in a joint that normally has a soft or firm end-feel	Chondromalacia Osteoarthritis Loose bodies in joint space Fracture
Empty	No real end-feel because end of motion is never reached owing to pain, muscular guarding, or disruption in ligamentous integrity	Acute joint inflammation Bursitis Abscess Fracture

neuromuscular efficiency will create further dysfunction, and ultimately further injury. Cookson and Kent (13) described physiologic and pathologic (abnormal) end-feels (Table 7-1).

TECHNIQUES AND PROCEDURES

Competency and proficiency in goniometric assessment requires the examiner to acquire the following knowledge and skills to produce reliable and valid measurements.

Knowledge of:

1. Recommended testing position
2. Alternative testing position
3. Anatomic bony landmarks
4. Normal end-feels
5. Instrument alignment
6. Stabilization techniques required
7. Joint structure and function

Required skills:

1. Move a part through the appropriate range of motion
2. Position and stabilize correctly
3. Palpate the appropriate bony landmarks
4. Align the goniometer correctly
5. Determine the end-feel of the ROM when performing passive ROM
6. Read the measurement correctly
7. Record the measurement correctly

GETTING YOUR FACTS STRAIGHT

Testing Reliability and Validity

Objective information gained through goniometric assessment must be both reliable and valid. *Reliability* refers to the amount of agreement between successive measurements. The higher the agreement of the values, the higher the reliability. Two types of reliability are important in goniometry. These are intratester and intertester reliability. *Intratester reliability* refers to the amount of agreement between goniometric values obtained by the same tester. *Intertester reliability* refers to the amount of agreement between goniometric values obtained by different testers. *Validity* of joint motion assessment reflects how closely the measurement represents the actual angle or total available ROM. An evaluation that truly represents either the actual joint angle or available ROM is valid. Two successive recordings may be reliable, but not always valid. Reliability and validity are each enhanced when assessments (intertester and intratester) are performed using identical applications and procedures.

Positioning

Positioning is an important part of goniometry. Proper positioning aligns the joints in a zero starting position and helps to increase reliability and validity of measurements. Positioning affects the amount of tension involving tissues that surround a joint before adjusting ROM assessment.

Stabilization

The proximal joint structures must be properly stabilized before the goniometric assessments. Without correct stabilization, the measurement's reliability and validity are decreased. This stabilization is often applied by the examiner, or through proper positioning and subject awareness and self-stabilization.

THE USE OF GONIOMETRIC MEASUREMENTS

Various devices for assessing joint ROM have been designed to accommodate variations in the size of the joints and the complexity of movements in articulations that involve more than one joint (14–16). Of these devices, the simplest and most widely used is the goniometer (Figure 7-3). The goniometer is one tool by which joint motion is measured (3). The use of goniometric measurements enables health and fitness professionals to objectively determine the available ROM at each particular joint. However, accurate measurement of the joint ROM takes some practice on the part of the health and fitness professional. By passively moving a client's joint to an end-range (point of no further motion or point of compensatory motion of that joint), the available motion a client has can be compared with normative ROM data to determine the amount of restriction if any at that joint. Table 7-2 lists normal active joint ROM.

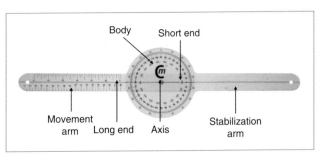

Figure 7.3 Goniometer.

Table 7.2	SUMMARY OF NORMAL JOINT END RANGES OF MOTION	
Joint	**Action**	**Degrees of Motion**
Shoulder	Flexion	160 degrees
	Extension	50 degrees
	Abduction	180 degrees
	Internal rotation	45 degrees
	External rotation	90 degrees
Elbow	Flexion	160 degrees
	Extension	0 degrees
Forearm	Pronation	90 degrees
	Supination	90 degrees
Wrist	Flexion	90 degrees
	Extension	70 degrees
	Radial deviation	20 degrees
	Ulnar deviation	30 degrees
Hip	Flexion	120 degrees
	Extension	0–10 degrees
	Abduction	40 degrees
	Adduction	15 degrees
	Internal rotation	45 degrees
	External rotation	45 degrees
Knee	Flexion	140 degrees
	Extension (hip neutral)	0 degrees
	Extension (hip flexed)	20 degrees
Ankle	Plantarflexion	45 degrees
	Dorsiflexion	20 degrees
Foot	Inversion	30 degrees
	Eversion	10 degrees

American Academy of Orthopaedic Surgeons. Joint Motion: Method of Measuring and Recording. Chicago, IL: AAOS; 1983.

Goniometric measurements can be highly effective in helping determine the cause and extent of restriction in joint ROM (3). This is especially true when an active ROM assessment such as an overhead squat or single-leg squat is performed before goniometric measurements (1,3). Furthermore, movement assessments and goniometric measurements should precede testing for muscle strength (manual muscle testing) to determine available ROM at the joint being tested (3). The use of goniometric measurements also provides the health and fitness professional with objective, reliable, and valid data necessary to develop an evidence-based corrective strategy (3).

A goniometer is essentially a large protractor with measurements in degrees. Goniometers come in different shapes and sizes, and are made of a variety of materials. However, they all adhere to the same basic design. A typical design for a goniometer includes a body, axis, stabilization arm, and movement arm.

- The body represents the arc of measurement. The goniometer in Figure 7-3 shows the measurement recorded in degrees of a circle (0–360 degrees).
- The *axis* (A) is the center of the goniometer and is the part that will be placed on the imaginary joint line (or axis of rotation for the joint).
- The *stabilization arm* (SA) is a structural part of the goniometer that is attached to the body. This part of the goniometer will be placed on the *stable*, nonmoving limb or bony segment that forms the joint being measured.
- The *movement arm* (MA) is the only moving component of the goniometer. It is placed on the *moving* limb of the joint being measure to provide the measurement reading.

For ease of measurement, the body, axis, and stabilizing arm should be placed directly on the client's joint and stable, nonmoving limb (or closest to the client's body), and the movement arm of the goniometer should remain on the outside, unimpeded and able to move freely. Reading the measurement on the goniometer will come from either the short end of the movement arm or the long end of the movement arm. The short end is considered the area from the axis to the bottom of the movement arm. The long end is considered the area from the axis upward toward the "ruler" looking section of the movement arm.

By aligning the two arms parallel to the longitudinal axis of the two segments involved in motion about a specific joint, it is possible to obtain relatively accurate measures of ROM.

In some cases, the health and fitness professional may use an inclinometer instead of a goniometer. (Figure 7-4). An inclinometer is a more precise measuring instrument with high reliability that has most often been used in research settings. Inclinometers are affordable and can easily be used to accurately measure ROM of all joints of the body from complex movements of the spine to simpler movements of the large joints of the extremities and the small joints of fingers and toes (17,18).

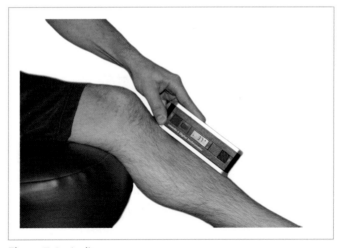

Figure 7.4   Inclinometer.

(*Text continues on page 164*)

NASM SELECTED GONIOMETRIC MEASUREMENTS

There are many joints in the body and most all are able to be measured goniometrically. However, NASM has only chosen a select number of joints to be measured. The following measurements were selected because of their overall importance to optimal human movement as well as their ability to correlate to the movement assessments. This following list is by no means intended to be exhaustive. Rather, its intent is to be very practical and used as part of an integrated assessment process.

➤ LOWER EXTREMITY

FOOT AND ANKLE COMPLEX

- Dorsiflexion

KNEE

- Extension (90-degree hip/90-degree knee position)

HIP COMPLEX

- Flexion (bent knee)
- Abduction
- Internal rotation
- External rotation
- Extension

➤ UPPER EXTREMITY

SHOULDER COMPLEX

- Shoulder flexion
- Glenohumeral internal rotation
- Glenohumeral external rotation

➤ FOOT AND ANKLE COMPLEX

DORSIFLEXION

1. Joint motion being assessed:
   a. Dorsiflexion of talocrural joint
2. Muscles being assessed:
   a. Gastrocnemius and soleus
   b. Posterior tibialis, peroneus longus, peroneus brevis, flexor hallucis longus, flexor digitorum longus, plantaris
3. Antagonists potentially underactive if ROM is limited:
   a. Anterior tibialis
   b. Extensor digitorum longus, extensor digitorum brevis, extensor hallucis longus, peroneus tertius
4. Normal Value (22): 20 degrees

Positioning The client is positioned supine with knee fully extended. The ankle is positioned in subtalar neutral (0 degrees of inversion and eversion at the subtalar joint). Pinch the talar neck with the thumb and index finger. Passively invert, then evert the foot until equal pressure is noted at the thumb and index finger. The foot will appear to be slightly inverted because it is in a nonweight-bearing position.

Continued on page 150

Dorsiflexion Assessment, Position

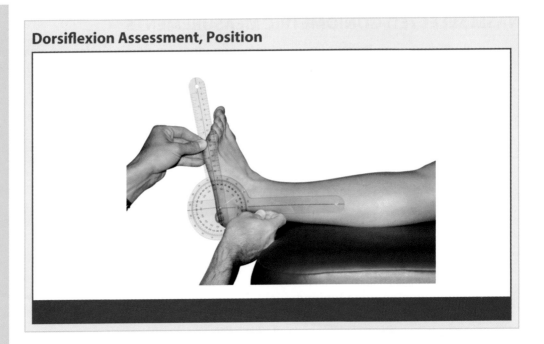

Execution

Place the goniometer as follows:

- **A:** Directly below the lateral malleolus near the base of the foot.
- **SA:** Lateral aspect of fibula.
- **MA:** Midline of fifth metatarsal.

Holding the plantar surface of the client's foot (just below the metatarsophalangeal joints, or "ball" of the foot), place the subtalar joint in neutral and guide the client as he or she actively dorsiflexes the ankle while passively assisting the path of motion to the point of first resistance or compensation. The primary compensations to look for are eversion of the ankle complex and/or flexing of the knee during dorsiflexion. Have the client hold the position and record measurement. Measurement is read at the long end of the movement arm on the upper red number between 0 and 20.

Dorsiflexion Assessment, Measurement

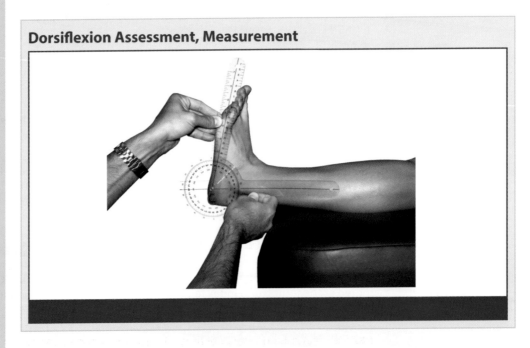

Common Errors Common errors that can occur during this measurement that must be avoided include failure of the health and fitness professional to maintain a subtalar neutral position.

Human Movement System Impairment This measurement is typically restricted in a person who demonstrates foot compensations (turning outward, flattening, or heels rising) and/or an excessive forward lean during an overhead squat assessment. Functional activities such as squatting into an average chair (the depth for an overhead squat assessment) and running require 20 degrees of dorsiflexion at the ankle, while normal walking requires up to approximately 15 degrees (19,20). A lack of dorsiflexion in the ankle has been shown to lead to knee injury (10).

➤ KNEE

EXTENSION (90 DEGREES OF HIP FLEXION, 90 DEGREES OF KNEE FLEXION)

1. Joint motion being assessed:
   a. Extension of the tibiofemoral joint
   b. Flexion of iliofemoral joint
2. Muscles being assessed:
   a. Hamstring complex, gastrocnemius, neural tissue (sciatic nerve)
3. Antagonists potentially underactive if ROM is limited:
   a. Hip flexor complex
   b. Quadriceps complex
4. Normal Value (22): 20 degrees

Positioning Client is positioned supine with the hip flexed at 90 degrees and knee flexed at 90 degrees. Hip is in neutral (0 degrees of rotation, abduction, and adduction).

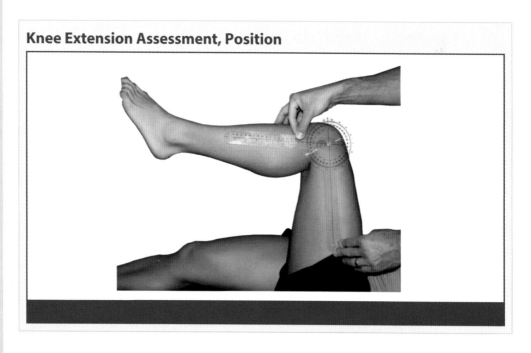

Knee Extension Assessment, Position

Execution Place the goniometer as follows:

- **A:** Center the goniometer at the lateral joint line of the tibiofemoral joint.
- **SA:** Lateral midline of the femur.
- **MA:** Lateral midline of the fibula.

Holding the client's lower leg with one hand and his or her thigh with the other hand, passively extend the knee until the first restriction or compensation. The primary

Continued on page 152

compensations to look for will be posterior tilting of the pelvis or hip extension. Have the client hold the position and record measurement. Measurement will be read from the short end of the movement arm on the middle black numbers.

Knee Extension Assessment, Measurement

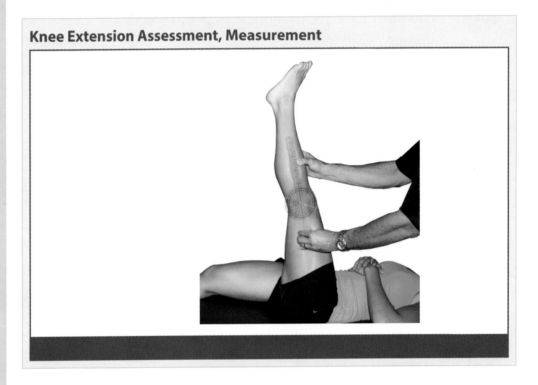

Common Errors

Common errors that can occur during this measurement that must be avoided include failure of the health and fitness professional to maintain a neutral hip or thigh position or moving the client into position too slowly, and an inability to see compensations.

Human Movement System Impairment

This measurement may be restricted in a person who demonstrates feet turned out (externally rotated), feet flattening, knee moving inward (short head of biceps femoris), knees moving outward (long head of biceps femoris), or low back rounding during the overhead squat or single-leg squat assessments.

➤ HIP COMPLEX

HIP FLEXION (BENT KNEE)

1. Joint motion being assessed:
   a. Flexion of iliofemoral joint
2. Muscles being assessed:
   a. Gluteus maximus, adductor magnus, upper portion of hamstring complex
   b. **NOTE:** If client reports a pinching sensation in the front of the hip during this assessment, the psoas and/or rectus femoris may be overactive.
3. Antagonists potentially underactive if ROM is limited:
   a. Hip flexor complex
   b. Hip extensor complex (gluteus maximus)
4. Normal Value (22): 120 degrees

Positioning

The client is positioned supine with the knee fully flexed, and the hip is in neutral (0 degrees of abduction, adduction, and rotation). The knee is flexed to shorten the hamstring complex, which may have a limiting effect on hip flexion.

Hip Flexion (Bent Knee) Assessment, Position

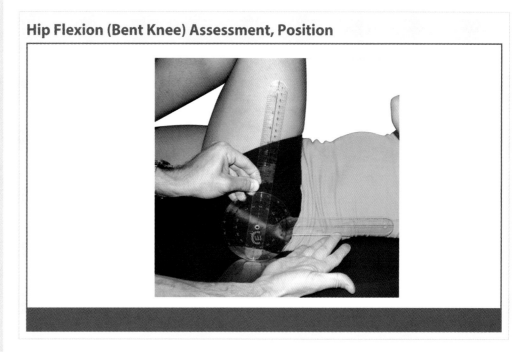

Execution

Place the goniometer as follows:

- **A:** Center the goniometer at the lateral thigh using the greater trochanter as a reference.
- **SA:** Lateral midline of the pelvis and midaxillary line of the trunk.
- **MA:** Lateral midline of the femur.

Holding the client's knee (tibial tuberosity), passively flex the hip to the point of first restriction or compensation. The primary compensation to look for is a posterior titling of the pelvis, lifting of the contralateral leg off the table, or abduction of the femur. Have the client hold the position and record measurement. Measurement is read at the short end of the movement arm on the middle black numbers.

Hip Flexion (Bent Knee) Assessment, Measurement

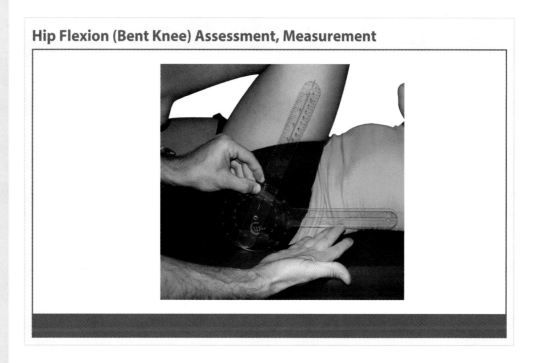

Continued on page 154

Common Errors

Common errors that can occur during this measurement that must be avoided include failure of the health and fitness professional to maintain a neutral hip or thigh position or moving the client into position too slowly, and an inability to see compensations.

Human Movement System Impairment

This measurement may be restricted in a person who demonstrates rounding of the low back during the overhead squat assessment. Sitting into a chair with an average seat height (the depth of an overhead squat) requires approximately 112 degrees of bent knee hip flexion, and squatting is said to require approximately 115 degrees (21).

HIP ABDUCTION

1. Joint motion being assessed:
   a. Abduction of iliofemoral joint
2. Muscles and ligaments being assessed:
   a. Adductor complex, pubofemoral ligament, iliofemoral ligament, medial hip capsule
   b. Medial hamstring complex
3. Antagonists potentially underactive if ROM is limited:
   a. Gluteus medius, gluteus minimus, tensor fascia latae (TFL), sartorius
   b. Biceps femoris
4. Normal Value (22): 40 degrees

Positioning

The client is positioned supine with the knee extended. The hip is in neutral (0 degrees of rotation, flexion, and extension).

Hip Abduction Assessment, Positioning

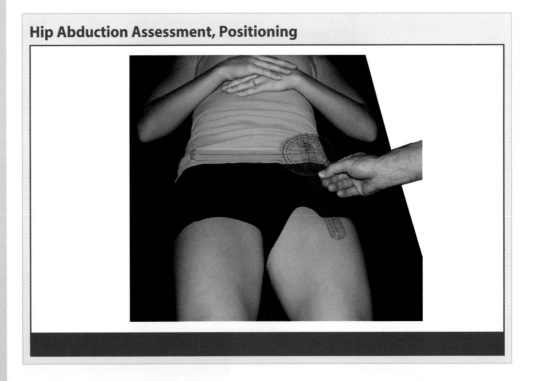

Execution

Place the goniometer as follows:

- **A:** Center the goniometer at the ASIS (anterior superior iliac spine) of the extremity being measured.
- **SA:** Imaginary line connecting one ASIS to the other ASIS.
- **MA:** Anterior midline of the femur, referencing the patellar midline.

Holding the client's lower leg, passively abduct the leg until the first restriction or compensation. The primary compensations to look for are motion in the opposite ASIS or lateral flexion of spine (or hip hike on the side of measurement). Have the client hold the position and record measurement. Measurement is read from the short end of the movement arm on the top red numbers between 0 and 40 degrees.

Hip Abduction Assessment, Measurement

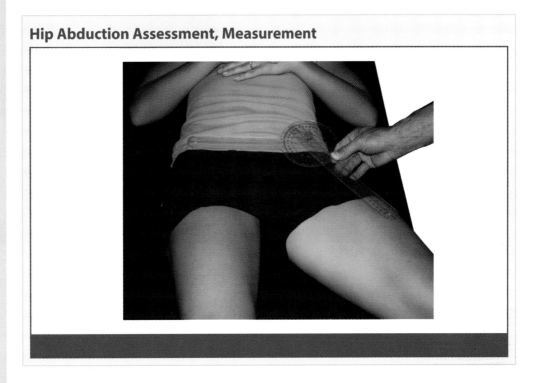

Common Errors

Common errors that can occur during this measurement that must be avoided include failure of the health and fitness professional to maintain a neutral hip or thigh position or moving the client into position too slowly, and an inability to see compensations.

Human Movement System Impairment

This measurement may be restricted in a person who demonstrates knees moving inward or an asymmetric weight shift during the overhead squat or single-leg squat assessments.

HIP INTERNAL ROTATION

1. Joint motion being assessed:
   a. Internal rotation of iliofemoral joint
2. Muscles and ligaments being assessed:
   a. Piriformis and hip external rotators (gemellus superior, gemellus inferior, obturator externus, obturator internus, quadratus femoris), adductor magnus (oblique fibers), ischiofemoral ligament
   b. Gluteus medius (posterior fibers), gluteus maximus
3. Antagonists potentially underactive if ROM is limited:
   a. Adductor magnus (longitudinal fibers), TFL, gluteus minimus, gluteus medius (anterior fibers), adductor longus, adductor brevis, pectineus, gracilis, medial hamstring complex
4. Normal Value (22): 45 degrees

Positioning

The client is positioned supine with the hip flexed to 90 degrees and 0 degrees of abduction and adduction. The knee is also flexed to 90 degrees.

Continued on page 156

Hip Internal Rotation Assessment, Positioning

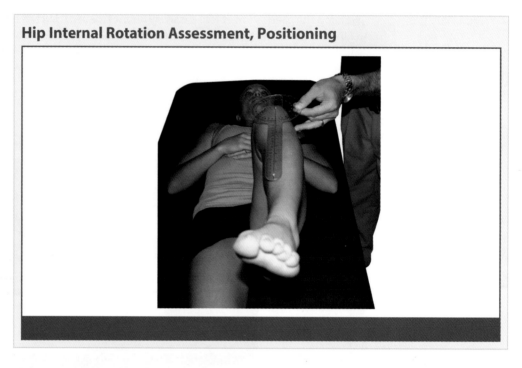

Execution

Place the goniometer as follows:

- **A:** Center the goniometer over the anterior aspect of the patella.
- **SA:** Parallel to an imaginary line down the center of the body.
- **MA:** Anterior midline of the lower leg, referencing the tibial tuberosity.

Holding the client's lower leg with one hand and the thigh with the other hand, passively rotate the femur internally until the first restriction or compensation. The primary compensation to look for is a hip hike (lateral flexion of spine) on the side of the measurement. Have the client hold the position and record measurement. Measurement is read from the long end of the movement arm on the middle black numbers.

Hip Internal Rotation Assessment, Measurement

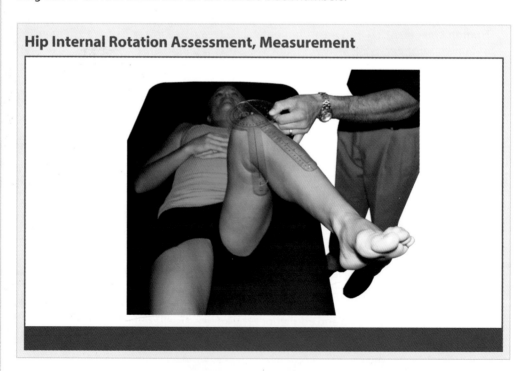

Common Errors

Common errors that can occur during this measurement that must be avoided include failure of the health and fitness professional to maintain a neutral hip or thigh position, moving the client into position too slowly, and an inability to see compensations or improper alignment of the stabilization arm.

Human Movement System Impairment

This measurement may be restricted in a person who demonstrates knees moving inward or outward or asymmetric weight shift during the overhead squat or single-leg squat assessments.

HIP EXTERNAL ROTATION

1. Joint motion being assessed:
   a. External rotation of iliofemoral joint
2. Muscles and ligaments being assessed:
   a. Adductor magnus (longitudinal fibers), iliofemoral ligament, pubofemoral ligament
   b. TFL, gluteus minimus, gluteus medius (anterior fibers)
3. Antagonists potentially underactive if ROM is limited:
   a. Piriformis and hip external rotators (gemellus superior, gemellus inferior, obturator externus, obturator internus, quadratus femoris), adductor magnus (oblique fibers)
   b. Gluteus medius (posterior fibers), gluteus maximus
4. Normal Value (22): 45 degrees

Positioning

The client is positioned supine with the hip flexed to 90 degrees and 0 degrees of abduction and adduction. The knee is also flexed to 90 degrees.

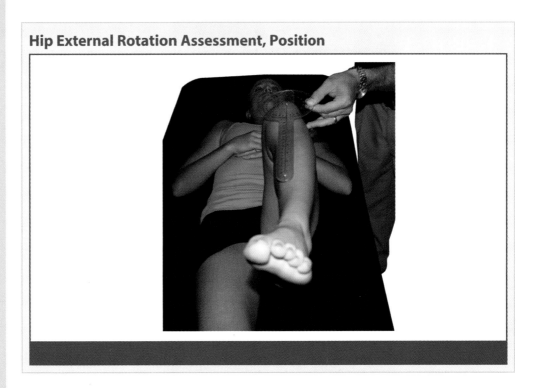

Hip External Rotation Assessment, Position

Execution

Place the goniometer as follows:

- **A:** Center the goniometer over the anterior aspect of the patella.
- **SA:** Parallel to an imaginary line down the center of the body.
- **MA:** Anterior midline of the lower leg, referencing the tibial tuberosity.

Continued on page 158

Holding the client's lower leg with one hand and the thigh with the other hand, passively rotate the femur externally until the first restriction or compensation. The primary compensation to look for is motion in the opposite ASIS. Have the client hold the position and record measurement. Measurement is read from the long end of the movement arm on the middle black numbers.

Hip External Rotation Assessment, Measurement

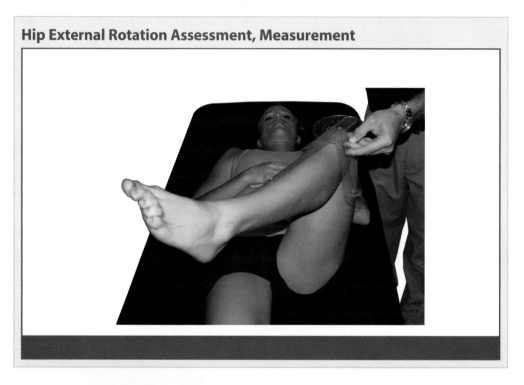

Common Errors

Common errors that can occur during this measurement that must be avoided include failure of the health and fitness professional to maintain a neutral hip or thigh position, moving the client into position too slowly, and inability to see compensations or improper alignment of the stabilization arm.

Human Movement System Impairment

This measurement may be restricted in a person who demonstrates the knees moving inward or asymmetric weight shift during the overhead squat or single-leg squat assessments.

HIP EXTENSION

1. Joint motion being assessed:
   a. Extension of iliofemoral joint
2. Muscles and tissues being assessed:
   a. Psoas, iliacus, rectus femoris, TFL, sartorius
   b. Adductor complex, anterior hip capsule
3. Antagonists potentially underactive if ROM is limited:
   a. Gluteus maximus, gluteus medius (posterior fibers)
   b. Hamstring complex, adductor magnus
4. Normal Value (22): 0–10 degrees

Positioning

The client is positioned supine with the pelvis off the table. The opposite hip is flexed to assist in flattening the low back against the table and rotating the pelvis posteriorly. The knee of the test leg should be flexed to almost 90 degrees.

Hip Extension Assessment, Position

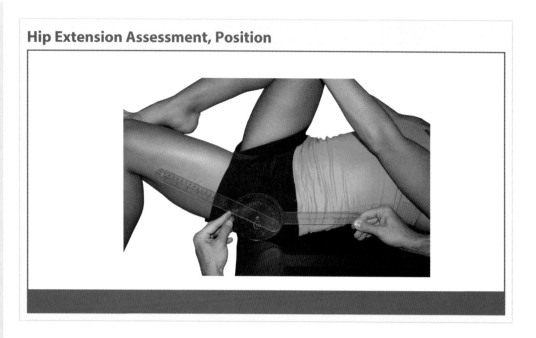

Execution

Place the goniometer as follows:

- **A:** Center the goniometer at the greater trochanter.
- **SA:** Lateral midline line of the trunk.
- **MA:** Lateral midline of the femur, referencing the lateral condyle.

Holding the client's thigh, passively allow the hip to extend until first restriction or compensation. The primary compensation to look for is anterior tilting of the pelvis or low back arching off the table. Have the client hold the position and record measurement. Measurement is read at the short end of the movement arm on the middle black numbers.

Hip Extension Assessment, Measurement

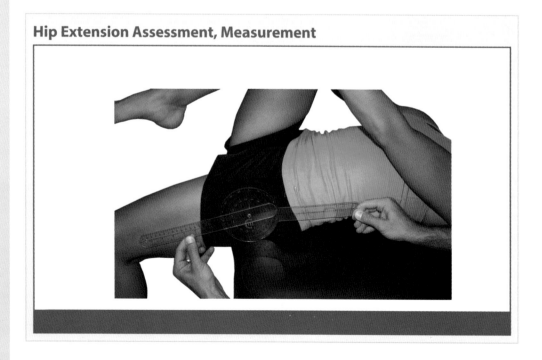

Continued on page 160

Variations

Many muscles can be implicated in this assessment and can be identified by the compensation noted at the hip and knee. Listed below are the possible scenarios for each muscle:

- If the *psoas* is the primary restriction the pelvis rotates anteriorly (low back begins to arch), the thigh stays in a neutral position, and the knee remains flexed.
- If the *rectus femoris* is the primary restriction, the pelvis rotates anteriorly, the thigh remains neutral, and the knee extends.
- If the *tensor fascia latae* is the primary restriction, the pelvis rotates anteriorly, the thigh abducts and internally rotates, and the knee extends via tension through the iliotibial band.
- If the *sartorius* is the primary restriction, the pelvis rotates anteriorly, the thigh abducts and externally rotates, and the knee remains flexed.
- If the *adductor complex* is the primary restriction, the pelvis rotates anteriorly, the thigh adducts, and the knee remains flexed.

Common Errors

Common errors that can occur during this measurement that must be avoided include failure of the health and fitness professional to maintain a neutral hip or thigh position (thigh tends to abduct) or moving the client into position too slowly, and an inability to see compensations.

Human Movement System Impairment

This measurement may be restricted in a person who demonstrates arching of the low back or excessive forward lean during the overhead squat or single-leg squat assessments.

➤ SHOULDER COMPLEX

SHOULDER FLEXION

1. Joint motion being assessed:
   a. Flexion of shoulder complex
2. Muscles being assessed:
   a. Latissimus dorsi, teres major, teres minor, infraspinatus, subscapularis, pectoralis major (lower fibers), triceps (long head)
3. Antagonists potentially underactive if ROM is limited:
   a. Anterior deltoid, pectoralis major (upper fibers, clavicular fibers), middle deltoid
   b. Lower and middle trapezius, rhomboids
4. Normal Value (22): 160 degrees

Positioning

The client is positioned supine with shoulder in neutral (0 degrees of abduction, adduction, and rotation).

Shoulder Flexion Assessment, Position

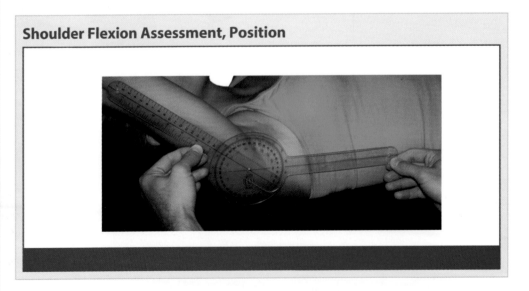

Execution   Place the goniometer as follows:

- ***A:*** Center the goniometer at the lateral shoulder, 1 inch distal to the acromion process.
- ***SA:*** Midaxillary line of the upper thorax.
- ***MA:*** Lateral midline of the humerus, referencing the lateral epicondyle of the humerus.

Holding the client's arm in external rotation, place the thumb on the lateral border of the scapula and passively flex the shoulder until excessive scapular movement is felt or the first resistance barrier is noted. Have the client hold the position and record measurement. Measurement is read at the long end of the measurement arm on the middle black numbers.

Shoulder Flexion Assessment, Measurement

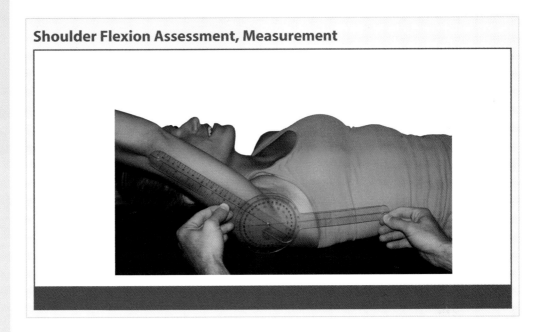

Common Errors   Common errors that can occur during this measurement that must be avoided include failure of the health and fitness professional to maintain a neutral shoulder position or moving the client into position too slowly, and an inability to see or feel compensations.

Human Movement System Impairment   This measurement may be restricted in a person who demonstrates arching of the low back or arms falling forward during the overhead squat assessment or shows restrictions in the shoulder flexion wall test.

GLENOHUMERAL JOINT INTERNAL ROTATION

1. Joint motion being assessed:
    a. Internal rotation of glenohumeral joint
2. Muscles being assessed:
    a. Infraspinatus, teres minor, posterior glenohumeral joint capsule
3. Antagonists potentially underactive if ROM is limited:
    a. Subscapularis, teres major, pectoralis major, latissimus dorsi, anterior deltoid
4. Normal Value (22): 45 degrees

Positioning   The client is positioned supine with the humerus abducted at 90 degrees and the elbow flexed at 90 degrees. The forearm is in also at 0 degrees of supination and pronation so that the palmar surface of the hand faces the ground during the measurement. The humerus can be supported by a towel to maintain a level position aligned with the acromion. Place the palm or heel of one hand on the client's anterior shoulder.

Continued on page 162

Glenohumeral Joint Internal Rotation, Position

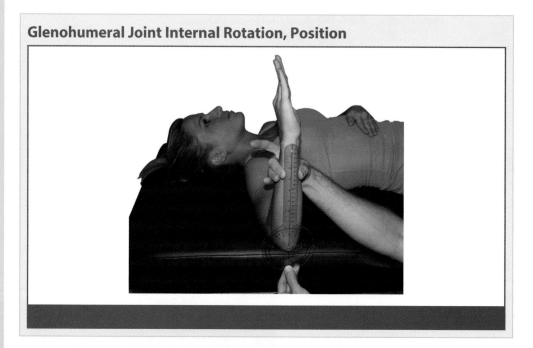

Execution   Place the goniometer as follows:

- **A:** Center the goniometer at the olecranon process of the elbow.
- **SA:** Align the arm to be perpendicular to the floor.
- **MA:** Align the arm with the lateral midline of the ulna, referencing the ulnar styloid and olecranon process.

Holding the client's arm, passively lower the humerus by applying downward pressure until the first resistance barrier or compensation is noted. The primary compensation to look for is an upward migration of the humeral head into the hand over the anterior shoulder. Have the client hold the position and record measurement. Measurement is read at the long end of the measurement arm on the middle black numbers.

Glenohumeral Joint Internal Rotation, Measurement

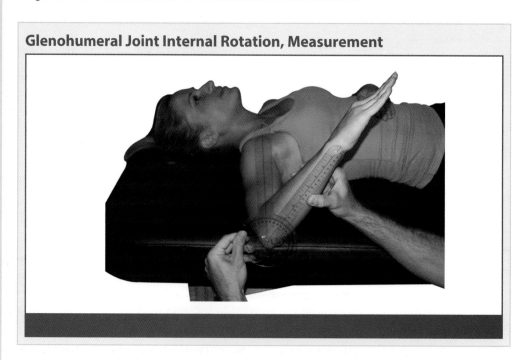

Common Errors   Common errors that can occur during this measurement that must be avoided include failure of the health and fitness professional to maintain a neutral shoulder position, moving the client into position too slowly, and an inability to see compensations.

Human Movement
System Impairment   This measurement may be restricted in a person who demonstrates arms falling forward during the overhead squat assessment or shows restrictions in the shoulder rotation wall test.

GLENOHUMERAL JOINT EXTERNAL ROTATION

1. Joint motion being assessed:
    a. External rotation of glenohumeral joint
2. Muscles and tissues being assessed:
    a. Subscapularis, latissimus dorsi, teres major, pectoralis major, anterior deltoid, anterior glenohumeral joint capsule
3. Antagonists potentially underactive if ROM is limited:
    a. Infraspinatus, teres minor
4. Normal Value (22): 90 degrees

Positioning   The client is positioned supine with the humerus abducted at 90 degrees and the elbow flexed at 90 degrees. The elbow is also at 0 degrees of supination and pronation so that the palmar surface of the hand faces the ceiling during the measurement. The humerus is supported by a towel to maintain a level position aligned with the acromion process. Place the palm or heel of one hand on the client's anterior shoulder.

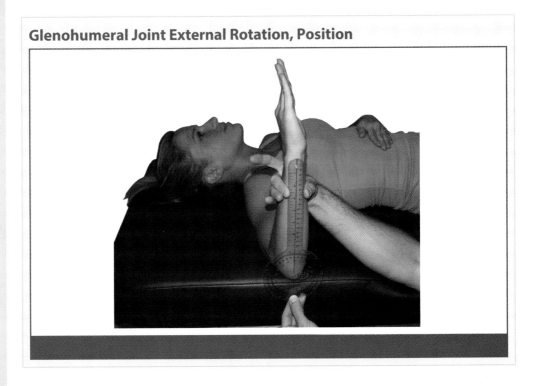

Glenohumeral Joint External Rotation, Position

Execution   Place the goniometer as follows:

- **A:** Center the goniometer at the olecranon process of the elbow.
- **SA:** Align the arm to be perpendicular to the floor.
- **MA:** Align the arm with the lateral midline of the ulna, referencing the ulnar styloid and olecranon process.

Holding the client's arm, passively lower the humerus into external rotation until the first resistance barrier or compensation is noted. The primary compensation to look for is an upward migration of the humeral head into the hand over the anterior shoulder. Have the

Continued on page 164

client hold the position and record measurement. Measurement is read at the long end of the measurement arm on the middle black numbers.

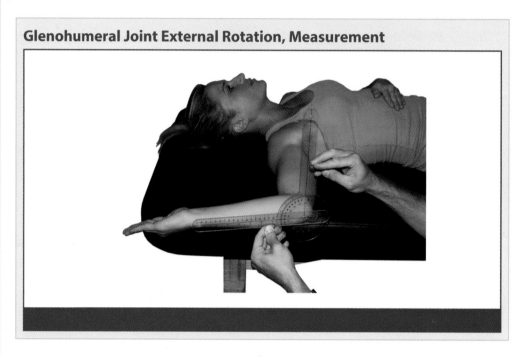

Glenohumeral Joint External Rotation, Measurement

Common Errors

Common errors that can occur during this measurement that must be avoided include failure of the health and fitness professional to maintain a neutral shoulder position, moving the client into position too slowly, and an inability to see or feel compensations.

Human Movement System Impairment

This measurement may be restricted in a person who demonstrates arms falling forward during the overhead squat assessment or shows restrictions in the shoulder rotation wall test.

SUMMARY • Measuring joint ROM is an important part in an integrated assessment process. Using ROM assessments through the use of a goniometer or inclinometer can help in confirming suspected reasons for movement compensations seen in the movement assessments. ROM assessments, in conjunction with movement and muscle strength assessments, can also help pinpoint specific regions of the body that must be addressed to assist the health and fitness professional in designing an individualized corrective exercise program that meets the needs of the client.

References

1. Sahrmann SA. Diagnosis and Treatment of Movement Impairment Syndromes. St. Louis, MO: Mosby; 2002.
2. Liebenson C. Integrated Rehabilitation Into Chiropractic Practice (blending active and passive care). In: Liebenson C, ed. Rehabilitation of the Spine. Baltimore, MD: Williams & Wilkins; 1996: 13–43.
3. Norkin CC, White DJ. Measurement of Joint Motion: A Guide to Goniometry. 3rd ed. Philadelphia, PA: FA Davis; 2003.
4. Comerford MJ, Mottram SL. Movement and stability dysfunction—contemporary developments. *Man Ther* 2001;6(1):15–26.
5. Panjabi MM. The stabilizing system of the spine. Part I: function, dysfunction, adaptation, and enhancement. *J Spinal Disord* 1992;5(4):383–9.
6. McCreary EK, Provance PG, Rogers MM, Rumani WA. Muscles: Testing and Function with Posture and Pain. 5th ed. Philadelphia, PA: Lippincott Williams & Wilkins; 2005.

7. Janda V. Evaluation of Muscle Imbalances. In: Liebenson C, ed. Rehabilitation of the Spine. Baltimore, MD: Williams & Wilkins; 1996:97–112.

8. Sahrmann SA. Posture and muscle imbalance: faulty lumbar-pelvic alignments. *Phys Ther* 1987;67:1840–4.

9. Lun V, Meeuwisse WH, Stergiou P, Stefanyshyn D. Relation between running injury and static lower limb alignment in recreational runners. *Br J Sports Med* 2004;38(5):576–80.

10. Powers CM. The influence of altered lower-extremity kinematics on patellofemoral joint dysfunction: a theoretical perspective. *J Orthop Sports Phys Ther* 2003;33(11):639–46.

11. Janda V. Muscle Strength in Relation to Muscle Length, Pain, and Muscle Imbalance. In: Harms-Ringdahl K, ed. International Perspectives in Physical Therapy 8. Edinburgh: Churchill Livingstone; 1993: 83–91.

12. Janda V. Muscles and Motor Control in Low Back Pain: Assessment and Management. In: Twomey LT, ed. Physical Therapy of the Low Back. Edinburgh: Churchill Livingstone; 1987:253–78.

13. Cookson JC, Kent BE. Orthopedic manual therapy—an overview: part I. *Phys Ther* 1979;59:136–46.

14. American Academy of Orthopaedic Surgeons. Joint Motion: Method of Measuring and Recording. Chicago, IL: AAOS; 1983.

15. Kersey R. Measurement of joint motion: a guide to goniometry. *Athl Ther Today* 2005;10(1):42.

16. American Medical Association. Guidelines to the Evaluation to Permanent Impairment. 3rd ed. Chicago, IL: AMA; 1988.

17. Clapis P, Davis SM, Davis RO. Reliability of inclinometer and goniometric measurements of hip flexor length used during the Thomas test. *J Orthop Sports Phys Ther* 2006;36(1):135–41.

18. Mullaney M, Johnson C, Banz J. Reliability of active shoulder range of motion comparing a goniometer to a digital level. *J Orthop Sports Phys Ther* 2006;36(1):A80.

19. McPoil TG, Cornwall MW. Applied Sports Mechanics in Rehabilitation Running. In: Zachazeweski JE, Magee DJ, Quillen WS, eds. Athletic Injuries and Rehabilitation. Philadelphia, PA: WB Saunders; 1996.

20. Ostrosky KM. A comparison of gait characteristics in young and old subjects. *Phys Ther* 1994;74(7):637–44.

21. Magee DJ. Orthopedic Physical Assessment. 4th ed. Philadelphia, PA: WB Saunders; 2002.

22. Greene WB, Heckman JD. American Academy of Orthopedic Surgeons. The Clinical Measurement of Joint Motion. Chicago, IL: AAOS; 1994.

23. Greene BL, Wolf SL. Upper extremity joint movement: comparison of two measurement devices. *Arch Phys Med Rehabil* 1989;70:288–90.

Strength Assessments

INTRODUCTION

Strength: the ability of the neuromuscular system to produce internal tension to overcome an external force.

To achieve optimal movement, muscles must be properly activated by the nervous system. The ability of the neuromuscular system to produce internal tension to overcome an external force is a simple definition of **strength** (1). Thus, the ability of the nervous system to recruit and activate muscles dictates muscle strength. Understanding muscle strength and how to assess it entails a comprehensive knowledge of human movement science, specifically functional anatomy, kinesiology, biomechanics, physiology, and motor control. The ability to identify accurate muscle strength is an important assessment tool for the health and fitness professional to develop a safe and effective corrective strategy for his or her clients. This chapter is intended to guide the health and fitness professional in the assessment of muscle strength through the use of manual muscle testing (MMT). It should be noted that one must be a qualified health and fitness professional (i.e., a licensed professional) to apply MMT techniques on clients.

THE SCIENTIFIC RATIONALE FOR MANUAL MUSCLE TESTING

Manual muscle testing (MMT) is a major component of a comprehensive and integrated assessment process (2–4). It involves the testing of muscle strength, which can provide an indication of neuromuscular recruitment, as well as the capability of the muscle to function during movement and provide stability (3).

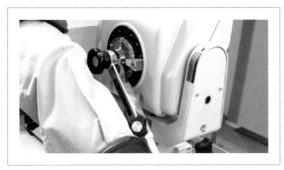

Figure 8.1 Isokinetic testing.

Isokinetic testing: muscle strength testing performed with a specialized apparatus that provides variable resistance to a movement, so that no matter how much effort is exerted, the movement takes place at a constant speed. Such testing is used to assess and improve muscular strength and endurance, especially after injury.

Dynamometry: the process of measuring forces at work using a handheld instrument (dynamometer) that measures the force of muscular contraction.

IT-band syndrome: continual rubbing of the IT band over the lateral femoral epicondyle leading to the area becoming inflamed.

Although other methods of evaluating muscle function exist that are more objective and reliable than MMT, such as **isokinetic testing** (Figure 8-1) or handheld **dynamometry**, MMT provides an opportunity to assess muscle function with low cost and little difficulty (3,5).

As mentioned in earlier chapters, each muscle must exhibit normal strength with proper neuromuscular control to effectively accelerate, decelerate, and stabilize the interconnected joints of the body and produce optimal human movement. Optimal muscle strength and recruitment can only be achieved through the integrated functioning of the skeletal, muscular, and nervous systems (chapter two) (1,2,6,7). When operating correctly, these three systems allow for optimal structural alignment, neuromuscular control (coordination and recruitment), and range of motion to occur at each joint (1,2,6,7). Coordination of these systems is essential to help ensure proper muscle balance and strength of each muscle (1–4,7,8).

However, for many reasons, such as repetitive stress, impact trauma, disease, and sedentary lifestyles, impairment to the human movement system can occur (2,3,8). When impairment of the human movement system occurs, muscle balance, muscle recruitment, and joint motion are altered (chapter three) (1,3,8,9). This impairment affects the ability of the muscular, nervous, and skeletal systems to function interdependently and effectively perform their functional tasks, which may ultimately result in injury (1,8–11). For example, research has demonstrated that weakness of hip abductors (i.e., gluteus medius) is associated with patellofemoral pain (10,11), iliotibial band (IT-band) syndrome (12), and overall lower extremity injury (13). Weakness of the gluteus medius, which is the primary frontal plane stabilizer of the femur, is also associated with overactivity (or synergistic dominance) of the tensor fascia lata (TFL) (2). The TFL attaches to the IT-band and onto the lateral aspect of the tibia via the IT-band. When overactive, the TFL can cause increased tension throughout the IT-band and lateral knee (**IT-band syndrome**) (Figure 8-2). Also, the TFL can cause external rotation of the tibia, placing increased stress on the tibiofemoral and patellofemoral joints, which may result in patellofemoral pain (14). The concept of human movement system impairment is important because it is what the health and fitness professional is helping to identify with MMT.

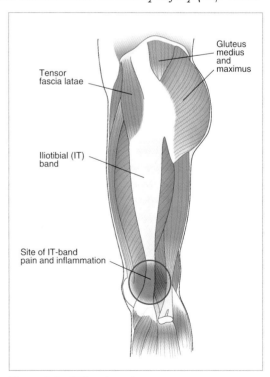

Tensor fascia latae

Gluteus medius and maximus

Iliotibial (IT) band

Site of IT-band pain and inflammation

Figure 8.2 IT-band syndrome.

THE NASM USE OF MANUAL MUSCLE TESTING

MMT is an assessment process used to test the recruitment capacity and contraction quality of individual muscles or movements (15). Although many motions are the result of more than one muscle working, emphasis can be placed on a particular muscle through proper positioning (3).

The premise behind MMT is to place the desired muscle in a position that will induce resistance against it. This can be done with gravity or manual pressure and through concentric or isometric muscle actions (3). The isometric MMT process has been termed a **break test** and is said to be the most common and easiest to perform (3). An isometric test is easier to perform and theoretically should be more reliable than a concentric test because confounding factors, such as speed of contraction and varying resistance in different positions and directions, are removed (15).

The ability of the client to withstand various levels of resistance will render a specific grade, usually numerical, on a 0 to 5 scale (Table 8-1) (3).

Although a variety of methods and grading systems exist for MMT, NASM has chosen to use a two-step isometric MMT process graded with a simple 3-point grading system (Table 8-2), as suggested by Kendall and colleagues (1). More extensive grading systems are recommended when the purpose of the MMT is to determine prognosis versus diagnosis or evaluation (3). The numerical grade of 3 represents a client who maintains good structural alignment and holds the end-range position against the assessor's pressure, which indicates a pure isometric contraction is present (15). A grade of 2 represents a client with good overall strength, but with compensations from other muscles or failure to maintain the isometric contraction. This will be evident by alteration of the body or limb position that occurs with increased pressure from the assessor. A grade of 1 indicates little to no ability of the client to withstand or resist pressure from the assessor.

The two-step process to assess muscle strength is used to help the health and fitness professional evaluate the possible cause of muscle weakness in a client, which will direct corrective exercise strategies. Muscle weakness can be attributable to several factors, but the most common factors in a healthy individual are atrophy or inhibition (16). An inhibited muscle always produces less counterpressure than requested by an examiner (15).

Step one of the NASM MMT process includes the following (Table 8-3):

- Place the joint in the desired position for the specific muscle to be tested.
- Ask the client to hold that position while applying pressure against the limb directly in the line of pull for the desired muscle.
- The pressure applied should be done in a ramping-up manner versus quickly applying maximum force.
- The client must hold that position and not allow the assessor to "break" the hold. This should be held for 4 seconds.

Break test: at the end of available range, or at a point in the range where the muscle is most challenged, the client is asked to hold that position and not allow the examiner to "break" the hold with manual resistance.

Table 8.1	MANUAL MUSCLE TESTING 6-POINT GRADING SYSTEM
Numerical Score	**Level of Strength**
5	Normal
4	Good
3	Fair
2	Poor
1	Trace activity
0	No activity

Table 8.2 NASM 3-POINT GRADING SYSTEM

Numerical Score	Level of Strength
3	Normal
2	Compensates (uses other muscles)
1	Weak (little to no activity)

- Determine and grade the client's level of strength.
- If the muscle tests normal with no compensation or movement, then the muscle is considered strong.
- If the position breaks (muscle assumes an eccentric contraction) or if compensations are observed, move to step two.

Step two involves the same process as step one, but involves lengthening of the muscle by placing the muscle in a midrange position. The reason for this second step involves simple joint mechanics. If muscles are shortening on one side of the joint, then muscles on the opposing side must be lengthening. If these lengthening muscles do not have the proper extensibility (ability to elongate), they will limit the functional capacity of the opposing muscle group (in this case the muscles being tested in the shortened position). This has been noted by several authors (2,3,7) and is known as altered reciprocal inhibition. It is important to note that although tight muscles may be the cause of a muscle's weakness in a shortened position, restrictions in skin, neural tissue, or articular ligaments and tissues can also result in muscle inhibition (15).

Overactivity of a shortened muscle will reciprocally inhibit its functional antagonist (2,3,8). This inhibition can lead to a false reading that a muscle is weak when in fact the strength impression is purely a factor of joint position. If the muscle tests normal (strong) in the midrange, then there is either a muscle length issue on the opposing side of the joint or possibly a joint restriction (15). In this situation, the health and fitness professional can easily assess muscle length through goniometric measurement, address the muscle with appropriate flexibility techniques (inhibit and lengthen), and retest the muscle strength.

An example of this can be seen in a weak or underactive gluteus medius. If the adductor complex is overactive and restricting proper hip abduction, extension, and external rotation, the gluteus medius will be limited (inhibited) in its functional ability. This will often lead to overactivity (synergistic dominance) of the TFL (2,9). When the adductor complex (and TFL, if necessary) is addressed with proper flexibility and the strength of the gluteus medius is

Table 8.3 NASM 2-STEP MANUAL MUSCLE TESTING PROCESS

Step 1	Step 2
- Place muscle in shortened position, or to point of joint compensation. - Ask client to hold that position while applying pressure. - Gradually increase pressure. - Client's strength is graded - If client can hold the position without compensation, then the muscle is noted as strong. - If the muscle is weak or compensates, move to step 2.	- Place muscle in midrange position and retest strength. - If muscle strength is normal in midrange, there may be opposing muscle overactivity or joint hypomobility—inhibit and lengthen. - If the muscle is weak or compensates in midrange position, the muscle is likely weak—reactivate and reintegrate.

regained, then the underlying problem may not be true muscle weakness, but altered reciprocal inhibition caused by an antagonist muscle group (adductors and TFL). If the muscle still tests weak or compensates in the midrange position, then it is likely that true muscle weakness exists. In this case, the health and fitness professional should reactivate the muscle and then reintegrate it back into its functional synergy.

NASM SELECTED MANUAL MUSCLE TESTS

There are many muscles in the body that can be evaluated with MMT. However, NASM has only chosen a select number of muscles to be tested (Table 8-4). The following muscles were selected because of their overall importance to optimal human movement, as well as their ability to correlate to the movement assessments and goniometric measurements. The following list is by no means intended to be exhaustive. Rather, its intent is to be very practical and used in an integrated assessment process. Refer to chapter two of this textbook for details on muscle location and integrated function.

Any MMT has limitations with variability and subjectivity. The health and fitness professional should remember that MMT only measures the force produced during a specific isometric movement in a specific position. To improve reliability and safety, as well as reduce errors with an MMT assessment, the following guidelines should be followed:

- The same health and fitness professional should be used with a single client to reduce intertester variability.
- Do not test a muscle in a fully lengthened position because it can lead to overstretching and injury.
- Ensure proper position of the joint before performing the test.
- Ensure proper stabilization to minimize compensations.
- Establish a time (4 seconds) for the client to hold the isometric muscle contraction.

Table 8.4 NASM SELECTED MANUAL MUSCLE TESTS		
Lower Extremity	**Trunk**	**Upper Extremity and Cervical Spine**
Foot/Ankle • Anterior tibialis • Posterior tibialis **Knee** • Medial hamstring complex • Biceps femoris **Hip** • Iliopsoas • Tensor fascia lata • Sartorius • Adductor complex • Gracilis • Adductor magnus • Gluteus medius • Hip external rotators • Gluteus maximus	• Rectus abdominis • Oblique abdominals	• Latissimus dorsi • Shoulder external rotators • Shoulder internal rotators • Rhomboids • Lower trapezius • Serratus anterior • Anterior neck flexors • Anterolateral neck flexors • Posterolateral neck extensors

- Provide gradual increases in pressure at a constant speed.
- Manual resistance should be applied at a 90-degree angle to the primary axis of a body part (17).
- Both the client and health and fitness professional should be in comfortable and stable positions.

(Text continues on page 195)

MANUAL MUSCLE TESTS

➤ FOOT AND ANKLE COMPLEX

ANTERIOR TIBIALIS

1. Joint position being tested:
   a. Dorsiflexion and inversion of ankle
2. Muscles being assessed:
   a. Anterior tibialis (prime mover)
   b. Extensor digitorum longus, extensor hallucis longus, peroneus tertius (synergists)
3. Potentially overactive muscles if strength is limited:
   a. Gastrocnemius, soleus, peroneus longus, peroneus brevis

Positioning   Client is supine with knee extended. Place ankle in dorsiflexion and inversion.

Execution
- Support the posterior lower leg just above the ankle.
- Instruct client to "hold" the position.
- Apply gradual and increasing pressure to the medial dorsal surface of the foot in the direction of plantarflexion and eversion.
- Look for compensations of the toes extending or foot everting.
- Grade client's strength: 3 = normal, 2 = compensates, 1 = weak.
- If graded 1 or 2, take client's foot or ankle into a midrange and retest.

Anterior Tibialis Assessment, Execution

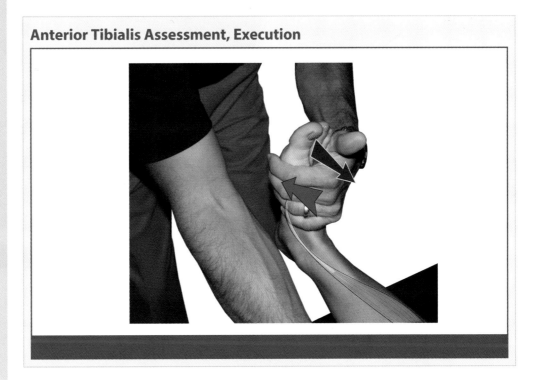

Continued on page 172

Human Movement System Impairment

This muscle may be weak in a person who demonstrates flattening of the feet (excessive pronation) during the overhead squat assessment. It may also appear weak at the end-range if there is limited dorsiflexion measured by goniometric measurement, which can be caused by overactivity in the gastrocnemius or soleus, as well as the peroneus longus and peroneus brevis.

POSTERIOR TIBIALIS

1. Joint position being tested:
   a. Plantarflexion and inversion of ankle
2. Muscles being assessed:
   a. Posterior tibialis
   b. Anterior tibialis, flexor digitorum longus, flexor hallucis longus, soleus, extensor hallucis longus
3. Potentially overactive muscles if strength is limited:
   a. Peroneus longus, brevis and tertius, extensor digitorum longus and brevis
   b. Lateral gastrocnemius

Positioning

Client is supine with knee extended. Place ankle in plantarflexion and inversion.

Execution

- Support the posterior lower leg just above the ankle.
- Instruct client to "hold" the position.
- Apply gradual and increasing pressure to the medial plantar surface of the foot in the direction of dorsiflexion and eversion.
- Look for compensations of the toes flexing or foot everting.
- Grade client's strength: 3 = normal, 2 = compensates, 1 = weak.
- If graded 1 or 2, take client's foot or ankle into a midrange and retest.

Posterior Tibialis Assessment, Execution

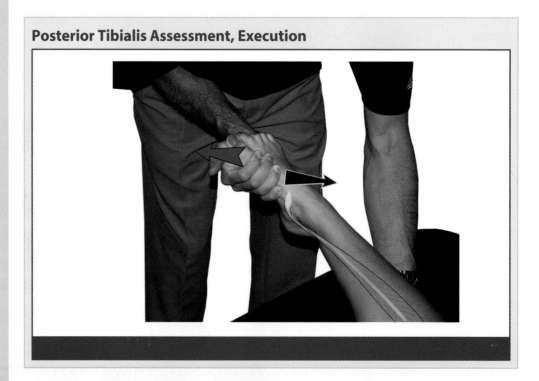

Human Movement System Impairment

This muscle may be weak in a person who demonstrates flattening of the feet (excessive pronation) during the overhead squat assessment. It may also appear weak at the end-range if there is limited dorsiflexion measured by goniometric measurement. Limited ankle dorsiflexion will not allow for proper sagittal plane motion at the ankle and will require compensatory movement in the frontal and transverse planes, which is eversion and excessive pronation.

➤ THE KNEE COMPLEX

MEDIAL HAMSTRING COMPLEX: SEMITENDONSUS, AND SEMIMEMBRANOSUS

1. Joint position being tested:
   a. Knee flexion
   b. Tibial internal rotation
2. Muscles being assessed:
   a. Semimembranosus, semitendinosus
   b. Gastrocnemius, popliteus, gracilis, sartorius, plantaris
3. Potentially overactive muscles if strength is limited:
   a. Quadriceps complex (rectus femoris, vastus lateralis, vastus medialis, vastus intermedius)
   b. Biceps femoris

Positioning

Client is prone with knee flexed approximately 50 to 70 degrees. Place thigh in slight internal rotation and internally rotate the tibia.

Execution

- Stabilize the upper leg just below the knee joint.
- Instruct client to "hold" the position.
- Apply gradual and increasing pressure to the posterior lower leg in the direction of knee extension and tibial external rotation.
- Look for compensations of ankle dorsiflexion, hip adduction, hip flexion, or spinal extension.
- Grade client's strength: 3 = normal, 2 = compensates, 1 = weak.
- If graded 1 or 2, take client's leg into a midrange and retest.

Medial Hamstrings Assessment, Execution

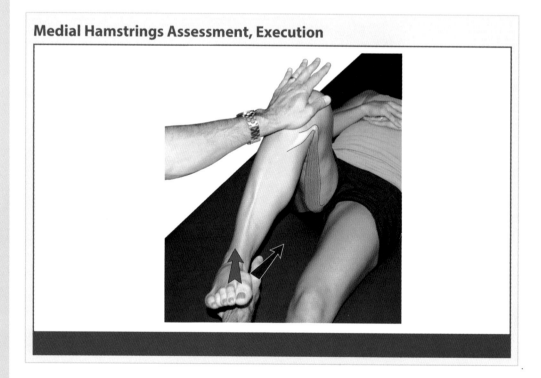

Human Movement System Impairment

These muscles may be weak in a person who demonstrates flattening of the feet (excessive pronation), low back arching, feet turning out, and/or knees moving inward during the overhead squat assessment. They may also appear weak at end-range if there is a limited goniometric measurement for hip extension (rectus femoris and/or TFL emphasis).

Continued on page 174

BICEPS FEMORIS

1. Joint position being tested:
   a. Knee flexion
   b. Tibial external rotation
2. Muscles being assessed:
   a. Biceps femoris
   b. Gastrocnemius, plantaris
3. Potentially overactive muscles if strength is limited:
   a. Quadriceps complex (rectus femoris, vastus lateralis, vastus medialis, vastus intermedius)
   b. Medial hamstring complex, popliteus, gracilis, sartorius

Positioning

Client is prone with knee flexed approximately 50 to 70 degrees. Place thigh in slight external rotation and externally rotate the tibia.

Execution

- Stabilize the upper leg anteriorly just below the knee joint.
- Instruct client to "hold" the position.
- Apply gradual and increasing pressure to the foot in the direction of knee extension and tibial internal rotation.
- Look for compensations of ankle dorsiflexion, hip abduction, hip flexion, and/or spinal extension.
- Grade client's strength: 3 = normal, 2 = compensates, 1 = weak.
- If graded 1 or 2, take client's leg into a midrange and retest.

Biceps Femoris Assessment, Execution

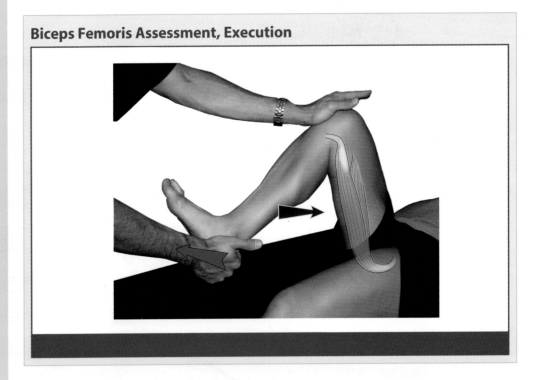

Human Movement System Impairment

This muscle may be weak in a person who demonstrates low back arching during the overhead squat assessment. It may also appear weak at end-range if there is a limited goniometric measurement for hip extension (rectus femoris emphasis).

➤ THE HIP COMPLEX

ILIOPSOAS: ILIACUS AND PSOAS MAJOR

1. Joint position being tested:
   a. Hip flexion
2. Muscles being assessed:
   a. Iliacus, psoas major
   b. Rectus femoris, sartorius, TFL, adductor longus, gluteus minimus, anterior fibers of gluteus medius
3. Potentially overactive muscles if strength is limited:
   a. Adductor magnus, medial hamstring complex
   b. Adductor longus, adductor brevis, pectineus, gracilis

Positioning

Client is supine with hip and knee flexed. Place thigh in slight external rotation and abduction.

Execution

- Stabilize the lower leg.
- Instruct client to "hold" the position.
- Apply gradual and increasing pressure at the distal end of the femur in the direction of hip extension.
- Look for compensations of knee flexion, hip abduction, hip internal rotation, and/or spinal extension.
- Grade client's strength: 3 = normal, 2 = compensates, 1 = weak.
- If graded 1 or 2, take client's leg into a midrange and retest.

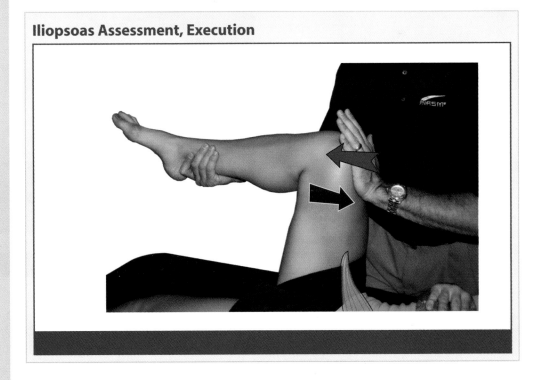

Iliopsoas Assessment, Execution

Human Movement System Impairment

This muscle may be weak in a person who demonstrates low back rounding during the overhead squat assessment. It may also appear weak at end-range if there is a limited goniometric measurement for knee extension (medial hamstring complex) or hip internal rotation (adductor magnus oblique fibers).

Continued on page 176

TENSOR FASCIA LATAE

1. Joint position being tested:
   a. Hip flexion, internal rotation, and abduction
2. Muscles being assessed:
   a. TFL
   b. Gluteus minimus, rectus femoris, sartorius, anterior fibers of gluteus medius
3. Potentially overactive muscles if strength is limited:
   a. Adductor magnus, biceps femoris

Positioning

Client is supine with hip flexed approximately 30 degrees and knee extended. Place thigh in slight internal rotation and abduction.

Execution

- Stabilize the opposite leg.
- Instruct client to "hold" the position.
- Apply gradual and increasing pressure to the medial foot or ankle in the direction of hip extension, adduction, and external rotation.
- Look for compensations of knee flexion, hip external rotation, and/or spinal extension.
- Grade client's strength: 3 = normal, 2 = compensates, 1 = weak.
- If graded 1 or 2, take client's leg into a midrange and retest.

Tensor Fascia Latae Assessment, Execution

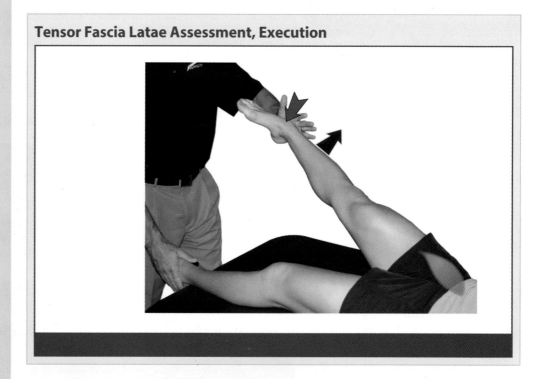

Human Movement System Impairment

This muscle may be weak in a person who demonstrates low back rounding during the overhead squat assessment. It may also appear weak at end-range if there is a limited goniometric measurement for knee extension (medial hamstring complex) and/or external rotation.

SARTORIUS

1. Joint position being tested:
   a. Hip flexion, external rotation, and abduction with knee flexion
2. Muscles being assessed:
   a. Sartorius
   b. Rectus femoris, iliopsoas, medial hamstring complex, gracilis, hip external rotators
3. Potentially overactive muscles if strength is limited:
   a. Adductor magnus
   b. Hamstring complex, adductor longus, adductor brevis, pectineus

Positioning Client is supine with hip and knee flexed. Place thigh in external rotation and abduction.

Execution
- Client may support self by holding on to the table.
- Support lower leg and knee in proper position.
- Instruct client to "hold" the position.
- Apply gradual and increasing pressure to the thigh and lower leg in the direction of hip extension, adduction, and internal rotation and knee extension.
- Look for compensations of knee extension, hip internal rotation, and/or spinal extension.
- Grade client's strength: 3 = normal, 2 = compensates, 1 = weak.
- If graded 1 or 2, take client's leg into a midrange and retest.

Sartorius Assessment, Execution

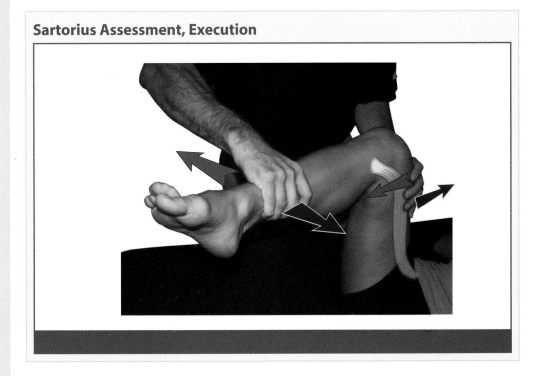

Human Movement System Impairment This muscle may demonstrate weakness in a person who demonstrates feet flattening, feet turning out, knees moving inward, and/or low back rounding during the overhead squat assessment. It may also appear weak at end-range if there is a limited goniometric measurement for hip abduction and/or internal rotation.

Continued on page 178

ADDUCTOR COMPLEX

1. Joint position being tested:
   a. Hip flexion, internal rotation, and adduction.
2. Muscles being assessed:
   a. Pectineus, adductor longus, adductor brevis
   b. Adductor magnus, gracilis
3. Potentially overactive muscles if strength is limited:
   a. Biceps femoris, piriformis, gluteus medius (posterior fibers), gluteus maximus

Positioning

Client is supine with hip flexed and knee extended. Place thigh in internal rotation and adduction.

Execution

- Stabilize the opposite leg on the table.
- Instruct client to "hold" the position.
- Apply gradual and increasing pressure to the lower leg in the direction of hip extension, abduction, and external rotation.
- Look for compensations of knee flexion, hip external rotation, and/or spinal extension.
- Grade client's strength: 3 = normal, 2 = compensates, 1 = weak.
- If graded 1 or 2, take client's leg into a midrange and retest.

Adductor Complex Assessment, Execution

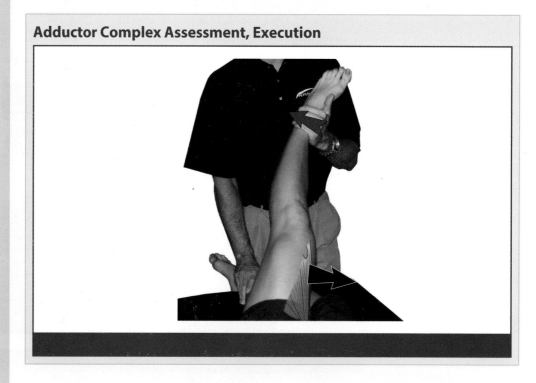

Human Movement System Impairment

This muscle may be weak in a person who demonstrates knees moving outward and/or low back rounding during the overhead squat assessment. It may also appear weak at end-range if there is a limited goniometric measurement for knee extension (biceps femoris) and/or hip internal rotation (piriformis).

GRACILIS

1. Joint position being tested:
   a. Hip adduction, knee internal rotation
2. Muscles being assessed:
   a. Gracilis
   b. Adductor longus, adductor brevis, adductor magnus, pectineus
3. Potentially overactive muscles if strength is limited:
   a. Biceps femoris, piriformis, gluteus medius (posterior fibers), gluteus maximus

Positioning Client is supine with hip in neutral and knee extended. Place thigh in internal rotation and adduction.

Execution
- Stabilize the opposite leg on the table.
- Instruct client to "hold" the position.
- Apply gradual and increasing pressure to the lower leg in the direction of abduction and external rotation.
- Look for compensations of knee flexion, hip external rotation, and/or spinal extension.
- Grade client's strength: 3 = normal, 2 = compensates, 1 = weak.
- If graded 1 or 2, take client's leg into a midrange and retest.

Gracilis Assessment, Execution

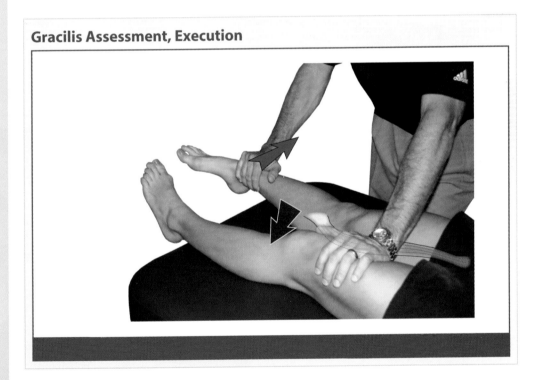

Human Movement System Impairment This muscle may be weak in a person who demonstrates feet turning out, knees moving outward, and/or low back rounding during the overhead squat assessment. It may also appear weak at end-range if there is a limited goniometric measurement for hip internal rotation.

Continued on page 180

ADDUCTOR MAGNUS

1. Joint position being tested:
   a. Hip extension, internal rotation, and adduction (vertical fibers)
   b. Hip extension, external rotation, and adduction (oblique fibers)
2. Muscles being assessed:
   a. Adductor magnus
   b. Adductor longus, adductor brevis, gracilis, pectineus
3. Potentially overactive muscles if strength is limited:
   a. Iliopsoas, rectus femoris, sartorius
   b. TFL, gluteus minimus

Positioning

Client is prone with hip and knee in extension. Place thigh in internal rotation and adduction for vertical fibers or external rotation and adduction for oblique fibers.

Execution

- Support the opposite hip.
- Instruct client to "hold" the position.
- For vertical fibers: apply gradual and increasing pressure to the lower leg in the direction of hip flexion and abduction.
- For oblique fibers: apply gradual and increasing pressure to the lower leg in the direction of hip flexion and abduction.
- Look for compensations of knee flexion, hip external rotation, and/or spinal extension.
- Grade client's strength: 3 = normal, 2 = compensates, 1 = weak.
- If graded 1 or 2, take client's leg into a midrange and retest.

Adductor Magnus Assessment, Execution

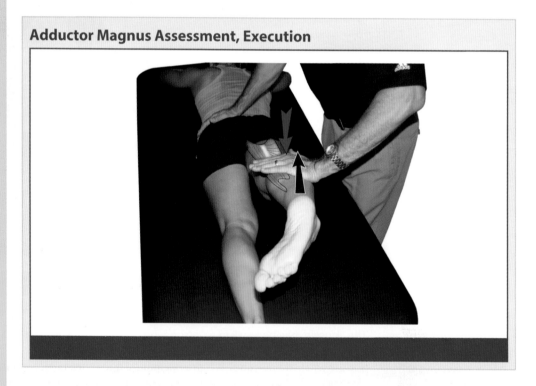

Human Movement System Impairment

This muscle may be weak in a person who demonstrates knees moving outward and/or low back arching during the overhead squat assessment. It may also appear weak at end-range if there is a limited goniometric measurement for hip extension.

GLUTEUS MEDIUS

1. Joint position being tested:
    a. Hip extension, external rotation, and abduction
2. Muscles being assessed:
    a. Gluteus medius
    b. Gluteus minimus, gluteus maximus (upper fibers), TFL
3. Potentially overactive muscles if strength is limited:
    a. Adductor brevis, adductor longus, pectineus, gracilis
    b. TFL, gluteus minimus, rectus femoris, iliopsoas

Positioning   Client is positioned in a side-lying position with hip slightly extended and knee extended. Place thigh in slight external rotation and abduction.

Execution
- Support the hip.
- Instruct client to "hold" the position.
- Apply gradual and increasing pressure to the lateral aspect of the lower leg just above the ankle joint in the direction of hip flexion and adduction.
- Look for compensations of knee flexion, hip flexion, hip internal rotation, and/or spinal extension.
- Grade client's strength: 3 = normal, 2 = compensates, 1 = weak.
- If graded 1 or 2, take client's leg into a midrange and retest.

Gluteus Medius Assessment, Execution

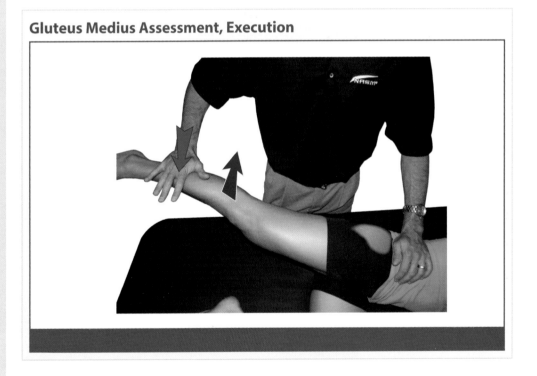

Human Movement System Impairment   This muscle may be weak in a person who demonstrates feet flattening, knees moving inward, and/or low back arching during the overhead squat or assessment It may also appear weak at end-range if there is a limited goniometric measurement for hip abduction (adductor complex) and/or hip extension (hip flexor complex).

Continued on page 182

HIP EXTERNAL ROTATORS: PIRIFORMIS, GEMELLUS SUPERIOR, GEMELLUS INFERIOR, OBTURATOR INTERNUS, OBTURATOR EXTERNUS

1. Joint position being tested:
   a. Hip flexion and external rotation
2. Muscles being assessed:
   a. Piriformis, gemellus superior, gemellus inferior, obturator internus, obturator externus
   b. Biceps femoris, gluteus medius (posterior fibers), gluteus maximus, sartorius, adductor magnus (oblique fibers), iliopsoas
3. Potentially overactive muscles if strength is limited:
   a. Adductor brevis, adductor longus, pectineus, gracilis
   b. Medial hamstring complex, TFL

Positioning   Client is supine with hip and knee flexed to 90 degrees. Place thigh in external rotation.

Execution   • Support the upper leg.
• Instruct client to "hold" the position.
• Apply gradual and increasing pressure to the lower leg in the direction of internal rotation.
• Look for compensations of knee flexion or extension and/or hip flexion.
• Grade client's strength: 3 = normal, 2 = compensates, 1 = weak.
• If graded 1 or 2, take client's leg into a midrange and retest.

Hip External Rotators Assessment, Execution

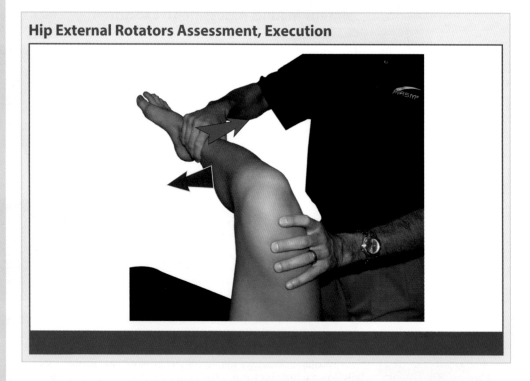

Human Movement System Impairment   This muscle may be weak in a person who demonstrates feet flattening or knees moving inward during the overhead squat or single-leg squat assessments. It may also appear weak at end-range if there is a limited goniometric measurement for hip abduction (adductor complex) and hip external rotation (adductor magnus vertical fibers).

GLUTEUS MAXIMUS

1. Joint position being tested:
   a. Hip extension, external rotation, and abduction
2. Muscles being assessed:
   a. Gluteus maximus
   b. Adductor magnus, hamstring complex, gluteus medius (posterior fibers)
3. Potentially overactive muscles if strength is limited:
   a. Iliopsoas, rectus femoris, adductor longus, adductor brevis, pectineus
   b. TFL, sartorius, gluteus minimus

Positioning

Client is prone with hip in extension and knee flexed. Place thigh into slight external rotation and abduction.

Execution

- Support the opposite hip.
- Instruct client to "hold" the position.
- Apply gradual and increasing pressure to the upper leg just above the knee in the direction of hip flexion, adduction, and internal rotation.
- Look for compensations of knee flexion, hip internal rotation, and/or spinal extension.
- Grade client's strength: 3 = normal, 2 = compensates, 1 = weak.
- If graded 1 or 2, take client's leg into a midrange and retest.

Gluteus Maximus Assessment, Execution

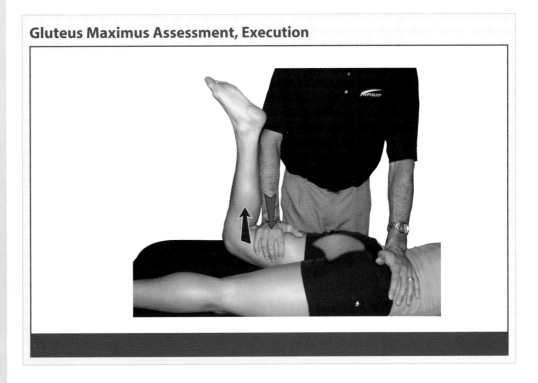

Human Movement System Impairment

This muscle may be weak in a person who demonstrates feet flattening, knees moving inward, and/or low back arching during the overhead squat assessments. It may also appear weak at end-range if there is a limited goniometric measurement for hip extension (hip flexor complex).

Continued on page 184

➤ **THE TRUNK**

RECTUS ABDOMINIS

1. Joint position being tested:
   a. Spinal (trunk) flexion
2. Muscles being assessed:
   a. Rectus abdominis
   b. External obliques, internal obliques
3. Potentially overactive muscles if strength is limited:
   a. Erector spinae
   b. Latissimus dorsi, iliopsoas, rectus femoris, TFL, sartorius, quadratus lumborum

Positioning Client is supine with trunk in flexion.

Execution
- Support the client's thighs.
- Instruct client to "hold" the position.
- Apply gradual and increasing pressure to the upper torso in the direction of spinal extension.
- Look for compensations of hip flexion or trunk rotation.
- Grade client's strength: 3 = normal, 2 = compensates, 1 = weak.
- If graded 1 or 2, take client into a midrange and retest.

Rectus Abdominis Assessment, Execution

Human Movement System Impairment This muscle may be weak in a person who demonstrates low back arching during the overhead squat assessments or if the low back arches (sags) during the push-up assessment.

OBLIQUE ABDOMINALS: EXTERNAL AND INTERNAL OBLIQUE

1. Joint position being tested:
   a. Spinal (trunk) flexion and rotation
2. Muscles being assessed:
   a. External obliques, internal obliques
   b. Rectus abdominis
3. Potentially overactive muscles if strength is limited:
   a. Erector spinae
   b. Latissimus dorsi, iliopsoas, rectus femoris, TFL, sartorius, quadratus lumborum, adductor longus, adductor brevis, adductor magnus, pectineus, gracilis

Positioning   Client is supine with trunk in flexion and rotation.

Execution
- Support the client's thighs.
- Instruct client to "hold" the position.
- Apply gradual and increasing pressure to the upper torso in the direction of opposite spinal rotation and extension.
- Look for compensations of hip flexion and/or hip adduction.
- Grade client's strength: 3 = normal, 2 = compensates, 1 = weak.
- If graded 1 or 2, take client into a midrange and retest.

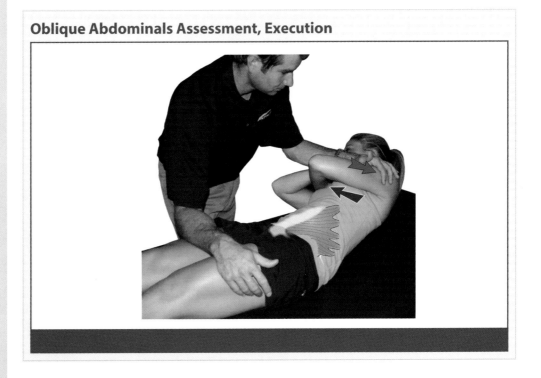

Oblique Abdominals Assessment, Execution

Human Movement System Impairment   This muscle may be weak in a person who demonstrates low back arching during the overhead squat assessment, inward or outward trunk rotation during the single-leg squat assessment, and/or if the low back arches (sags) during the push-up assessment.

Continued on page 186

➤ THE SHOULDER COMPLEX

LATISSIMUS DORSI

1. Joint position being tested:
   a. Shoulder extension, adduction, and internal rotation
2. Muscles being assessed:
   a. Latissimus dorsi
   b. Posterior deltoid, teres major, triceps brachii (long head), lower trapezius, rhomboids, mid-trapezius
3. Potentially overactive muscles if strength is limited:
   a. Anterior deltoid, upper trapezius, pectoralis major, pectoralis minor, biceps brachii (long head), infraspinatus, teres minor
   b. Biceps femoris, medial hamstrings, adductor magnus, rectus abdominis, oblique abdominal complex

Positioning Client is prone with shoulder complex in extension, adduction, and internal rotation.

Execution
- Support the client's opposite shoulder.
- Instruct client to "hold" the position.
- Apply gradual and increasing pressure to the forearm in the direction of shoulder flexion and abduction.
- Look for compensations of trunk extension, shoulder elevation, or scapular adduction.
- Grade client's strength: 3 = normal, 2 = compensates, 1 = weak.
- If graded 1 or 2, take client's arm into a midrange and retest.

Latissimus Dorsi Assessment, Execution

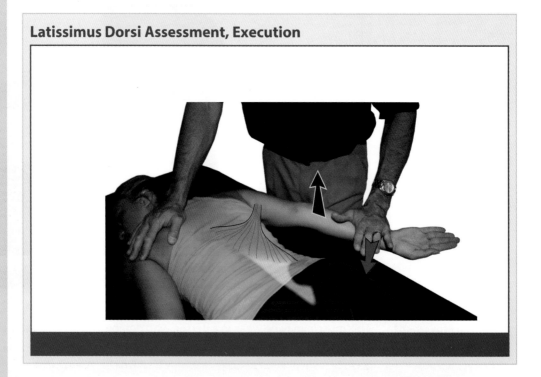

Human Movement System Impairment This muscle may be tight in a person who demonstrates arms falling forward and/or low back arching during the overhead squat. Low back rounding during the overhead squat may indicate weakness. It may also appear weak at end-range if there is a limited goniometric measurement for glenohumeral external rotation.

SHOULDER EXTERNAL ROTATORS: INFRASPINATUS AND TERES MINOR

1. Joint position being tested:
   a. Shoulder external rotation
2. Muscles being assessed:
   a. Infraspinatus, teres minor
   b. Posterior deltoid, middle deltoid
3. Potentially overactive muscles if strength is limited:
   a. Subscapularis
   b. Latissimus dorsi, teres major, pectoralis major, pectoralis minor

Positioning

Client is seated, maintaining proper posture with the arm to the side with the elbow at 90 degrees.

Execution

- Support the client's opposite shoulder.
- Instruct client to "hold" the position.
- Apply gradual and increasing pressure to the lower arm just above the wrist in the direction of shoulder internal rotation.
- Look for compensations of shoulder elevation and/or scapular adduction.
- Grade client's strength: 3 = normal, 2 = compensates, 1 = weak.
- If graded 1 or 2, take client's arm into a midrange and retest.

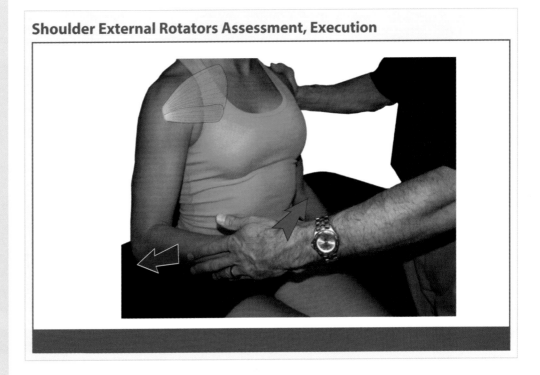

Shoulder External Rotators Assessment, Execution

Human Movement System Impairment

This muscle may be weak in a person who demonstrates arms falling forward during the overhead squat and overhead pressing assessment or whose shoulders elevate during the push-up or pulling assessments. It may also appear weak at end-range if there is a limited goniometric measurement for shoulder internal rotation (subscapularis and teres major).

Continued on page 188

SHOULDER INTERNAL ROTATORS: SUBSCAPULARIS AND TERES MAJOR

1. Joint position being tested:
   a. Shoulder internal rotation
2. Muscles being assessed:
   a. Subscapularis, teres major
   b. Anterior deltoid, latissimus dorsi, pectoralis major
3. Potentially overactive muscles if strength is limited:
   a. Posterior deltoid
   b. Infraspinatus, teres minor

Positioning

Client is seated, maintaining proper posture with the arm to the side with the elbow at 90 degrees.

Execution

- Support the client's shoulder.
- Instruct client to "hold" the position.
- Apply gradual and increasing pressure to the lower arm just above the wrist in the direction of shoulder external rotation.
- Look for compensations of shoulder elevation and/or scapular adduction.
- Grade client's strength: 3 = normal, 2 = compensates, 1 = weak.
- If graded 1 or 2, take client's arm into a midrange and retest.

Shoulder Internal Rotators Assessment, Execution

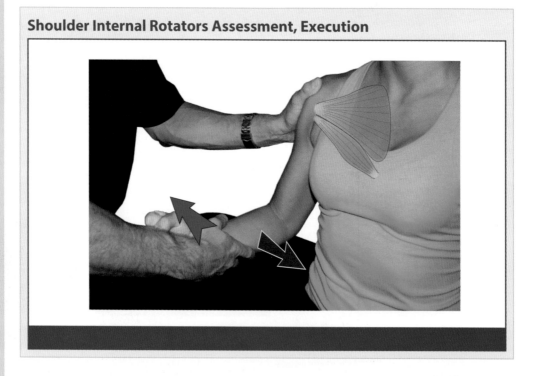

Human Movement System Impairment

This muscle may be weak in a person who demonstrates arms falling forward during the overhead squat and overhead pressing assessments or whose shoulders elevate during the push-up or pulling assessments. It may also appear weak at end-range if there is a limited goniometric measurement for shoulder external rotation (infraspinatus and teres minor).

RHOMBOIDS

1. Joint position being tested:
   a. Scapular adduction and downward rotation
2. Muscles being assessed:
   a. Rhomboids
   b. Middle trapezius, upper trapezius, levator scapulae
3. Potentially overactive muscles if strength is limited:
   a. Serratus anterior, pectoralis minor
   b. Latissimus dorsi, pectoralis major, anterior deltoid

Positioning Client is prone, elbow flexed, and shoulder complex in scapular adduction and slight elevation. Place shoulder in 90 degrees of abduction and slight internal rotation.

Execution
- Support the client on opposite scapula.
- Instruct client to "hold" the position.
- Apply gradual and increasing pressure to the distal humerus just above the elbow in a downward direction toward the floor.
- Look for a shoulder elevation compensation.
- Grade client's strength: 3 = normal, 2 = compensates, 1 = weak.
- If graded 1 or 2, take client's arm into a midrange and retest.

Rhomboids Assessment, Execution

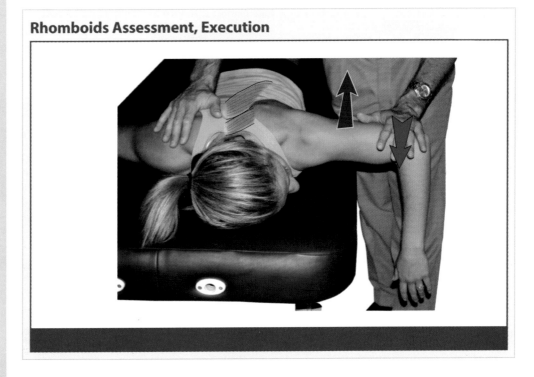

Human Movement
System Impairment This muscle may be weak in a person who demonstrates arms falling forward during the overhead squat, the shoulders round during pulling assessments, and/or the scapulae wing during the push-up test.

Continued on page 190

LOWER TRAPEZIUS

1. Joint position being tested:
    a. Adduction and depression of scapula with outward rotation (inferior angle of scapula is displaced laterally on the thorax)
2. Muscles being assessed:
    a. Lower trapezius
    b. Middle trapezius
3. Potentially overactive muscles if strength is limited:
    a. Pectoralis minor, upper trapezius, levator scapula
    b. Pectoralis major, latissimus dorsi, anterior deltoid

Positioning

Client is prone with elbow extended and shoulder complex in scapular adduction and depression. Place shoulder in approximately 145 degrees of abduction and external rotation.

Execution

- Support the client's opposite shoulder.
- Instruct client to "hold" the position.
- Apply gradual and increasing pressure to the lower arm just above the wrist in a downward direction toward the floor.
- Look for compensations of shoulder elevation.
- Grade client's strength: 3 = normal, 2 = compensates, 1 = weak.
- If graded 1 or 2, take client's arm into a midrange and retest.

Lower Trapezius Assessment, Execution

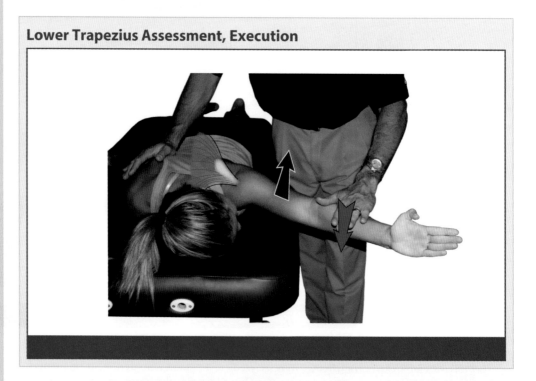

Human Movement System Impairment

This muscle may be weak in a person who demonstrates arms falling forward during the overhead squat, the shoulders elevate during pushing and pulling assessments, and or the scapulae wing during the push-up test.

SERRATUS ANTERIOR

1. Joint position being tested:
   a. Scapular upward rotation and abduction
2. Muscles being assessed:
   a. Serratus anterior
3. Potentially overactive muscles if strength is limited:
   a. Pectoralis minor
   b. Middle trapezius
   c. Rhomboids

Positioning Client is seated with shoulder flexed 120 to 130 degrees with neutral rotation and pro-tracted scapula.

Execution • Support the client on lateral aspect of scapula.
• Instruct client to "hold" the position.
• Apply gradual pressure to the upper arm and against the lateral scapular border in the direction of medial scapular rotation to assist in tracking the movement of the scapula.
• Look for compensations of shoulder elevation or trunk flexion.
• Grade client's strength: 3 = normal, 2 = compensates, 1 = weak
• If graded 1 or 2, take client's arm into a midrange and retest.

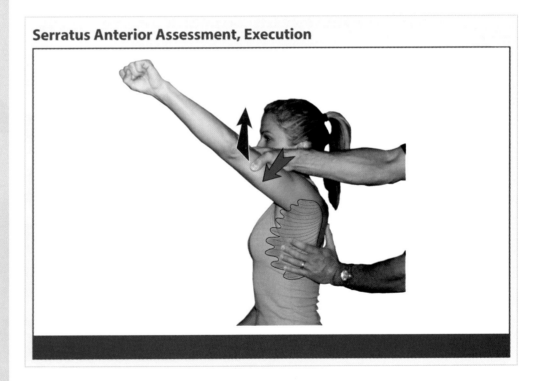

Serratus Anterior Assessment, Execution

Human Movement System Impairment This muscle may be weak in a person who demonstrates scapular winging during the push-up assessment.

Continued on page 192

➤ THE CERVICAL SPINE

ANTERIOR NECK FLEXORS

1. Joint position being tested:
   a. Cervical flexion
2. Muscles being assessed:
   a. Longus capitis
   b. Longus coli
   c. Rectus capitis
3. Potentially overactive muscles if strength is limited:
   a. Sternocleidomastoid
   b. Scalenes
   c. Upper trapezius

Positioning   Client is supine with the elbows bent, hands overhead resting on table, and the cervical spine flexed (chin tucked toward chest).

Execution

- Instruct client to "hold" the position.
- Apply gradual pressure to the forehead in the direction of cervical extension.
- Look for compensations of hyperextension of the cervical spine (forward head position).
- Grade client's strength: 3 = normal, 2 = compensates, 1 = weak.
- If graded 1 or 2, take client's head into a midrange and retest.

Anterior Neck Flexor Assessment, Execution

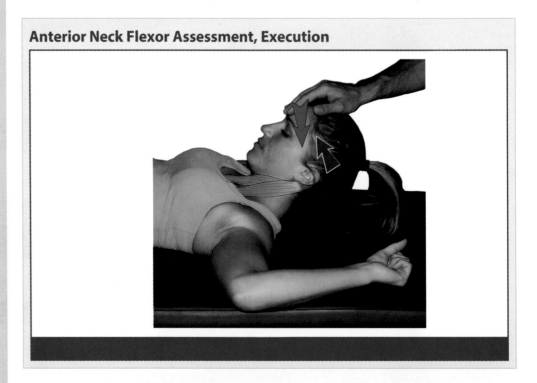

Human Movement System Impairment   These muscles may be weak in a person who demonstrates a forward head posture during pushing, pulling, and pressing movement assessments.

ANTEROLATERAL NECK FLEXORS

1. Joint position being tested:
   a. Cervical flexion and rotation
2. Muscles being assessed:
   a. Sternocleidomastoid
   b. Scalenes
3. Potentially overactive muscles if strength is limited:
   a. Upper trapezius

Positioning

Client is supine with the elbows bent, hands overhead resting on table, and the cervical spine flexed and rotated.

Execution

- Instruct client to "hold" the position.
- Apply gradual pressure to the side of the head (temporal region) in an obliquely posterior direction.
- Look for compensations of the shoulders elevating or lifting away from the table.
- Grade client's strength: 3 = normal, 2 = compensates, 1 = weak.
- If graded 1 or 2, take client's arm into a midrange and retest.

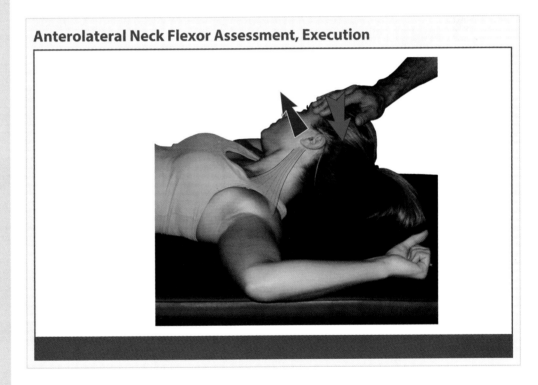

Anterolateral Neck Flexor Assessment, Execution

Human Movement System Impairment

These muscles may be weak in a person who demonstrates a forward head posture.

Continued on page 194

POSTEROLATERAL NECK EXTENSORS

1. Joint position being tested:
   a. Cervical extension and rotation
2. Muscles being assessed:
   a. Transversospinalis cervicis and capitis divisions
3. Potentially overactive muscles if strength is limited:
   a. Upper trapezius

Positioning Client is prone with the elbows bent, hands overhead resting on table, and the cervical spine extended and rotated.

Execution
- Instruct client to "hold" the position.
- Apply gradual pressure to the posterolateral aspect of the head in an anterolateral direction.
- Look for compensations of the shoulders elevating.
- Grade client's strength: 3 = normal, 2 = compensates, 1 = weak.
- If graded 1 or 2, take client's arm into a midrange and retest.

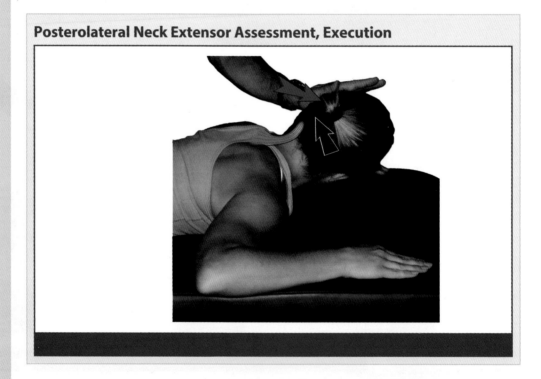

Posterolateral Neck Extensor Assessment, Execution

Human Movement System Impairment These muscles may be weak in a person who demonstrates a forward head posture or if the shoulders elevate during pushing and pulling assessments.

SUMMARY • Health and fitness professionals should be able to accurately and reliably assess muscle strength to understand human movement dysfunctions. Following the NASM guidelines for evaluating muscle strength will enable the individual to understand possible causes of weakness caused by muscle imbalances or altered length-tension relationships. It is crucial that the health and fitness professional is qualified to perform these techniques on clients. Using these techniques along with movement and range of motion assessments will enhance the health and fitness professional in determining the specific areas of focus when designing a corrective exercise program.

References

1. Clark MA, Lucett SC, Corn RJ. NASM Essentials of Personal Fitness Training. 3rd ed. Baltimore, MD: Lippincott Williams & Wilkins; 2008.
2. Sahrmann S. Diagnosis and Treatment of Movement Impairment Syndromes. St. Louis, MO: Mosby; 2002.
3. Kendall F, McCreary E, Provance P, Rodgers M, Romani. Muscles: Testing and Function With Posture and Pain. 5th ed. Philadelphia, PA: Lippincott Williams & Wilkins; 2005.
4. Liebenson C. Integrated Rehabilitation Into Chiropractic Practice (blending active and passive care). In: Liebenson C, ed. Rehabilitation of the Spine. Baltimore, MD: Williams & Wilkins; 1996:13–43.
5. Schwartz S, Cohen ME, Herbison GJ, Shah A. Relationship between two measures of upper extremity strength: manual muscle test compared to hand-held myometry. *Arch Phys Med Rehabil* 1992;73(11):1063–8.
6. Panjabi M. The stabilizing system of the spine. Part I. Function, dysfunction, adaptation, and enhancement. *J Spinal Disord* 1992;5(4):383–9.
7. Comerford M, Mottram S. Movement and stability dysfunction—contemporary developments. *Man Ther* 2001;6(1):3–14.
8. Janda V. Evaluation of Muscle Imbalances. In: Liebenson C, ed. Rehabilitation of the Spine. Baltimore, MD: Williams & Wilkins; 1996:97–112.
9. Janda V. Muscle Strength in Relation to Muscle Length, Pain, and Muscle Imbalance. In Harms-Ringdahl, ed.: International Perspectives in Physical Therapy VIII. Edinburgh: Churchill Livingstone; 1993:83–91.
10. Ireland ML, Willson JD, Ballantyne BT, Davis IM. Hip strength in females with and without patellofemoral pain. *J Orthop Sports Phys Ther* 2003;33(11):671–6.
11. Powers CM. The influence of altered lower-extremity kinematics on patellofemoral joint dysfunction: a theoretical perspective. *J Orthop Sports Phys Ther* 2003;33(11):639–46.
12. Janda V. Muscles and Motor Control in Low Back Pain: Assessment and Management. In: Twomey L, ed. Physical Therapy of the Low Back. Edinburgh: Churchill Livingstone; 1987:253–78.
13. Edgerton V, Wolf S, Levendowski D, Roy R. Theoretical basis for patterning EMG amplitudes to assess muscle dysfunction. *Med Sci Sports Exerc* 1996;28(6):744–51.
14. Fredericson M, Cookingham CL, Chaudhari AM, Dowdell BC, Oestreicher N, Sahrmann SA. Hip abductor weakness in distance runners with iliotibial band syndrome. *Clin J Sport Med* 2000;10(3):169–75.
15. Leetun D, Ireland ML, Wilson J, Ballantyne B, Davis I. Core stability measures as risk factors for lower extremity injury in athletes. *Med Sci Sports Exerc* 2004;36(6):926–34.
16. Vasilyeva L, Lewit K. Diagnosis of Muscular Dysfunction by Inspection. In: Liebenson C, ed. Rehabilitation of the Spine. Baltimore, MD: Williams & Wilkins; 1996:113–42.
17. Warmerdam A. Manual Therapy: Improve Muscle and Joint Functioning. Wantagh, NY: Pine Publications; 1998.
18. Hurley MV. The effects of joint damage on muscle function, proprioception and rehabilitation. *Man Ther* 1997;2(1):11–7.
19. Hislop H. Daniels and Worthingham's Muscle Testing: Techniques of Manual Examination. 8th ed. Philadelphia, PA: Saunders; 2007.
20. Bitter NL, Clisby EF, Jones MA, Magarey ME, Jaberzadeh S, Sandow MJ. Relative contributions of infraspinatus and deltoid during external rotation in healthy shoulders. *J Shoulder Elbow Surg* 2007;16(5):563–8.

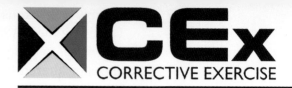

SECTION 3

THE CORRECTIVE EXERCISE CONTINUUM

CHAPTER 9

Inhibitory Techniques: Self-Myofascial Release

INTRODUCTION

THE first phase in the Corrective Exercise Continuum (Figure 9-1) is to inhibit. More specifically, the term inhibit refers to decreasing overactivity of neuromyofascial tissue. The primary technique used here is **self-myofascial release** (SMR), although many other manual techniques are also used (positional release, myopractic, soft tissue release, active release, joint mobilization, and so forth).

Self-myofascial release: a flexibility technique used to inhibit overactive muscle fibers.

SELF-MYOFASCIAL RELEASE

During the past decade the use of a self-induced neuromyofascial release techniques (i.e., foam-rolling muscles as in Figure 9-2) has emerged to become a relatively common and practical flexibility technique used within the health and fitness environment. This technique is termed self-myofascial release (SMR). Interestingly, there is little current research specific to SMR and its effects on flexibility or tissue response. This may lead many critics to question its usefulness or efficacy in a typical training environment. However, evidence supporting the rationale for using SMR for flexibility purposes is derived from research on ischemic compression and myofascial release techniques (1–8). The NASM position and rationale will be reviewed in the following sections.

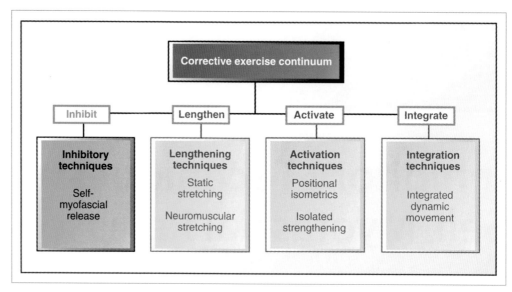

Figure 9.1 The corrective exercise continuum.

SELF-MYOFASCIAL RELEASE AND THE CUMULATIVE INJURY CYCLE

It is essential for the health and fitness professional to understand that poor posture and repetitive movements can create dysfunction within the connective tissue of the human movement system (9–16). This dysfunction is treated by the body as an injury and will initiate a repair process termed the cumulative injury cycle (Figure 9-3) (10,13). This process was introduced in chapter three, but will be reviewed in further detail in this chapter as it has a direct correlation for the use of SMR.

Any trauma to the tissue of the body creates inflammation. Inflammation in turn activates the body's pain receptors and initiates a protective mechanism, increasing muscle tension and causing muscle spasm. These muscle spasms are not like a calf cramp. Heightened activity of muscle spindles in particular areas of the muscle create, in essence, a microspasm. As a result of the spasm, adhesions ("knots" or "trigger points") will begin to form in the soft tissue. These adhesions form a weak, inelastic (unable to stretch) matrix that decreases normal elasticity of the soft tissue (9,10,13–16)

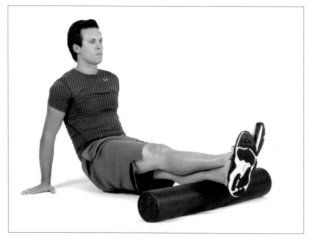

Figure 9.2 Foam rolling.

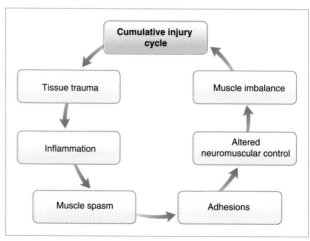

Figure 9.3 Cumulative injury cycle.

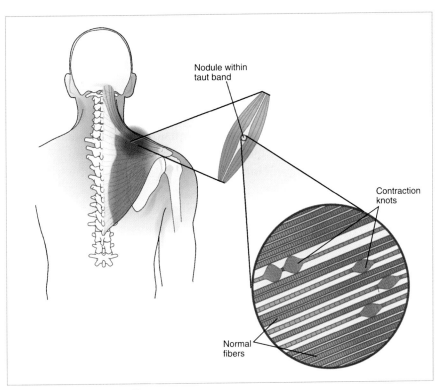

Figure 9.4 Myofascial adhesions.

(Figure 9-4). The result is altered length-tension relationships (leading to altered reciprocal inhibition), altered force-couple relationships (leading to synergistic dominance), and arthrokinetic dysfunction (leading to altered joint motion) (17–19). Left unchecked, these adhesions can begin to form permanent structural changes in the soft tissue that are evident by **Davis's law**.

Davis's law states that soft tissue will model along the lines of stress (9,10). Soft tissue remodels or rebuilds itself with an inelastic collagen matrix that forms in a random fashion. This simply means that it usually does not run in the same direction as the muscle fibers. If the muscle fibers are lengthened, these inelastic connective tissue fibers are acting as roadblocks, not allowing the muscle fibers to move properly. This creates alterations in normal tissue extensibility and causes **relative flexibility** (17). Relative flexibility is the phenomenon of the human movement system seeking the path of least resistance during functional movement patterns (or movement compensation) (17). Continued movement compensation can lead to further muscle imbalances and potential injury.

Self-myofascial techniques may help in "releasing" the microspasms that develop in traumatized tissue and "break up" the fascial adhesions that are created through the cumulative injury cycle process, thus potentially improving the tissue's ability to lengthen through stretching techniques. This will be reviewed in greater detail in the next chapter.

> **Davis's law:** states that soft tissue will model along the lines of stress.

> **Relative flexibility:** the phenomenon of the human movement system seeking the path of least resistance during functional movement patterns (or movement compensation).

SCIENTIFIC RATIONALE FOR SELF-MYOFASCIAL RELEASE

SMR can be used for two primary reasons:

1. To alleviate the side effects of active or latent trigger points
2. To influence the autonomic nervous system

Self-Myofascial Release and Trigger Points

External pressure stimulates receptors located throughout the muscle, fascia, and connective tissues of the human movement system to override the dysfunctional yet protective mechanism caused by the cumulative injury cycle. The Golgi tendon organ (GTO) (or other Golgi receptors) is one proposed receptor that responds to tension. It has been shown that static tension placed on the musculotendinous unit activates the GTO, which is suggested to produce **autogenic inhibition** (muscle inhibited by its own receptors) (20). However, others suggest that the GTO is mostly sensitive to tension via muscle contraction and not tension via muscle stretch (9,21) and that the GTO is assisted by other receptors (low-threshold joint capsule and cutaneous) to produce autogenic inhibition (22). Researchers have also identified interstitial receptors (type III and IV) and Ruffini endings (type II) located throughout the fascia that are specifically responsive to slow, deep, sustained pressure (5,6).

SMR is therefore believed to stimulate the aforementioned receptors through sustained pressure at a specific intensity, amount, and duration to produce an inhibitory response to the muscle spindle and decrease **gamma loop** activity (Figure 9-5). This concept has been supported in a randomized controlled trial study by Hou and colleagues (2), who reported that ischemic compression (pressure from an object) at a high intensity (maximal pain tolerance) for a low duration (30 seconds) or at a low intensity (minimal pain threshold) for a longer duration (90 seconds) significantly reduced pain and trigger point sensitivity. Furthermore, when applied in conjunction with stretching techniques, it was shown to significantly increase range of motion (2).

In an earlier study by Hanten and colleagues (1), it was demonstrated that ischemic compression and static stretching as a home program was significantly effective at reducing trigger point pain and sensitivity in individuals with neck and upper back pain.

The practical significance is that by holding pressure on the tender areas of tissue (trigger points) for a sustained period, trigger point activity can be diminished. This will then allow the application of a stretching (or lengthening) technique such as static stretching to increase muscle extensibility of the

> **Autogenic inhibition:** inhibition of the muscle spindle resulting from the Golgi tendon organ stimulation.

> **Gamma loop:** the reflex arc consisting of small anterior horn nerve cells and their small fibers that project to the intrafusal bundle and produce its contraction, which initiates the afferent impulses that pass through the posterior root to the anterior horn cells, inducing, in turn, reflex contraction of the entire muscle.

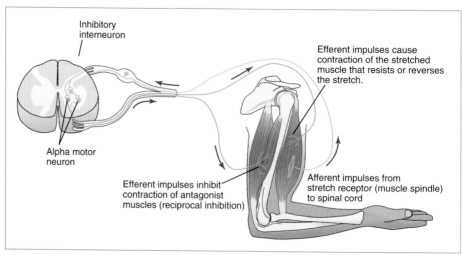

Figure 9.5 Gamma loop.

shortened muscles and provides for optimal length-tension relationships. With optimal length-tension relationships, subsequent use of corrective activation and integrated strengthening exercises will ensure an increase in intramuscular and intermuscular coordination, endurance strength, and optimal force-couple relationships that will produce proper arthrokinematics. Collectively, these processes enable the human movement system to reestablish neuromuscular efficiency. This is the NASM rationale for establishing and using corrective flexibility as a component of a complete corrective exercise programming system.

Self-Myofascial Release and Influencing the Autonomic Nervous System

It should come as no surprise that manipulating one aspect of the human movement system (nervous system, muscular system, and skeletal system) can have profound effects on the others. However, beyond the three listed systems of the human movement system there exist many support systems, which include the cardiorespiratory system and endocrine system (23). When discussing the application of pressure and tension on the muscular system, it should be expected that there can and will be a concomitant effect on not only the nervous and skeletal systems, but ultimately on all systems of the body. In fact, this is true with the application of pressure to the muscular system as seen in SMR and how it impacts many aspects of the human movement system.

Some textbooks detail the functions of the type I and type II sensory receptors, which include the muscle spindle, GTO, Pacini corpuscles, and Ruffini endings (9). However, these receptors are noted as only composing about 20% of the receptor pool (6). The remaining 80% is composed of type III and type IV receptors that are called interstitial receptors and are often thought of as merely pain receptors. Their ability to respond to mechanical pressure and tension, however, has been noted and this constitutes a mechanoreceptor function (6).

These type III and type IV receptors (interstitial receptors) in conjunction with Ruffini endings have also been shown to have autonomic functions that include changes in heart rate, blood pressure, and respiration, as well as lowering of sympathetic tone (via the anterior lobe of the hypothalamus), which reduces overall muscle tonus, vasodilation, and local fluid dynamics, which in turn changes viscosity of tissue (6,24).

Neuromechanically, these effects are significant to help decrease the overall effects of stress (emotional or physical) on the human movement system:

- Increasing vasodilation, the tissue can receive adequate amounts of oxygen and nutrients as well as removal of waste byproducts (via blood) to facilitate tissue recovery and repair. Healthy tissue may be less predisposed to alter muscle recruitment patterns that may cause injuries (25).
- Changing the viscosity of the tissue allows for better tissue dynamics, which may provide better overall muscle contraction and joint motion (4,6).
- Decreasing sympathetic tone reduces the prolonged faulty contraction of muscle tissue that can lead to the cumulative injury cycle (6,13).

- Affecting respiration can lead to better oxygen content in blood as well as decrease feelings of anxiety and fatigue (26). It has been noted that faulty breathing patterns (shallow chest breathing versus proper diaphragmatic breathing) can alter carbon dioxide and oxygen content of blood, which perpetuates dysfunctional breathing and leads to synergistic dominance of secondary breathing muscles (26).

The importance of the effect neuromyofascial release or pressure and tension has on the autonomic nervous system is that it influences (6):

1. The fluid properties of tissue that affects the viscosity (resistance to flow or motion).
2. The hypothalamus, which increases vagal tone and decreases global muscle tonus.
3. Smooth muscle cells in fascia that may be related to regulation of fascial pretension.

THE EFFECTS OF TISSUE PRESSURE

Figure 9-6 demonstrates the integrated process involved in tissue changes. Sustained or slow tissue pressure stimulates mechanoreceptors that send information to the central and autonomic nervous systems. In turn, the central nervous system response changes the muscle tonus (or decreases hypertonicity) in skeletal muscle. The autonomic nervous system response also changes global muscle tonus as well as fluid dynamics to decrease viscosity and the tonus of the smooth muscle cells located in fascia.

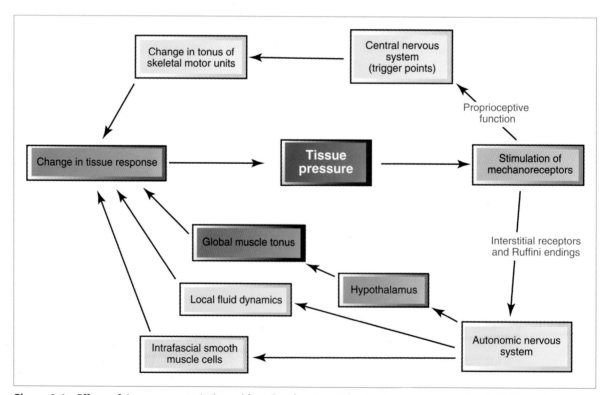

Figure 9.6   Effects of tissue pressure. (Adapted from Bandy WD, Sanders B. Therapeutic exercise: Techniques for intervention. Philadelphia, PA: Lippincott Williams & Wilkins; 2001.)

(Text continues on page 209)

APPLICATION GUIDELINES FOR SELF-MYOFASCIAL RELEASE

➤ SELF-MYOFASCIAL RELEASE TOOLS

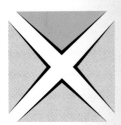

There are a variety of tools to use in the application of SMR. Tools will have varying effects depending on their size and construction. Those made of softer, less rigid materials will have an effect on more superficial layers of the fascia, whereas tools that are harder and more rigid will increase pressure on soft tissue structures and access deeper layers of the fascia (27).

ROLLERS (CYLINDRICAL)

Rollers are constructed from a variety of different materials and come in different lengths and diameters. One should begin using a softer foam roller, which offers less penetration into the soft tissue because of its increased compressibility. For individuals who have never performed SMR, a foam roller will more than likely be all they can initially handle and should be the modality of choice to start. Over time, one can progress to using a stiffer roller that compresses and deforms less and works deeper into the soft tissue. A larger diameter roller will not penetrate as deeply into the soft tissue as a smaller diameter roller. Begin with a large diameter roller and progress to one with a smaller diameter. A six-inch diameter roller is a good size to begin with.

Softer rollers, must be used on a firm surface such as the floor. More rigid rollers made of three-inch diameter PVC (polyvinyl chloride) with a ¼-inch wall or rollers constructed from steel pipe inherently resist bending and compression. Foam rollers are considered less expensive and the method of use is easy to learn. However, it is more difficult to control the depth of penetration into the soft tissue with a roller in comparison with other SMR tools.

SMR with Foam Roller

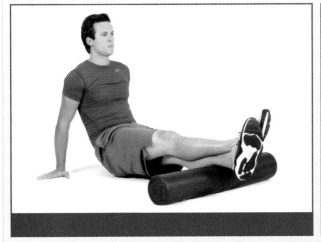

SMR with PVC pipe

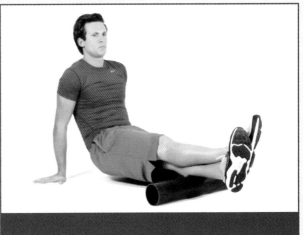

BALLS

Like rollers, balls used for SMR are constructed from a variety of different materials and come in different diameters. Progression should be made by beginning with a large diameter ball (e.g., medicine ball) to a smaller diameter, firmer ball (e.g., tennis ball, softball, baseball, golf ball). Balls are considered less expensive, and the method of use is easy to learn and can be a progression from the foam roller. However, like rollers, it is more difficult to control depth of penetration into the soft tissue with a ball than with other SMR tools.

Continued on page 204

SMR with Medicine ball

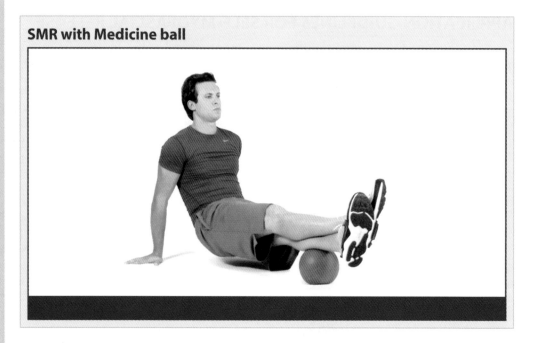

HANDHELD ROLLERS

There are a variety of handheld rollers on the market. Some are stiff and resist bending whereas others are more flexible and bend considerably while being used. The user controls the amount of force that the handheld roller puts on the soft tissue. The greater the force applied, the deeper the penetration. Flexible handheld rollers offer more surface area contact, but will require more force to penetrate as deeply as a stiff roller. These modalities are also good alternatives for individuals who may have a hard time getting up and down from the floor, such as with some seniors or individuals who may be overweight. Handheld rollers are considered less expensive, and the method of use is easy to learn. It is easier to control depth of penetration into the soft tissue with a handheld roller in comparison with traditional foam rollers or balls.

SMR with Handheld Roller

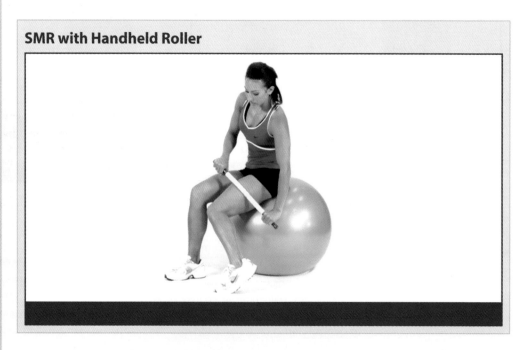

INSTRUMENT-ASSISTED SOFT TISSUE MOBILIZATION

A variety of handheld instruments can be used to release soft tissue. These instruments come in different shapes and sizes and are constructed from different materials, including plastic, ceramic, and stainless steel. Many of these instruments are especially useful to address hard to reach areas, such as the lumbar spine, as well as areas where other SMR modalities may not be suitable, such as the neck region. They are also designed to provide the user with a better mechanical advantage to apply pressure comfortably. The user controls the amount of force that the handheld instrument puts on the soft tissue. The instrument is typically held on the localized region that needs to be addressed until discomfort subsides. Increased pressure on the instrument will penetrate deep into the soft tissue whereas light pressure will affect more superficial structures. The area treated can be very precise depending on the size and shape of the instrument.

SMR to Low Back with Instrument Assisted Device

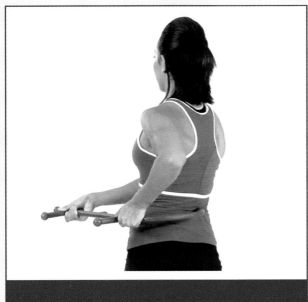

SMR to Neck Region with Instrument Assisted Device

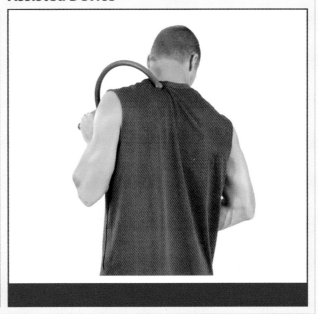

VIBRATION OR PERCUSSION DEVICES

Some handheld percussive massagers are strong enough to create a vibration in the soft tissue that travels from the treatment site into the surrounding area and are used to mobilize tissue. Vibration or percussive devices are considered more expensive, but the method of use is easy to learn. Although these devices can be self-applied, they typically require a second individual to apply the massager to the desired regions while the client is lying down relaxed to ensure optimal results.

Continued on page 206

SMR with Vibration Device

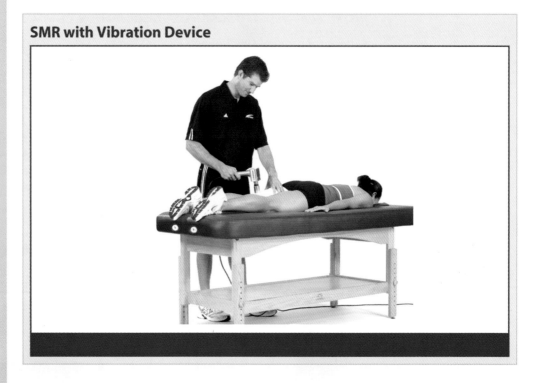

➤ KEY APPLICATION POINTS FOR SELF-MYOFASCIAL RELEASE

1. Make sure the client maintains proper postural alignment while performing SMR.

2. Instruct the client to maintain the drawing-in maneuver (pulling the navel in toward the spine) at all times to provide stability to the lumbo-pelvic-hip complex during treatment.

3. The client may use his or her extremities to alter the amount of weight on the treatment area to decrease or increase pressure on the soft tissue. For example, when foam rolling the calves, the client may cross the free leg over the treated leg to increase pressure or keep the legs uncrossed to decrease pressure.

4. The client should roll the device slowly over the treatment area. He or she should not roll the device over the area quickly to decrease the risk of further tissue excitation. Remember, the goal is to inhibit the overactive tissue.

5. Instruct the client to relax and not tighten up while working on an area. Tension in the tissue being treated will prevent the roller from penetrating into the deeper layers of soft tissue.

6. Instruct the client to pause the rolling action over painful areas until a "release" is felt in the area or the pain subsides and the tissue softens (roughly 30 seconds with maximal pain tolerance and 90 seconds for lower pain tolerance) (2).

7. Areas that have myofascial restrictions will be more painful to mobilize. As soft tissue restrictions break down with subsequent sessions, treatment will become less painful.

➤ PRECAUTIONS AND CONTRAINDICATIONS

Anyone using SMR techniques should follow the same precautionary measures as those established for massage or myofascial release. As is the case with any form of exercise, an appropriately licensed medical professional should be consulted for further information and direction. SMR should be cautioned or avoided by people with congestive heart failure, kidney failure or any organ failure such as the liver and pancreas, bleeding disorders, and contagious skin conditions (28). If a client has cancer, you should consult with the physician before using SMR because under certain circumstances such treatments should not be applied. For example, sometimes massage, pressure, or tension can damage tissue that is fragile from chemotherapy or radiation treatments (28). Other contraindications for SMR are shown in the table below (4,29).

CONTRAINDICATIONS FOR SELF-MYOFASCIAL RELEASE	
Malignancy	Goiter (enlarged thyroid)
Osteoporosis	Eczema and other skin lesions
Osteomyelitis (infection of bone tissue)	Hypersensitive skin conditions
Phlebitis (infection of superficial veins)	Open wounds
Cellulitis (infection of soft tissue)	Healing fractures
Acute rheumatoid arthritis	Obstructive edema
Blood clot	Advanced diabetes
Aneurysm	Hematoma or systemic or localized infection
Anticoagulant therapy	Febrile state
Bursitis	Advanced degenerative changes
Sutures	Organ failure
Congestive heart failure	
Bleeding disorders	

➤ ACUTE VARIABLES

To be effective, SMR must follow sound acute variables (see the accompanying table). At the current time, there are no known reasons that SMR cannot be performed on a daily basis. This is the current practice of NASM with apparently healthy individuals. However, this will ultimately be determined by the client, any possible precautions that exist, and the advice of a licensed medical professional. One set per noted body region or muscle group is sufficient. As mentioned earlier, one should hold the foam roller (or other SMR modality) on the tender area for roughly 30 seconds at high intensity (maximal pain tolerance) and 90 seconds for lower intensity (minimal pain tolerance) before moving to the next region (2).

ACUTE VARIABLES FOR SELF-MYOFASCIAL RELEASE			
Frequency	**Sets**	**Repetitions**	**Duration**
Daily (unless specified otherwise)	1	n/a	Hold tender spots for 30 to 90 seconds depending on intensity of application

n/a = not applicable.

Continued on page 208

Example Self-Myofascial Release Exercises

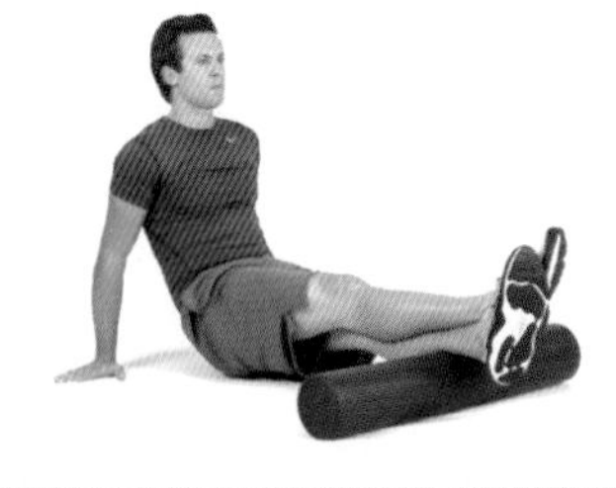

Calves

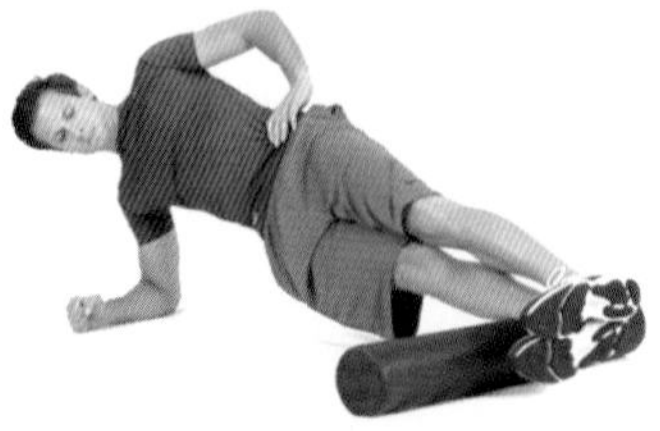

Peroneals

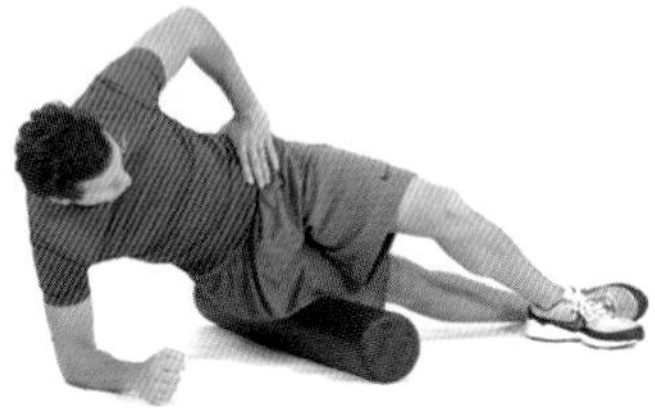

IT-band

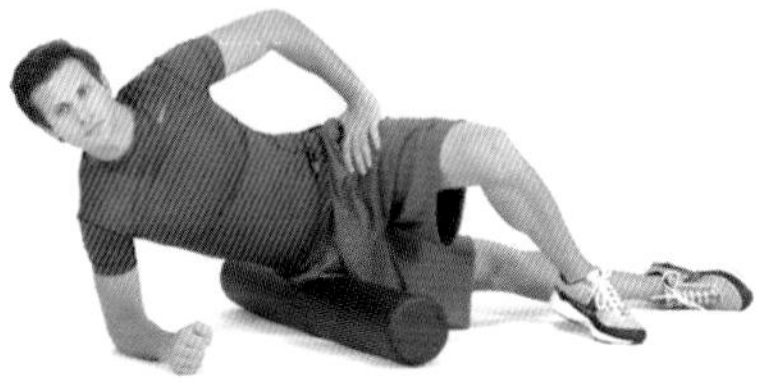

TFL

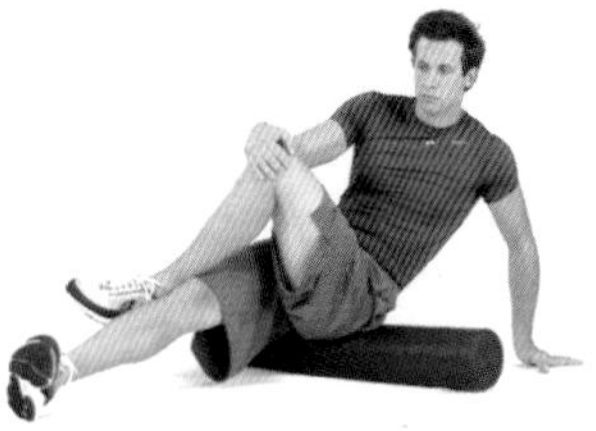

Piriformis

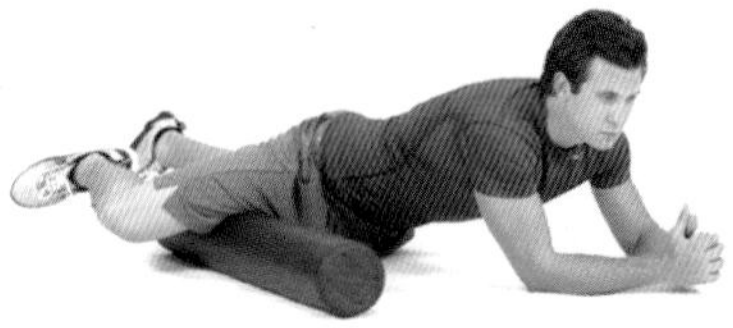

Adductors

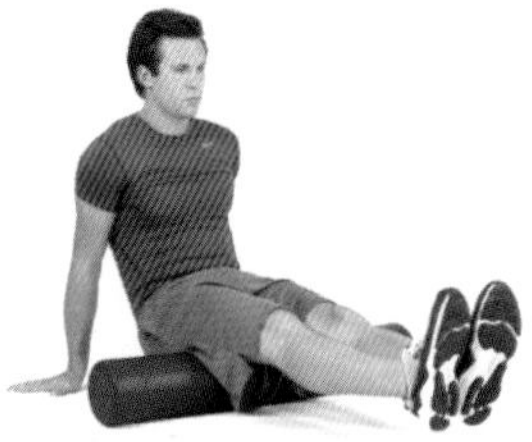

Hamstrings

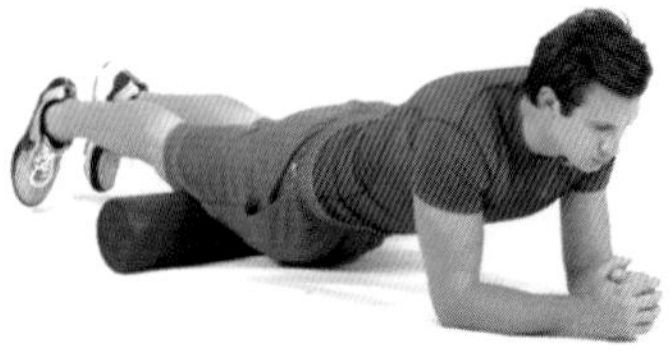

Quadriceps

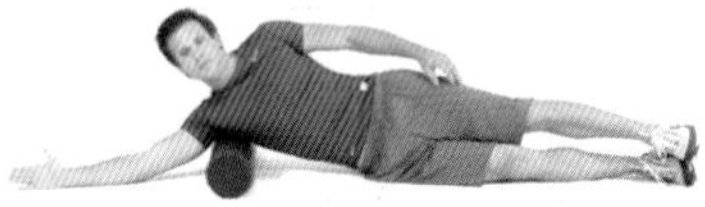

Latissimus dorsi

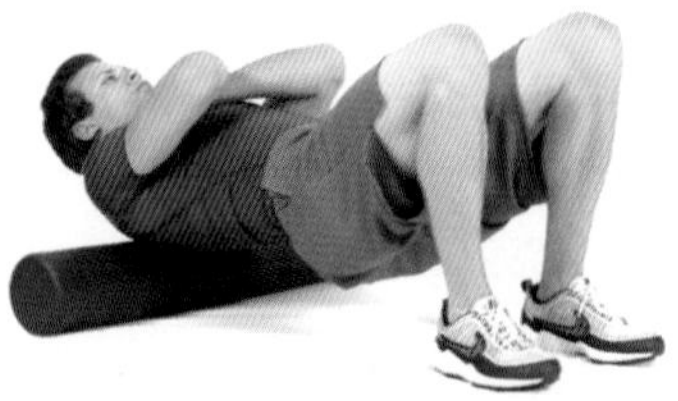

Thoracic spine

SUMMARY • Self-myofascial release is the primary inhibitory technique used in the first phase of the Corrective Exercise Continuum. SMR is used to release tension or decrease activity of overactive neuromyofascial tissues in the body. There are a variety of SMR tools to choose from depending on the intended soft tissue structures to be mobilized. SMR tools will have varying effects depending on their size, shape, and construction. More rigid SMR tools can influence the level of pressure exerted on the soft tissue and allow the patient to access deeper layers of the fascia. Additional considerations when choosing an SMR tool are expense, ease of use, and ability to control depth of penetration into soft tissue. Clients will achieve the desired effect of soft tissue mobilization, reestablish neuromuscular efficiency in the body, and avoid injury after they have been properly instructed in and follow the correct application of SMR.

References

1. Hanten WP, Olson SL, Butts NL, Nowicki AL. Effectiveness of a home program of ischemic pressure followed by sustained stretch for treatment of myofascial trigger points. *Phys Ther* 2000;80:997–1003.

2. Hou C-R, Tsai L-C, Cheng K-F, Chung K-C, Hong C-Z. Immediate effects of various therapeutic modalities on cervical myofascial pain and trigger-point sensitivity. *Arch Phys Med Rehabil* 2002;83:1406–14.

3. Simons DG, Travell JG, Simons LS. Myofascial Pain and Dysfunction: The Trigger Point Manual, The Upper Extremities. 2nd ed. Baltimore, MD: Williams & Wilkins; 1999.

4. Barnes JF. Myofascial Release. In: Hammer WI, ed. Functional Soft Tissue Examination and Treatment by Manual Methods. 2nd ed. Gaithersburg, MD: Aspen Publishers; 1999.533-547

5. Schleip R. Facial plasticity—a new neurobiological explanation: Part 1. *J Bodyw Mov Ther* 2003;7(1):11–9.

6. Schleip R. Facial plasticity—a new neurobiological explanation: Part 2. *J Bodyw Mov Ther* 2003;7(2):104–16.

7. Arroyo-Morales M, Olea N, Martinez M, Moreno-Lorenzo C, Díaz-Rodríguez L, Hidalgo-Lozano A. Effects of myofascial release after high-intensity exercise: a randomized clinical trial. *J Manipulative Physiol Ther* 2008;31(3):217–23.

8. Aguilera FJ, Martín DP, Masanet RA, Botella AC, Soler LB, Morell FB. Immediate effect of ultrasound and ischemic compression techniques for the treatment of trapezius latent myofascial trigger points in healthy subjects: a randomized controlled study. *J Manipulative Physiol Ther* 2009;32(7):515–20.

9. Alter MJ. Science of Flexibility. 2nd ed. Champaign, IL: Human Kinetics; 1996.

10. Chaitow L. Muscle Energy Techniques. New York, NY: Churchill Livingstone; 1997.

11. Grant R. Physical Therapy of the Cervical and Thoracic Spine. Edinburgh: Churchill Livingstone; 1988.

12. Lewitt K. Manipulation in Rehabilitation of the Locomotor System. London: Butterworths; 1993.

13. Leahy PM. Active Release Techniques: Logical Soft Tissue Treatment. In: Hammer WI, ed. Functional Soft Tissue Examination and Treatment by Manual Methods. Gaithersburg, MD: Aspen Publishers; 1999.549-560

14. Menéndez CC, Amick BC 3rd, Jenkins M, et al. Upper extremity pain and computer use among engineering graduate students: a replication study. *Am J Ind Med* 2009;52(2):113–23.

15. Smith J. Moving beyond the neutral spine: stabilizing the dancer with lumbar extension dysfunction. *J Dance Med Sci* 2009;13(3):73–82.

16. Beach TA, Parkinson RJ, Stothart JP, Callaghan JP. Effects of prolonged sitting on the passive flexion stiffness of the in vivo lumbar spine. *Spine* 2005;5(2):145–54.

17. Gossman MR, Sahrman SA, Rose SJ. Review of length-associated changes in muscle: experimental evidence and clinical implications. *Phys Ther* 1982;62:1799–808.

18. Janda V. Muscle spasm—a proposed procedure for differential diagnosis. *Man Med* 1991;6(4):136–9.

19. Clark MA, Lucett SL, Corn RJ. *NASM Essentials of Personal Fitness Training*. 3rd Edition. Baltimore, MD: Lippincott, Williams and Wilkins: 2008.

20. Bandy WD, Sanders B. Therapeutic Exercise: Techniques for Intervention. Philadelphia, PA: Lippincott Williams & Wilkins; 2001.

21. Jami L. Golgi tendon organs in mammalian skeletal muscle: functional properties and central actions. *Physiol Rev* 1992;73(3):623–66.

22. Moore JC. The Golgi tendon organ: a review and update. *Am J Occup Ther* 1984;38(4):227–36.

23. Sahrmann S. Diagnosis and Treatment of Movement Impairment Syndromes. St. Louis, MO: Mosby; 2002.

24. Delaney JP, Leong KS, Watkins A, Brodie D. The short-term effects of myofascial trigger point massage therapy on cardiac autonomic tone in healthy subjects. *J Adv Nurs* 2002;37(4):364–71.

25. Edgerton VR, Wolf SL, Levendowski DJ, Roy RR. Theoretical basis for patterning EMG amplitudes to assess muscle dysfunction. *Med Sci Sports Exerc* 1996;28(6):744–51.

26. Timmons B. Behavioral and Psychological Approaches to Breathing Disorders. New York, NY: Plenum Press; 1994.

27. Curran PF, Fiore RD, Crisco JJ. A comparison of the pressure exerted on soft tissue by 2 myofascial rollers. *J Sport Rehabil* 2008;17:432–42.

28. Ramsey SM. Holistic manual therapy techniques. *Primary Care* 1997;24(4):759–86.

29. Harris RE, Clauw DJ. The use of complementary medical therapies in the management of myofascial pain disorders. *Curr Pain Headache Rep* 2002;6(5):370–4.

CHAPTER 10

Lengthening Techniques

OBJECTIVES *Upon completion of this chapter, you will be able to:*

➤ Understand the various methods for stretching and lengthening muscular and connective tissue.

➤ Describe the scientific rationale supporting the use of lengthening techniques in a comprehensive corrective exercise program.

➤ Properly apply lengthening techniques to improve range of motion and inhibit overactive, tight structures as part of a comprehensive corrective exercise program.

INTRODUCTION

As reviewed in the previous chapter, inhibitory techniques are used in the first phase of the Corrective Exercise Continuum to decrease overactivity of neuromyofascial tissue and thus prepare the tissue for other corrective exercise techniques. The second phase in the Corrective Exercise Continuum is to now lengthen those overactive or tight neuromyofascial tissues (Figure 10-1). Lengthening refers to the elongation of mechanically shortened muscle and connective tissue necessary to increase range of motion (ROM) at the tissue and joint. There are several stretching methods available to accomplish this; however, for the purpose of this text we will focus on two of the most common methods of stretching: static stretching and neuromuscular stretching (Table 10-1). Although the goal of each form of stretching is the same (improving available ROM at a joint, increasing tissue extensibility, and enhancing neuromuscular efficiency), each method can be used separately or integrated with other techniques to achieve program goals.

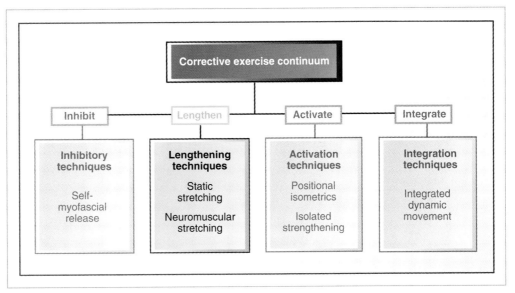

Figure 10.1   Corrective exercise continuum.

Table 10.1 DESCRIPTION OF STRETCHING TECHNIQUES	
Technique	**Description**
Static Stretching	Static stretching combines low force with long duration using autogenic inhibition. This form of stretching allows for relaxation and concomitant elongation of muscle. To properly perform static stretching, the stretch is held at the first point of tension or resistance barrier for 30 seconds. It is theorized that this form of flexibility decreases muscle spindle activity and motor neuron excitability.
Neuromuscular Stretching	Neuromuscular stretching (commonly called proprioceptive neuromuscular facilitation, or PNF) involves taking the muscle to its end ROM (point of joint compensation), actively contracting the muscle to be stretched for 7–15 seconds, then passively moving the joint to a new end ROM and holding this position for 20–30 seconds. This can be repeated several times to achieve a change in joint ROM. Typically neuromuscular stretching involves the aid of a partner to provide a resistance to the active muscle contraction, and passively stretch the joint into the new ROM.

TYPES OF LENGTHENING TECHNIQUES

Static Stretching

Arguably, during the last half century static stretching has been the most common flexibility training technique used by health and fitness professionals (1,2). Static stretching is a flexibility technique used to increase the extensibility of muscle and connective tissue (lengthening) and thus ROM at a joint (1,2). Although the exact mechanisms responsible for the efficacy of static stretching are not fully understood, it is believed that static stretching may produce both mechanical and neural adaptations that result in increased ROM (1,3–5).

Mechanically, static stretching appears to affect the viscoelastic component of neuromyofascial tissue (6,7). More specifically, there is a probable decrease in the passive resistance a muscle has to a stretch force throughout most of the ROM and not the rate at which the muscle-tendon unit increases its stiffness (8–10).

In other words, although a muscle may not be as resistant to being stretched (allowing for better extensibility), it still maintains the rate of increase in stiffness in response to stimuli (the ability to respond to a stretch force).

Neurologically, static stretching of neuromyofascial tissue to the end ROM appears to decrease motor neuron excitability, possibly through the inhibitory effects from the Golgi tendon organs (autogenic inhibition) as well as possible contributions from the Renshaw recurrent loop (**recurrent inhibition**) (6). Recurrent inhibition is a feedback circuit that can decrease the excitability of motor neurons via the interneuron called the Renshaw cell (11) (Figure 10-2). Collectively, these may decrease the responsiveness of the **stretch reflex** (Figure 10-3) and increase the tolerance a person has to stretch and thus allow for increased ROM.

> Recurrent inhibition: a feedback circuit that can decrease the excitability of motor neurons via the interneuron called the Renshaw cell.

> Stretch reflex: a muscle contraction in response to stretching within the muscle.

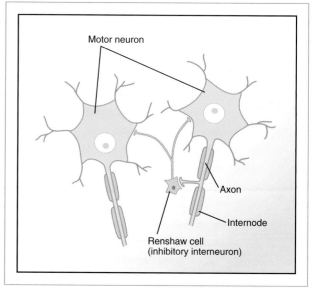

Figure 10.2   Renshaw cells and recurrent inhibition.

In general, it is thought that static stretching of 20 to 30 seconds causes an acute viscoelastic stress relaxation response, allowing for an immediate increase in ROM. Long-term, the increases in maximal joint ROM may be caused by increased tolerance to stretch and not necessarily changes in the viscoelastic properties of myofascial tissue (5,12) or a possible increase in muscle mass and added sarcomeres in series (4).

In practice, static stretching is characterized by (1,2):

* The elongation of neuromyofascial tissue to an end-range and statically holding that position for a period of time
* Maximal control of structural alignment
* Minimal acceleration into and out of the elongated (stretch) position

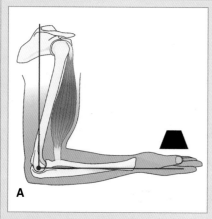

Figure 10.3A   Stretch reflex.

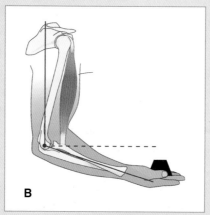

Figure 10.3B   Stretch reflex.

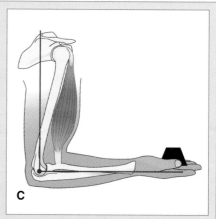

Figure 10.3C   Stretch reflex.

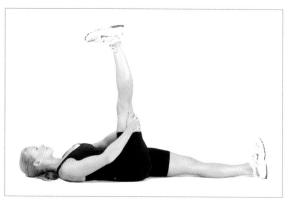

Figure 10.4   Static stretching.

The ability of individuals to perform static stretching on their own and the slow-minimal to no motion required has led this form of flexibility training to be associated with the lowest risk for injury during the stretching routine and deemed it to be the safest to use (13). In addition, static stretching is typically performed solo (without the aid of another person), so it can be easily incorporated into any integrated exercise program (Figure 10-4).

Neuromuscular Stretching

Neuromuscular stretching (NMS) has received greater attention during the past 20 years as a method for lengthening neuromyofascial tissues. Many clinicians and researchers believe that this form of stretching combines the benefits of both static and active stretching while keeping the risk of tissue injury low (14–16). Most of the current research has demonstrated that NMS stretching is equally effective at increasing ROM when compared with static stretching (14,15,17), and some studies have shown NMS to be more effective and impact muscular power less than static stretching (18,19). NMS is usually characterized by:

1. Taking the muscle to its end ROM (point of joint compensation)
2. Active contraction of the muscle to be stretched
3. Passively (or actively) moving to a new end ROM
4. Statically holding new position for 20–30 seconds and repeating 3 times

NMS is a technique that involves a process of isometrically contracting a desired muscle in a lengthened position to induce a relaxation response on the tissue, allowing it to further elongate (1,15). It is believed that the isometric contraction used during NMS decreases motor neuron excitability as a result of stimulation to the Golgi tendon organ and that this leads to autogenic inhibition, resulting in decreased resistance to a change in length (or ability to increase length of tissue) (15). After the isometric contraction, there is a "latency period" characterized by a substantial decrease in motor neuron excitability that is said to last up to 15-seconds (20). The premise behind NMS is very similar to static stretching; however, NMS usually requires the assistance of another person, thus it is traditionally used under the supervision of a health and fitness professional (Figure 10-5).

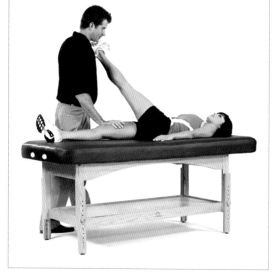

Figure 10.5   Neuromuscular stretching.

SCIENTIFIC RATIONALE FOR STRETCHING

Traditional Theory Behind Stretching

Stretching has been the subject of debate for several decades, leading researchers to continue to study the effects, duration, and methodologies behind stretching. To date, this subject might be one of the most widely diverse and profusely studied topics related to human performance. The traditional thought is that regular stretching improves flexibility, which results in a decreased risk of injury and improved performance (21–23). Consequently, regular stretching is a recommended component of exercise programs, such as during a warm-up or cool-down. The proposed mechanism for the use of stretching as it relates to muscle injury risks is illustrated in Figure 10-6. The compliance (or flexibility) of the musculotendinous unit affects the relative amount of energy absorbed by the muscle and tendon (24):

- High compliance (↑ flexibility) = ↓ Muscle energy absorption
- Low compliance (↓ flexibility) = ↑ Muscle energy absorption
- ↑ Muscle energy absorption = ↑ force and trauma to muscle fibers

Thus, increasing musculotendinous flexibility through stretching will lead to a decrease in muscle energy absorption and trauma to muscle fibers with a decrease in injury risk being the potential result.

The proposed mechanism for the use of stretching as it relates to performance is illustrated in Figure 10-7. The stiffness of the musculotendinous unit influences the work required to move the limb:

- High stiffness (↓ flexibility) → ↑ Work required
- Low stiffness (↑ flexibility) → ↓ Work required
- ↓ Flexibility limits joint range of motion = decreased performance

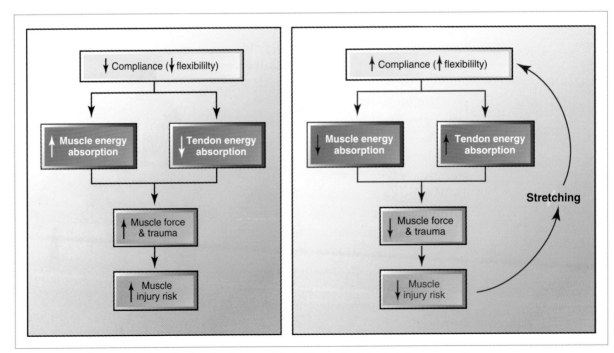

Figure 10.6   The proposed mechanism for the use of stretching as it relates to injury prevention.

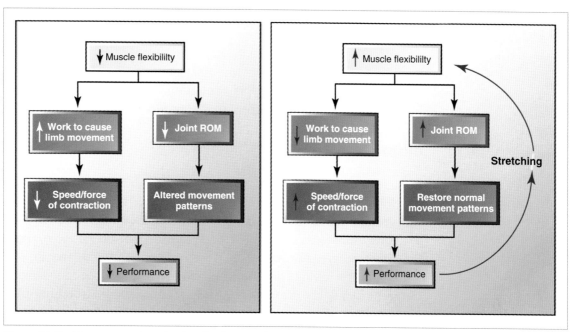

Figure 10.7   The proposed mechanism for the use of stretching as it relates to performance.

Thus, decreasing muscle stiffness through stretching will decrease the work required to perform a particular activity and potentially increase overall performance.

Conversely, recent research has also indicated that prestretching negatively impacts force production (performance) and may not influence injury risk; however, the physiologic basis for this is not well understood. The proposed mechanism for how stretching can negatively affect force production is illustrated in Figure 10-8. The general theory is that stretching can affect the structural and neurologic components of muscle, which can lead to an inability of the muscle to effectively generate force.

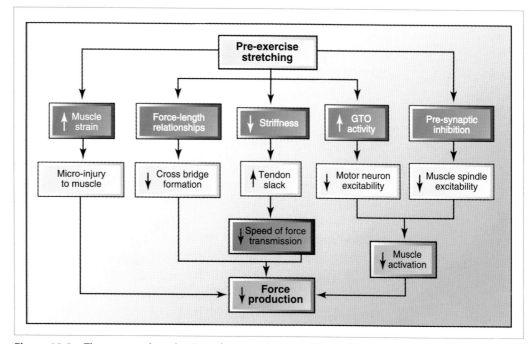

Figure 10.8   The proposed mechanism of preexercise stretching and force production.

Conflict between traditional theory and recent research on preexercise stretching has created confusion between professionals and the industry, with the common question being asked "should stretching be performed to improve performance and decrease the risk of injury?" The following section will review what the evidence has shown on the effect of stretching on improving ROM, performance enhancement, and injury prevention.

Improving ROM

Stretching exercises are primarily used to increase the available ROM at a particular joint, specifically if the ROM at that joint is limited by tight neuromyofascial tissues. The scientific literature strongly supports the use of stretching exercises to achieve this goal (16,25–49). Several excellent literature reviews have found that stretching, both acutely and chronically, increase the ROM at the target joint (50,51). This appears to be particularly true for the hamstring complex, one of the most widely examined muscle groups in the stretching literature. Other muscle groups do not appear to respond as favorably to stretching (specifically static stretching), but the scientific evidence is not as extensive (nor as well controlled) for other joints and muscle groups in the body (43,52,53). Several researchers suggest that each joint and muscle group may respond differently to stretching protocols; thus, each tissue to be stretched should be carefully evaluated, and the stretching protocol may need to be different for each ROM limitation found. For instance, a 6-week stretching program for the hamstring complex effectively increased ROM, but the same program applied to the gastrocnemius muscle did not result in a change of ROM (25,49,53). Clinicians should carefully evaluate each tissue through appropriate assessments, and frequently reevaluate movement, to determine whether a protocol is effective at changing ROM.

Most of the debate surrounding the use of stretching protocols has involved the necessary duration and frequency of stretching to produce a change in ROM. Excellent studies by Bandy and colleagues found that static hamstring stretches need to be held for 30 seconds, and performed 5 times a week for 6 weeks, to produce significant changes in knee extension ROM (25,49). The majority of other studies have found durations of 15 to 30 seconds produce significant changes in ROM, both acutely and chronically (16,27,41). However, researchers have yet to fully investigate how weekly stretching frequency may impact chronic gains in ROM. It is still unclear whether stretching should be performed daily or can be performed as few as 3 times a week to produce significant changes (25,27,28,49). Additionally, the chronic duration of the ROM gains (how long the increased ROM persists) has yet to be fully investigated. Although some studies suggest that ROM improvements are negated after 4 weeks of no stretching (54), others have found that stretching does improve long-lasting ROM (55). Finally, the majority of this research has been performed using static stretching, so the durations, frequencies, and long-term changes that are attributable to active or NMS stretching need further study. Some initial evidence suggests that NMS or active stretching protocols can produce greater gains in ROM compared with static stretching, and that these gains may occur more quickly (33,35,43,44,56). However, other studies have found no differences in ROM gains between active, NMS, or static stretching (26,29,31,46,57,58).

Recently researchers have examined the impact of stretching on not only the tissues that are lengthened during joint movement, but also the agonists to the movement. For instance, the resting position of the pelvis may significantly impact the available ROM at the hip joint. A tight or shortened hip flexor group may create an anterior pelvic tilt, which will cause the hamstring complex to be lengthened under normal, resting positions. This may inhibit normal hip flexion ROM. Clark and colleagues examined how stretching tight ipsilateral quadriceps and hip flexor musculature would impact hip flexion ROM (59). The authors found that lengthening the quadriceps and hip flexors significantly improved hip flexion ROM, suggesting that multiple soft tissues surrounding the joint impact the available ROM. Sullivan and colleagues also found that the tilt position of the pelvis influenced ROM gains more than stretching alone, further suggesting that the overall movement of a joint is dependent on the optimal length and positioning of all tissues (60). This provides further evidence that a comprehensive evaluation through movement, ROM, and strength assessments should be performed on all clients to address the specific needs of the entire movement system.

Improving Athletic Performance

The research that has investigated changes in athletic performance caused by stretching protocols is less clear than the literature supporting changes in ROM caused by flexibility protocols. First, the term "athletic performance" may encompass changes in muscular strength, power, or performance of jumping, sprinting, or agility activities. Reviews of the best available research suggest that, acutely, stretching may have a detrimental effect on muscular strength and power (18,61–63). A number of studies have found that preexercise stretching causes a loss of one-repetition maximal strength, as well as vertical jump height and sprint speed, when compared with a no-stretching control (18,19,61,63–67). This effect generally appears to last less than 10 minutes, but some studies have found that strength may be impaired up to one hour after the stretching protocol (61,68). However, several studies have also found that preexercise stretching does not impair strength or power production acutely (69–71). The effect of stretching on acute changes in strength and power may be partially explained by the type of stretching protocol used. In general, static stretching held for at least 30 seconds does appear to decrease muscular strength and power, whereas ballistic or NMS stretching does not have the same effect (19,72,73). Thus, more research needs to examine whether alternative forms of stretching may be more appropriate before athletic activity. A second consideration may be the presence (or absence) of a ROM limitation in the muscle. Very few studies have examined how stretching a tight or shortened muscle may impact strength or power, or more overall tests of athletic ability (such as sprinting, agility, or vertical jump). It is possible that the negative changes in strength or power are seen primarily in individuals who do not have functional ROM limitations, and thus may not be candidates for stretching programs. This illustrates how important a comprehensive and evidence-based approach may be when examining the human body.

Chronic, long-term stretching protocols have produced varied effects on athletic performance. Although ROM is typically improved in the tested muscle, other variables such as muscular strength, power, vertical jump, sprint speed, agility, or balance have not found the same consistent response. Although one study found a decrease in vertical jump performance, sprint speed, or reaction time (66), most have demonstrated increases in vertical jump, muscular strength, power, and balance ability after a regular stretching program (5,74–79).

Prevention of Injury

Many coaches and athletes perform stretching as part of a routine "warm-up" before activity, prompted by the belief that stretching can prevent certain injuries. The current evidence suggests that preexercise stretching does not have a significant impact on injury risk or rates (80–82), although the effects of chronic, long-term stretching protocols tend to lead to decreased injury rates (21,80–85). Several authors and researchers have shown that regular, long-term stretching can lead to a decreased incidence of injury and decreased cost of time lost from injury, and that fewer severe muscle/tendon injuries occurred in the stretched subjects compared with control subjects (21,83,84). In these studies, injury rates were decreased by 18 to 43% (21,83,84). In all of the studies cited, there does not appear to be any negative consequences relative to injury risk when implementing a regular or preexercise stretching program.

GETTING YOUR FACTS STRAIGHT

Is a Warm-Up Necessary Before Stretching?

Most individuals believe that a muscle must be warmed up by performing a low- to moderate-intensity aerobic activity before any stretching exercise (1,2). This is supposedly to increase the temperature of the tissue, reducing the viscosity (resistance to force) and decreasing the resistance of the tissue to stretching (1). However, this belief is primarily based on animal tissue studies at unrealistic tissue temperatures (temperatures that are unlikely to exist within the human body) (1–3). More recent research suggests that ROM can be improved by the application of heat or ice (either heating or cooling the tissue), suggesting that warming up tissues is not necessary to improve ROM (4,5). Other studies have found that neither passive nor active warm-up exercises result in significant changes in the efficacy of stretching exercises (5,6). A study by Magnusson and colleagues found that a 10-minute warm-up (running at 70% VO_{2max}) did not change the viscosity of the target tissue, even though it elevated the tissue's temperature (3). Furthermore, this study found that four different static stretches did produce changes in the viscoelastic properties of the tissue. Although these stretches were held longer than is typically practiced (90 seconds), this study does suggest that stretching is more effective than short-term endurance exercise at changing the properties of the tissue, making it more compliant and less resistant to lengthening. Thus, an active warm-up may not be necessary before stretching when an improvement of ROM is the goal.

1. Alter MJ. Science of Flexibility. Champaign, IL: Human Kinetics; 2004.
2. Weijer VC, Gorniak GC, Shamus E. The effect of static stretch and warm-up exercise on hamstring length over the course of 24 hours. *J Orthop Sports Phys Ther* 2003;33(12):727–33.
3. Magnusson SP, Aagaard P, Nielson JJ. Passive energy return after repeated stretches of the hamstring muscle-tendon unit. *Med Sci Sports Exerc* 2000;32(6):1160–4.
4. Brodowicz GR, Welsh R, Wallis J. Comparison of stretching with ice, stretching heat, or stretching alone on hamstring flexibility. *J Athl Train* 1996;31:324–7.
5. Peres SE, Draper DO, Knight KL, Ricard MD. Pulsed shortwave diathermy and prolonged long-duration stretching increase dorsiflexion range of motion more than identical stretching without diathermy. *J Athl Train* 2002;37(1):43–50.
6. DeWeijer VC, Gorniak GC, Shamus E. The effect of static stretch and warm-up exercise on hamstring length over the course of 24 hours. *J Orthop Sports Phys Ther* 2003;33(12):727–33.

Summary of the Evidence

As indicated by the aforementioned review of research and literature surrounding flexibility, the following has been determined:

- There is moderate evidence to indicate that regular stretching improves ROM, strength, and performance and decreases injury risk in healthy individuals without identified limitations in flexibility.
- There is moderate evidence to indicate that acute, preexercise stretching performed in isolation decreases strength and performance and does not affect injury risk in healthy individuals without identified limitations in flexibility.

Limitations of the Research and Improving Effectiveness

In review of the literature surrounding stretching, some limitations surfaced. These limitations include:

1. Research was not performed on individuals with limited flexibility.
    a. Preexercise stretching may have positive effects on performance and injury risk in those who are inflexible.
2. Research focused primarily on stretching as the sole exercise.
    a. Flexibility is only one piece to maximizing performance and decreasing injury risk.
    b. An integrated continuum may have different results.
        i. Inhibit → Stretch → Activate → Integrate into Functional Movement
3. Address an individual's specific needs based on the assessment.
    a. Research has taken a "one size fits all" approach.
    b. Research needs to investigate the effects of preexercise stretching on inflexible muscle groups.
4. A customized corrective exercise strategy may be most effective in improving performance and decreasing the risk of injury.

GETTING YOUR FACTS STRAIGHT

Psychological Benefits of Stretching

Although most clinicians and patients focus on the physical changes produced by stretching, the psychological benefits may be just as great. Several researchers have studied the effects of stretching programs on muscle tension (measured by electromyographic [EMG] activity), self-reported emotions, feelings of muscle tension, and levels of stress-related hormones within the saliva (1–4). These studies have found that stretching reduces both physiologic (EMG) and self-reported muscle tension, results in a decreased feeling of sadness, and can decrease the levels of stress-related hormones (1–4). Anecdotally, many individuals report similar feelings of reduced tension after routine stretching, and feel that this "mentally prepares" them for physical activity. Thus, although stretching itself may not significantly impact athletic performance, the psychological benefit may be an important consideration when working with clients.

1. Carlson CR, Collins FL, Nitz AJ, Sturgis ET, Rogers JL. Muscle stretching as an alternative relaxation training procedure. *J Behav Ther Exp Psychiatry* 1990;21(1):29–38.
2. Carlson CR, Curran SL. Stretch-based relaxation training. *Patient Educ Couns* 1994;23(1):5–12.
3. Hamaguchi T, Fukudo S, Kanazawa M, et al. Changes in salivary physiological stress markers induced by muscle stretching in patients with irritable bowel syndrome. *Biopsychosoc Med* 2008;2:20.
4. Sugano A, Nomura T. Influence of water exercise and land stretching on salivary cortisol concentrations and anxiety in chronic low back pain patients. *J Physiol Anthropol Appl Human Sci* 2000;19(4):175–80.

(*Text continues on page 227*)

APPLICATION GUIDELINES FOR LENGTHENING TECHNIQUES

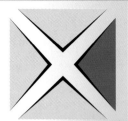

The use of stretching, like any other form of exercise, should be pursued with an understanding of any potential risks involved. Certain precautions and contraindications exist and can be seen in the table below. The precautions and contraindications listed may prevent stretching from being used only in a particular muscle or muscle group and not necessarily for all possible muscles for a client. Care should be taken at all times that pain is not felt during the stretching protocol. Mild discomfort from the stretch may be experienced, but this should be explained by the health and fitness professional to the client.

PRECAUTIONS AND CONTRAINDICATIONS FOR STRETCHING	
Precautions	**Contraindications**

Special populations
   Seniors
    Hypertensive patients
 Neuromuscular disorders
 Joint replacements
	Acute injury or muscle strain or tear of the muscle being stretched
	 Acute rheumatoid arthritis of the effected joint
	 Osteoporosis (NMS)

➤ STATIC STRETCHING ACUTE VARIABLES

Most research studies on static stretching have shown a frequency of five days per week using 1–4 repetitions for the duration of 15–30 seconds to be most beneficial for the apparently healthy population between the ages of 15 and 45 years of age (3,5,16, 25–27,36,49,52,60,85–87). Although there is a range in time, 20 to 30 seconds of stretch duration may in fact produce more reliable, and possibly quicker, results (25,26,88). In a population of clients at least 65 years of age, it has been shown that longer durations of 60 seconds may produce better and longer-lasting results (16). In a corrective exercise program, static stretching should only be applied to muscles that have been determined to be overactive or tight during the assessment.

ACUTE VARIABLES FOR STATIC STRETCHING			
Frequency (per week)	**Sets**	**Repetitions**	**Duration of Each Repetition**
Daily (unless specified otherwise)	n/a	1–4	20- to 30-seconds hold
			60-seconds hold for older patients (≥65 years)

n/a = not applicable.

Example Static Stretches

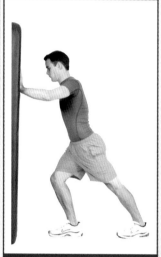

Static Gastrocnemius Stretch

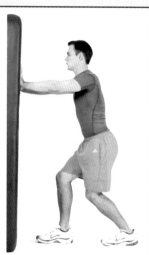

Static Soleus Stretch

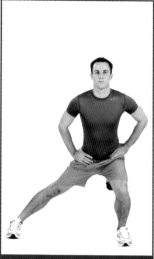

Static Standing Adductor Stretch

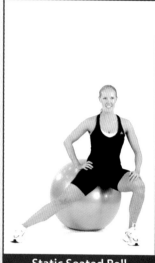

Static Seated Ball Adductor Stretch

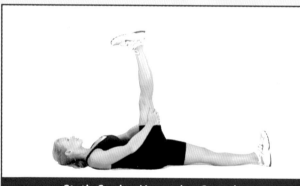

Static Supine Hamstring Stretch

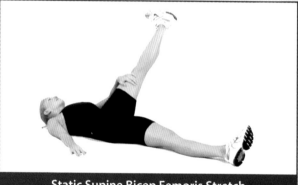

Static Supine Bicep Femoris Stretch

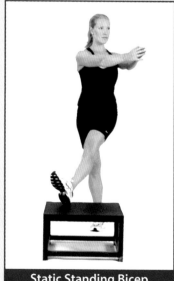

Static Standing Bicep Femoris Stretch

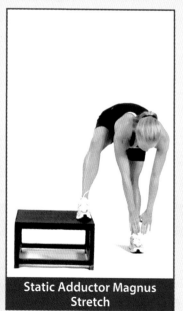

Static Adductor Magnus Stretch

Continued on page 222

Example Static Stretches

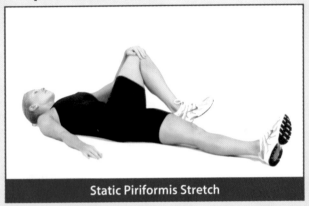
Static Piriformis Stretch

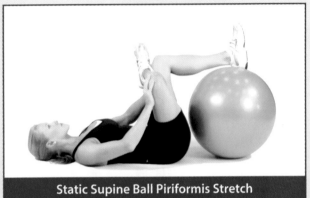
Static Supine Ball Piriformis Stretch

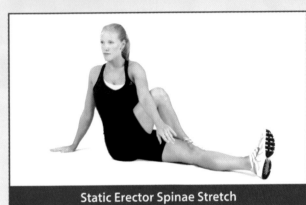
Static Erector Spinae Stretch

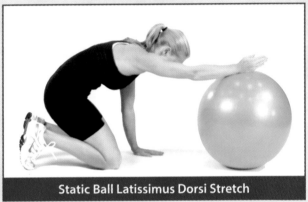
Static Ball Latissimus Dorsi Stretch

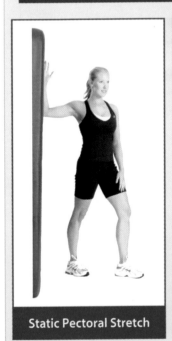
Static Pectoral Stretch

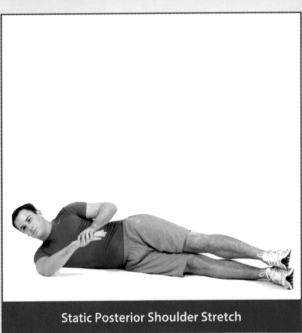
Static Posterior Shoulder Stretch

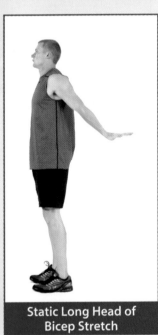
Static Long Head of Bicep Stretch

Example Static Stretches

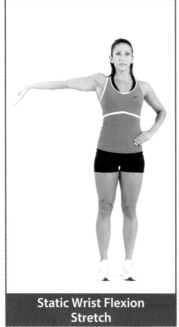

Static Wrist Flexion Stretch

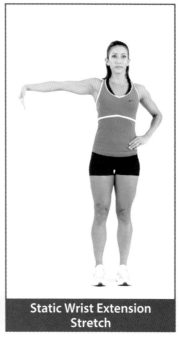

Static Wrist Extension Stretch

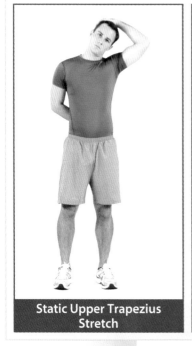

Static Upper Trapezius Stretch

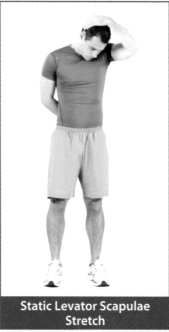

Static Levator Scapulae Stretch

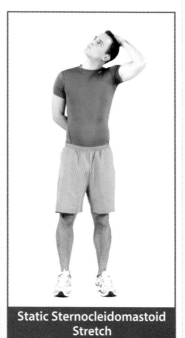

Static Sternocleidomastoid Stretch

Continued on page 224

Example Static Stretches: Static Kneeling Hip Flexor Stretch

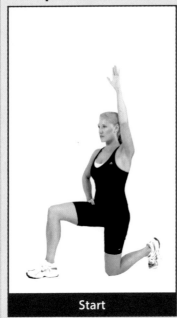

Start

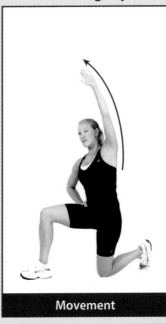

Movement

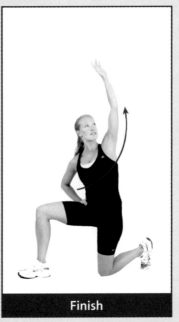

Finish

Example Static Stretches: Static Standing Hip Flexor Stretch

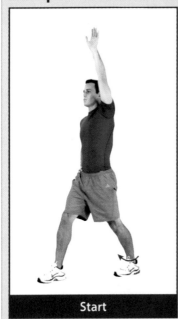

Start

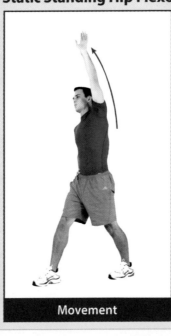

Movement

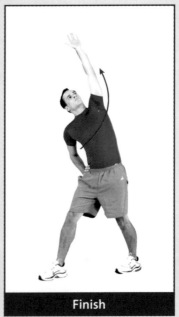

Finish

Example Static Stretches: Static TFL Stretch

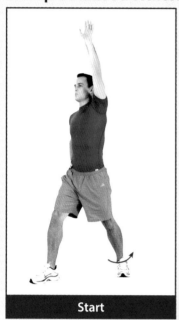
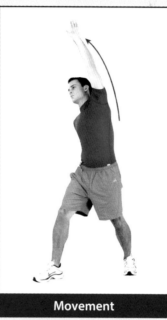
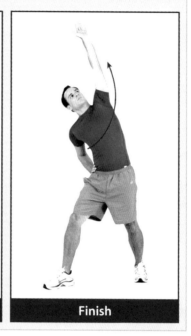

| Start | Movement | Finish |

➤ NEUROMUSCULAR STRETCHING ACUTE VARIABLES

NMS can be performed daily unless otherwise stated. Typically one to three repetitions or cycles (contract, relax) are used per stretch with a contraction time ranging from 7 to 15 seconds, with at least 10 seconds being ideal (6,14,31,42). If using some of the static stretching research, then holding the passive stretch for 20 to 30 seconds may produce the greatest results. Acutely, it appears that there is no significant difference between three-, six-, and ten-second holds (isometric contractions) (14). However for chronic gains, it appears that longer durations produce better results (42). Research has also shown that a submaximal contraction intensity of 20% was effective to produce significantly increased ROM (36). Like static stretching, NMS should only be applied to muscles that have been determined to be overactive or tight during the assessment. See the figure for examples of neuromuscular stretches.

ACUTE VARIABLES FOR NEUROMUSCULAR STRETCHING			
Frequency (per week)	**Sets**	**Repetitions**	**Duration of Each Repetition**
Daily (unless specified otherwise)	n/a	1–3	**Contraction**: 7 to 15 seconds
			Stretch: 20–30 seconds
			Intensity: submaximal, approximately 20–25% of maximal contraction

n/a = not applicable.

Continued on page 226

Example Neuromuscular Stretches

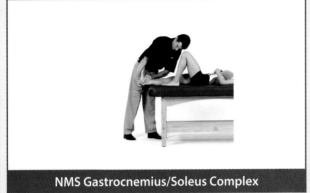

NMS Gastrocnemius/Soleus Complex

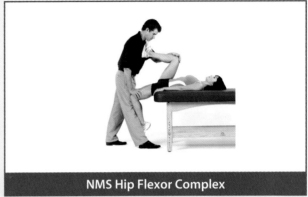

NMS Hip Flexor Complex

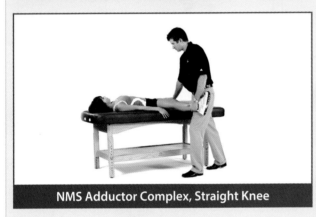

NMS Adductor Complex, Straight Knee

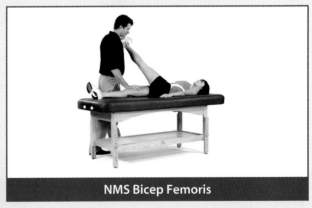

NMS Adductors Complex, Bent Knee

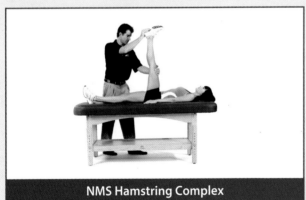

NMS Hamstring Complex

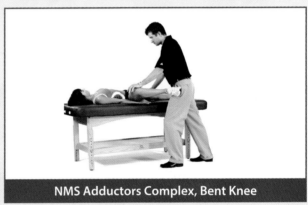

NMS Bicep Femoris

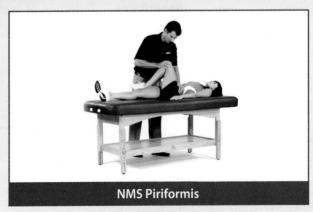

NMS Piriformis

SUMMARY • Stretching is one of the most commonly used modalities by health and fitness professionals, yet it is still widely misused and misunderstood. As with all components of the Corrective Exercise Continuum, proper application of stretching depends on the needs of the patient and the goals of the fitness program. Stretching should be used to correct faulty movement patterns (found during the functional movement assessment), specifically to lengthen shortened neuromyofascial tissues. Stretching should not be used without conducting a movement assessment first. The different types of stretching techniques (static or NMS) can each produce improvements in ROM. When integrated with inhibition, activation, and integration exercises, stretching can be used to effectively enhance the fitness and well-being of patients.

References

1. Alter MJ. Science of Flexibility. 3rd ed. Champaign, IL: Human Kinetics; 2004.
2. Nelson RT, Bandy WD. An update on flexibility. *Strength Cond J* 2005;27(1):10-6.
3. Guissard N, Duchateau J. Effect of static stretch training on neural and mechanical properties of the human plantar-flexor muscles. *Muscle Nerve* 2004;29(2):248-55.
4. Reid DA, McNair PJ. Passive force, angle, and stiffness changes after stretching of hamstring muscles. *Med Sci Sports Exerc* 2004;36(11):1944-8.
5. Shrier I. Does stretching improve performance? A systematic and critical review of the literature. *Clin J Sport Med* 2004;14(5):267-73.
6. Guissard N, Duchateau J, Hainaut K. Mechanisms of decreased motoneurone excitation during passive muscle stretching. *Exp Brain Res* 2001;137(2):163-9.
7. Magnusson SP, Simonsen EB, Aagaard P, Kjaer M. Biomechanical responses to repeated stretches in human hamstring muscle in vivo. *Am J Sports Med* 1996;24(5):622-8.
8. Cornwell A, Nelson AG, Sidaway B. Acute effects of stretching on the neuromechanical properties of the triceps surae muscle complex. *Eur J Appl Physiol* 2002;86(5):428-34.
9. Kubo K, Kanehisa H, Fukunaga T. Is passive stiffness in human muscles related to the elasticity of tendon structures? *Eur J Appl Physiol* 2001;85(3-4):226-32.
10. Kubo K, Kanehisa H, Fukunaga T. Effect of stretching training on the viscoelastic properties of human tendon structures in vivo. *J Appl Physiol* 2002;92(2):595-601.
11. Enoka RM. Neuromechanics of Human Movement. 3rd ed. Champaign, IL: Human Kinetics; 2002.
12. Magnusson SP, Aagaard P, Nielson JJ. Passive energy return after repeated stretches of the hamstring muscle-tendon unit. *Med Sci Sports Exerc* 2000;32(6):1160-4.
13. Smith CA. The warm-up procedure: to stretch or not to stretch. A brief review. *J Orthop Sports Phys Ther* 1994;19(1):12-7.
14. Bonnar BP, Deivert RG, Gould TE. The relationship between isometric contraction durations during hold-relax stretching and improvement of hamstring flexibility. *J Sports Med Phys Fitness* 2004;44(3):258-61.
15. Burke DG, Culligan CJ, Holt LE. The theoretical basis of proprioceptive neuromuscular facilitation. *J Strength Cond Res* 2000;14(4):496-500.
16. Feland JB, Myrer JW, Schulthies SS, Fellingham GW, Measom GW. The effect of duration of stretching of the hamstring muscle group for increasing range of motion in people aged 65 years or older. *Phys Ther* 2001;81(5):1110-7.
17. Higgs F, Winter SL. The effect of a four-week proprioceptive neuromuscular facilitation stretching program on isokinetic torque production. *J Strength Cond Res* 2009;23(5):1442-7.
18. Marek SM, Cramer JT, Fincher AL, et al. Acute effects of static and proprioceptive neuromuscular facilitation stretching on muscle strength and power output. *J Athl Train* 2005;40(2):94-103.
19. Young W, Elliott S. Acute effects of static stretching, proprioceptive neuromuscular facilitation stretching, and maximum voluntary contractions on explosive force production and jumping performance. *Res Q Exerc Sport* 2001;72(3):273-9.
20. Chaitow L. Muscle Energy Techniques. London: Churchill Livingstone; 1999.
21. Hartig DE, Henderson JM. Increasing hamstring flexibility decreases lower extremity overuse injuries in military basic trainees. *Am J Sports Med* 1999;27(2):173-6.
22. Witvrouw E, Bellemans J, Lysens R, Danneels L, Cambier D. Intrinsic risk factors for the development of patellar tendinitis in an athletic population. A two-year prospective study. *Am J Sports Med* 2001;29(2):190-5.
23. Witvrouw E, Danneels L, Asselman P, D'Have T, Cambier D. Muscle flexibility as a risk factor for developing muscle injuries in male professional soccer players. A prospective study. *Am J Sports Med* 2003;31(1):41-6.
24. Safran MR, Seaber AV, Garrett WE Jr. Warm-up and muscular injury prevention. An update. *Sports Med* 1989;8(4):239-49.
25. Bandy WD, Irion JM, Briggler M. The effect of time and frequency of static stretching on flexibility of the hamstring muscles. *Phys Ther* 1997;77(10):1090-6.

26. Bandy WD, Irion JM, Briggler M. The effect of static stretch and dynamic range of motion training on the flexibility of the hamstring muscles. *J Orthop Sports Phys Ther* 1998;27(4):295–300.

27. Ford GS, Mazzone MA, Taylor K. The effect of 4 different durations of static hamstring stretching on passive knee-extension range of motion. *J Sport Rehabil* 2005;14(2):95–107.

28. Godges JJ, MacRae PG, Engelke KA. Effects of exercise on hip range of motion, trunk muscle performance, and gait economy. *Phys Ther* 1993;73(7):468–77.

29. Gribble PA, Guskiewicz KM, Prentice WE, Shields EW. Effects of static and hold-relax stretching on hamstring range of motion using the FlexAbility LE1000. (Effets de l'etirement statique et relache sur l'amplitude des mouvements des ischio-jambiers en utilisant l'appareil "Flexability LE 100".). *J Sport Rehabil* 1999;8(3):195–208.

30. Chan SP, Hong Y, Robinson PD. Flexibility and passive resistance of the hamstrings of young adults using two different static stretching protocols. *Scand J Med Sci Sports* 2001;11(2):81–6.

31. Davis DS, Ashby PE, McCale KL, McQuain JA, Wine JM. The effectiveness of 3 stretching techniques on hamstring flexibility using consistent stretching parameters. *J Strength Cond Res* 2005;19(1):27–32.

32. de Weijer VC, Gorniak GC, Shamus E. The effect of static stretch and warm-up exercise on hamstring length over the course of 24 hours. *J Orthop Sports Phys Ther* 2003;33(12):727–33.

33. Decicco PV, Fisher MM. The effects of proprioceptive neuromuscular facilitation stretching on shoulder range of motion in overhand athletes. *J Sports Med Phys Fitness* 2005;45(2):183–7.

34. Depino GM, Webright WG, Arnold BL. Duration of maintained hamstring flexibility after cessation of an acute static stretching protocol. *J Athl Train* 2000;35(1):56–9.

35. Etnyre BR, Lee EJ. Chronic and acute flexibility of men and women using three different stretching techniques. (La souplesse chronique et aigue chez des hommes et des femmes utilisant trois techniques d' etirement differentes.). *Res Q Exerc Sport* 1988;59(3):222–8.

36. Feland JB, Marin HN. Effect of submaximal contraction intensity in contract-relax proprioceptive neuromuscular facilitation stretching. *Br J Sports Med* 2004;38(4):E18.

37. Hubley CL, Kosey JW, Stanish WD. The effects of static stretching exercises and stationary cycling on range of motion at the hip joint. *J Orthop Sports Phys Ther* 1984;6(2):104–9.

38. McNair PJ, Stanley SN. Effect of passive stretching and jogging on the series elastic muscle stiffness and range of motion of the ankle joint. *Br J Sports Med* 1996;30(4):313–8.

39. Nelson RT, Bandy WD. Eccentric training and static stretching improve hamstring flexibility of high school males. *J Athl Train* 2004;39(3):254–8.

40. Osternig LR, Robertson RN, Troxel RK, Hansen P. Differential responses to proprioceptive neuromuscular facilitation (PNF) stretch techniques. *Med Sci Sports Exerc* 1990;22(1):106–11.

41. Roberts JM, Wilson K. Effect of stretching duration on active and passive range of motion in the lower extremity. *Br J Sports Med* 1999;33(4):259–63.

42. Rowlands AV, Marginson VF, Lee J. Chronic flexibility gains: effect of isometric contraction duration during proprioceptive neuromuscular facilitation stretching techniques. *Res Q Exerc Sport* 2003;74(1):47–51.

43. Sady SP, Wortman M, Blanke D. Flexibility training: ballistic, static or proprioceptive neuromuscular facilitation? *Arch Phys Med Rehabil* 1982;63(6):261–3.

44. Schuback B, Hooper J, Salisbury L. A comparison of a self-stretch incorporating proprioceptive neuromuscular facilitation components and a therapist-applied PNF-technique on hamstring flexibility. *Physiotherapy* 2004;90(3):151–7.

45. Wallin D, Ekblom B, Grahn R, Nordenborg T. Improvement of muscle flexibility. A comparison between two techniques. *Am J Sports Med* 1985; 13(4):263–8.

46. Webright WG, Randolph BJ, Perrin DH. Comparison of nonballistic active knee extension in neural slump position and static stretch techniques on hamstring flexibility. *J Orthop Sports Phys Ther* 1997;26(1):7–13.

47. Williford HN, East JB, Smith FH, Burry LA. Evaluation of warm-up for improvement in flexibility. (Evaluation de l' utilite de l' echauffement pour ameliorer la souplesse.). *Am J Sports Med* 1986;14(4):316–9.

48. Winters MV, Blake CG, Trost JS, et al. Passive versus active stretching of hip flexor muscles in subjects with limited hip extension: a randomized clinical trial. *Phys Ther* 2004;84(9):800–7.

49. Bandy WD, Irion JM. The effect of time on static stretch on the flexibility of the hamstring muscles (including commentary by Walker JM with author response). *Phys Ther* 1994;74(9):845–52.

50. Decoster LC, Cleland J, Altieri C, Russell P. The effects of hamstring stretching on range of motion: a systematic literature review. *J Orthop Sports Phys Ther* 2005;35(6):377–87.

51. Radford JA, Burns J, Buchbinder R, Landorf KB, Cook C. Does stretching increase ankle dorsiflexion range of motion? A systematic review. *Br J Sports Med* 2006;40(10):870–5.

52. Nelson AG, Kokkonen J, Arnall DA. Acute muscle stretching inhibits muscle strength endurance performance. *J Strength Cond Res* 2005;19(2):338–43.

53. Youdas JW, Krause DA, Egan KS, Therneau TM, Laskowski ER. The effect of static stretching of the calf muscle-tendon unit on active ankle dorsiflexion range of motion. *J Orthop Sports Phys Ther* 2003;33(7):408–17.

54. Willy RW, Kyle BA, Moore SA, Chleboun GS. Effect of cessation and resumption of static hamstring muscle stretching on joint range of motion. *J Orthop Sports Phys Ther* 2001;31(3):138–44.

55. Harvey L, Herbert R, Crosbie J. Does stretching induce lasting increases in joint ROM? A systematic review. *Physiother Res Int* 2002;7(1):1–13.

56. Fasen JM, O'Connor AM, Schwartz SL, et al. A randomized controlled trial of hamstring stretching: comparison of four techniques. *J Strength Cond Res* 2009;23(2):660–7.

57. Lucas RC, Koslow R. Comparative study of static, dynamic, and proprioceptive neuromuscular facilitation stretching techniques on flexibility. *Percept Mot Skills* 1984;58(2):615–8.

58. Winters MV, Blake CG, Trost JS, et al. Passive versus active stretching of hip flexor muscles in subjects with limited hip extension: a randomized clinical trial. *Phys Ther* 2004;84(9):800–7.

59. Clark S, Christiansen A, Hellman DF, Hugunin JW, Hurst KM. Effects of ipsilateral anterior thigh soft tissue stretching on passive unilateral straight-leg raise. *J Orthop Sports Phys Ther* 1999;29(1):4–12.

60. Sullivan MK, Dejulia JJ, Worrell TW. Effect of pelvic position and stretching method on hamstring muscle flexibility. *Med Sci Sports Exerc* 1992;24(12):1383–9.

61. Fowles JR, Sale DG, MacDougall JD. Reduced strength after passive stretch of the human plantarflexors. *J Appl Physiol* 2000;89(3):1179–88.

62. Knudson D, Noffal G. Time course of stretch-induced isometric strength deficits. *Eur J Appl Physiol* 2005;94(3):348–51.

63. Kokkonen J, Nelson AG, Cornwell A. Acute muscle stretching inhibits maximal strength performance. *Res Q Exerc Sport* 1998;69(4):411–5.

64. Young WB, Behm DG. Effects of running, static stretching and practice jumps on explosive force production and jumping performance. *J Sports Med Phys Fitness* 2003;43(1):21–7.

65. Beckett JR, Schneiker KT, Wallman KE, Dawson BT, Guelfi KJ. Effects of static stretching on repeated sprint and change of direction performance. *Med Sci Sports Exerc* 2009;41(2):444–50.

66. Chaouachi A, Chamari K, Wong P, et al. Stretch and sprint training reduces stretch-induced sprint performance deficits in 13- to 15-year-old youth. *Eur J Appl Physiol* 2008;104(3):515–22.

67. Behm DG, Bambury A, Cahill F, Power K. Effect of acute static stretching on force, balance, reaction time, and movement time. *Med Sci Sports Exerc* 2004;36(8):1397–402.

68. Power K, Behm D, Cahill F, Carroll M, Young W. An acute bout of static stretching: effects on force and jumping performance. *Med Sci Sports Exerc* 2004;36(8):1389–96.

69. Bazett-Jones DM, Winchester JB, McBride JM. Effect of potentiation and stretching on maximal force, rate of force development, and range of motion. *J Strength Cond Res* 2005;19(2):421–6.

70. Unick J, Kieffer HS, Cheesman W, Feeney A. The acute effects of static and ballistic stretching on vertical jump performance in trained women. *J Strength Cond Res* 2005;19(1):206–12.

71. Torres EM, Kraemer WJ, Vingren JL, et al. Effects of stretching on upper-body muscular performance. *J Strength Cond Res* 2008;22(4):1279–85.

72. Bacurau RF, Monteiro GA, Ugrinowitsch C, Tricoli V, Cabral LF, Aoki MS. Acute effect of a ballistic and a static stretching exercise bout on flexibility and maximal strength. *J Strength Cond Res* 2009;23(1):304–8.

73. Papadopoulos G, Siatras T, Kellis S. The effect of static and dynamic stretching exercises on the maximal isokinetic strength of the knee extensors and flexors. *Isokinetics Exerc Sci* 2005;13(4):285–91.

74. Hunter JP, Marshall RN. Effects of power and flexibility training on vertical jump technique. *Med Sci Sports Exerc* 2002;34(3):478–86.

75. Gajdosik RL, Vander Linden DW, McNair PJ, Williams AK, Riggin TJ. Effects of an eight-week stretching program on the passive-elastic properties and function of the calf muscles of older women. *Clin Biomech (Bristol, Avon)* 2005;20(9):973–83.

76. Kokkonen J, Nelson AG, Eldredge C, Winchester JB. Chronic static stretching improves exercise performance. *Med Sci Sports Exerc* 2007;39(10):1825–31.

77. Wilson GJ, Elliott BC, Wood GA. Stretch shorten cycle performance enhancement through flexibility training. *Med Sci Sports Exerc* 1992;24(1):116–23.

78. LaRoche DP, Lussier MV, Roy SJ. Chronic stretching and voluntary muscle force. *J Strength Cond Res* 2008;22(2):589–96.

79. Bazett-Jones DM, Gibson MH, McBride JM. Sprint and vertical jump performances are not affected by six weeks of static hamstring stretching. *J Strength Cond Res* 2008;22(1):25–31.

80. Andrish JT, Bergfeld JA, Walheim J. A prospective study on the management of shin splints. *J Bone Joint Surg Am* 1974;56(8):1697–700.

81. Pope R, Herbert R, Kirwan J. Effects of ankle dorsiflexion range and pre-exercise calf muscle stretching on injury risk in Army recruits. *Aust J Physiother* 1998;44(3):165–72.

82. Pope RP, Herbert RD, Kirwan JD, Graham BJ. A randomized trial of preexercise stretching for prevention of lower-limb injury. *Med Sci Sports Exerc* 2000;32(2):271–7.

83. Amako M, Oda T, Masuoka K, Yokoi H, Campisi P. Effect of static stretching on prevention of injuries for military recruits. *Mil Med* 2003;168(6):442–6.

84. Hilyer JC, Brown KC, Sirles AT, Peoples L. A flexibility intervention to reduce the incidence and severity of joint injuries among municipal firefighters. *J Occup Med* 1990;32(7):631–7.

85. Thacker SB, Gilchrist J, Stroup DF, Kimsey CD Jr. The impact of stretching on sports injury risk: a systematic review of the literature. *Med Sci Sports Exerc* 2004;36(3):371–8.

86. Knudson D, Bennett K, Corn R, Leick D, Smith C. Acute effects of stretching are not evident in the kinematics of the vertical jump. *J Strength Cond Res* 2001;15(1):98–101.

87. Nelson AG, Guillory IK, Cornwell C, Kokkonen J. Inhibition of maximal voluntary isokinetic torque production following stretching is velocity-specific. *J Strength Cond Res* 2001;15(2):241–6.

88. Shrier I, Gossal K. Myths and truths of stretching. Individualized recommendations for healthy muscles. *Physician Sportsmed* 2000;28(8). Available at: http://www.physsportsmed.com/issues/2000/08_00/shrier.htm. Accessed Jun 13, 2005.

Activation and Integration Techniques

INTRODUCTION

PHASES one and two of the Corrective Exercise Continuum addresses the overactive myofascial tissue that can restrict optimal joint range of motion (ROM) and ultimately decrease movement ability. The third phase of the Corrective Exercise Continuum is activation (Figure 11-1). Activation refers to the stimulation (or reeducation) of underactive myofascial tissue. Because HMS impairments (muscle imbalances) include both overactive and underactive muscles, a comprehensive corrective strategy must also address the underactive muscles.

The fourth and final phase of the Corrective Exercise Continuum culminates with integration techniques (Figure 11–1). Integration techniques are used to reeducate the human movement system back into a functional synergistic movement pattern. The use of multiple joint actions and multiple muscle synergies helps to reestablish neuromuscular control, promoting coordinated movement among the involved muscles. This chapter will review the science and application of these last two phases of the Corrective Exercise Continuum.

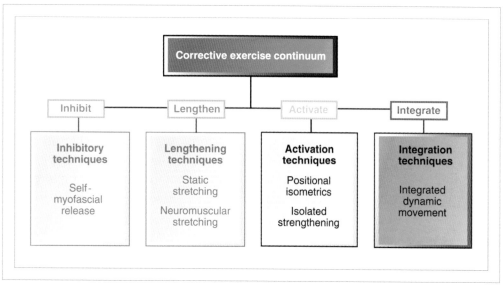

Figure 11.1   Corrective exercise continuum.

ACTIVATION TECHNIQUES

Isolated Strengthening

Intramuscular coordination: the ability of the neuromuscular system to allow optimal levels of motor unit recruitment and synchronization within a muscle.

Isolated strengthening exercises are used to isolate particular muscles to increase the force production capabilities through concentric and eccentric muscle actions. These exercises are applied to potentially underactive or "weak" muscles as indicated through the assessment process.

SCIENTIFIC RATIONALE FOR ISOLATED STRENGTHENING

Isolated strengthening is a technique used to increase **intramuscular coordination** of specific muscles. This is achieved through a combination of enhanced **motor unit activation**, **synchronization**, and **firing rate**. Each of these parameters is known to increase the strength of a muscle contraction (1). Intramuscular coordination is known to be developed through traditional resistance exercises focusing on a particular muscle (2). More importantly, however, is the increased activation of the muscle throughout the full ROM of a joint or joints associated with the particular muscle. This is important to achieve before performing integrated exercises to avoid overcompensation of synergistic muscles (synergistic dominance).

Motor unit activation: the progressive activation of a muscle by successive recruitment of contractile units (motor units) to accomplish increasing gradations of contractile strength.

Isolated strengthening exercises can be performed immediately after inhibitory and lengthening techniques. Although there is no specific scientific evidence to support this claim, clinically it has produced favorable results. An example of an isolated strengthening exercise is a standing cable hip adductor exercise as shown in Figure 11.2. The idea is to position the client and the resistance in the best line of action for an optimal recruitment of each desired muscle. In the case of the standing cable hip adductor

Synchronization: the synergistic activation of multiple motor units.

Firing rate: the frequency at which a motor unit is activated.

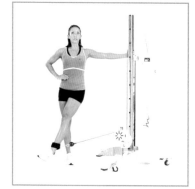

Figure 11.2   Hip Adduction Isolated Strengthening Exercise.

exercise, the movement desired is hip adduction, thus the resistance must be set up to directly oppose this motion (hip abduction). These exercises can be performed with manual resistance (proprioceptive neuromuscular facilitation [PNF] patterns, positional isometrics), cables, elastic tubing, dumbbells, and machines.

The eccentric component involved with isolated strengthening has been proven to play a role in the recovery of muscle injury, tendinopathies, and in preparation for integrated training (3–6). Greater strength gains were also made with groups training with concentric and eccentric versus concentric only in vertical jump and squat movements (7). Eccentric training has also been shown to be more effective at increasing total strength and muscle mass possibly because of higher forces developed during this form of training (8).

GETTING YOUR FACTS STRAIGHT

Clinical Scenario: Muscle Weakness and Lower Extremity Injuries

Patellofemoral problems are commonly addressed with open and closed chain strengthening exercises. A study comparing the efficacy of both type of exercises found that open and closed chain exercises improved subjective and clinical outcomes in patients with patellofemoral pain syndrome (1). Considerable research has been done to investigate the involvement of associated hip weakness with patellofemoral problems leading to the importance of recognition and treatment of hip weakness (2–5). Clinical research has also made reference to isolated weakness of the gluteus maximus and medius with ankle injuries (6,7).

1. Herrington L, Al-Sherhi A. A controlled trial of weight-bearing versus non-weight-bearing exercises for patellofemoral pain. J Orthop Sports Phys Ther 2007;37(4):155–60.
2. Piva SR, Goodnite EA, Childs JD. Strength around the hip and flexibility of soft tissue in individuals with and without patellofemoral pain syndrome. J Orthop Sports Phys Ther 2005;35(12):793–801.
3. Bolgla LA, Malone TR, Umberger BR, Uhl TL. Hip strength and hip and knee kinematics during stair descent in females with and without patellofemoral pain syndrome. J Orthop Sports Phys Ther 2008;38(1):12–8.
4. Souza RB, Powers CM. Differences in hip kinematics, muscle strength and muscle activation between subjects with and without patellofemoral pain. J Orthop Sports Phys Ther 2009;29(1):12–9.
5. Boling MC, Padua DA, Alexander CR. Concentric and eccentric torque of the hip musculature in individuals with and without patellofemoral pain. J Athl Train 2009;44(1):7–13.
6. Friel K, McLean N, Myers C, Caceres M. Ipsilateral hip abductor weakness after ankle inversion sprain. J Athl Train 2006;41(1):74–8.
7. Bullock-Saxton JE, Janda V, Bullock MI. The influence of ankle sprain injury on muscle activation during hip extension. Int J Sports Med 1994;15(6):330–4.

(*Text continues on page 241*)

APPLICATION GUIDELINES FOR ISOLATED STRENGTHENING TECHNIQUES

➤ PRECAUTIONS AND CONTRAINDICATIONS

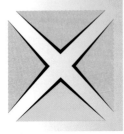

Precautions for isolated strengthening exercises follow those for most forms of training (see accompanying table).

PRECAUTIONS AND CONTRAINDICATIONS FOR ISOLATED STRENGTHENING	
Precautions	**Contraindications**
Special populations Neuromuscular disorders Clients with poor core stabilization strength	Acute injury or muscle strain or tear of the muscle being strengthened Acute rheumatoid arthritis of the affected joint Impaired joint motion Pain produced during the movement

Acute Variables   Isolated strengthening can be performed three to five days per week depending on the intensity and volume used. One to two sets of 10 to 15 repetitions is suitable before an integrated exercise program. Each repetition will consist of a two-second isometric hold at end ROM and a four-second eccentric component (see table below) (9). Examples of isolated strengthening exercises follow.

ACUTE VARIABLES FOR ISOLATED STRENGTHENING			
Frequency	**Sets**	**Repetitions**	**Duration of Rep**
3–5 days per week	1–2	10–15	2 seconds isometric hold at end-range and 4 seconds eccentric

MENNELL'S FOUR BASIC TRUISMS

Mennell's truisms provide a theoretical basis for the hypothesis that attempting to strengthen muscles when joint motion restriction is present will provide less than optimal results and limited joint ROM needs to be considered during any exercise application (1).

1. When a joint is not free to move, the muscles that move it cannot be free to move it.
2. Muscles cannot be restored to normal if the joints that they move are not free to move.

3. Normal muscle function is dependent on normal joint movement.
4. Impaired muscle function perpetuates and may cause deterioration in abnormal joints.

These four truisms are some of the reasons to perform inhibitory and lengthening techniques (first two phases of the corrective exercise continuum) before isolated strengthening exercises.

1. Mendell J. Joint Pain: Diagnosis and Treatment Using Manipulative Techniques. Boston, MA: Little, Brown; 1964.

Example Isolated Strengthening Exercises: Foot and Ankle

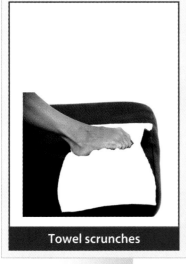

Towel scrunches

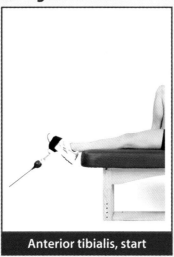

Anterior tibialis, start

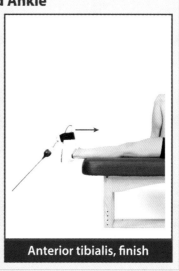

Anterior tibialis, finish

Continued on page 234

Example Isolated Strengthening Exercises: Knee

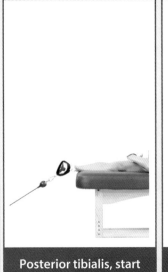

Posterior tibialis, start

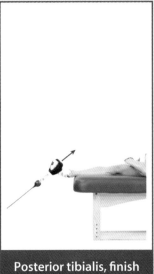

Posterior tibialis, finish

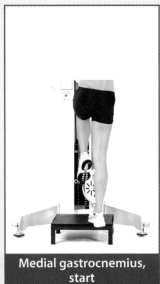

Medial gastrocnemius, start

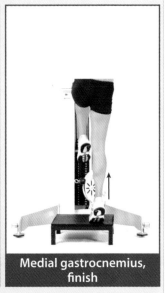

Medial gastrocnemius, finish

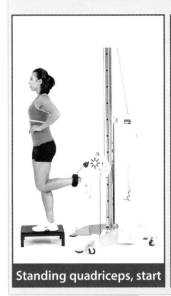

Standing quadriceps, start

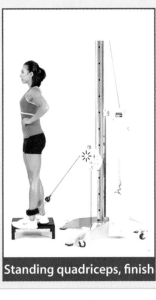

Standing quadriceps, finish

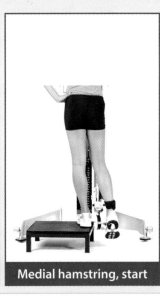

Medial hamstring, start

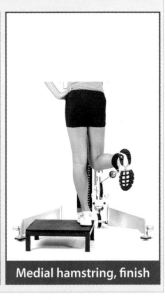

Medial hamstring, finish

Example Isolated Strengthening Exercises: Hip

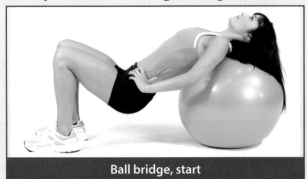

Ball bridge, start

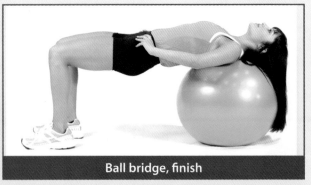

Ball bridge, finish

Example Isolated Strengthening Exercises: Hip

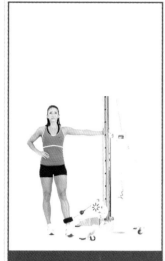

Standing adductor, start

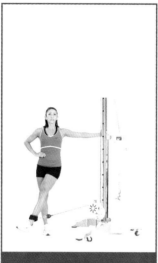

Standing adductor, finish

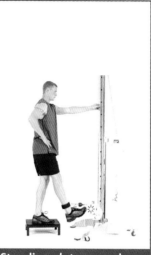

Standing gluteus maximus, start

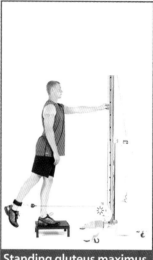

Standing gluteus maximus, finish

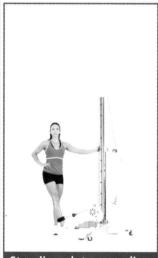

Standing gluteus medius, start

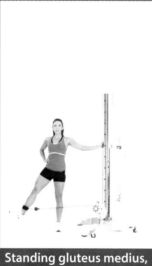

Standing gluteus medius, finish

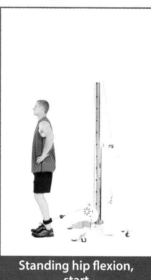

Standing hip flexion, start

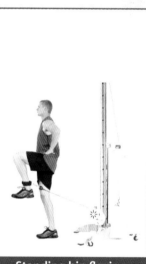

Standing hip flexion, finish

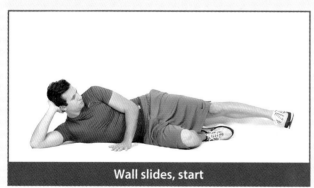

Wall slides, start

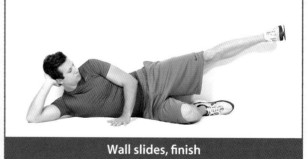

Wall slides, finish

Continued on page 236

Example Isolated Strengthening Exercises: Abdominals/Intrinsic Core Stabilizers

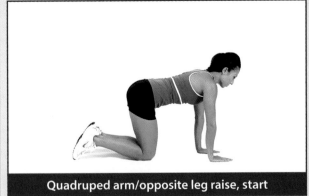

Quadruped arm/opposite leg raise, start

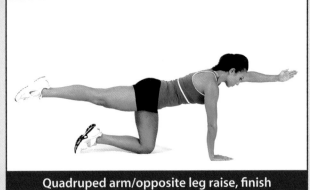

Quadruped arm/opposite leg raise, finish

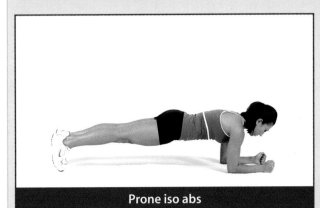

Prone iso abs

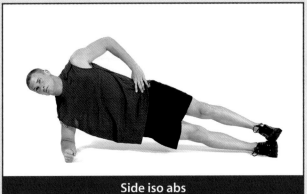

Side iso abs

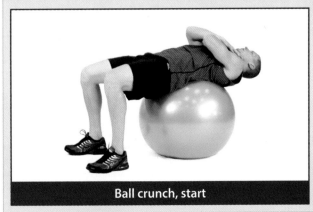

Ball crunch, start

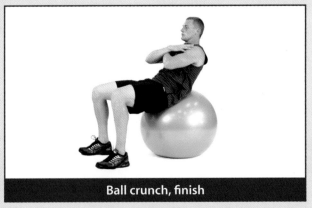

Ball crunch, finish

Example Isolated Strengthening Exercises: Shoulder

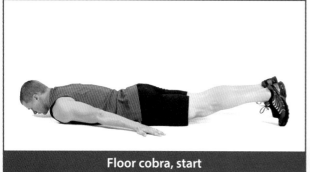

Floor cobra, start

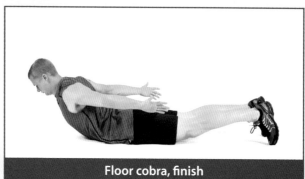

Floor cobra, finish

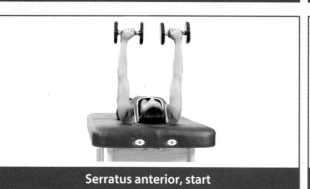

Serratus anterior, start

Serratus anterior, finish

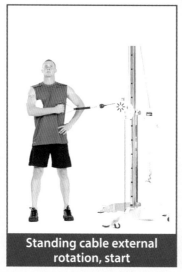

Standing cable external
rotation, start

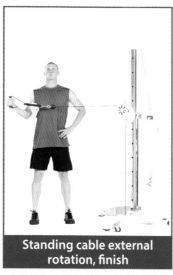

Standing cable external
rotation, finish

Continued on page 238

Example Isolated Strengthening Exercises: Shoulder

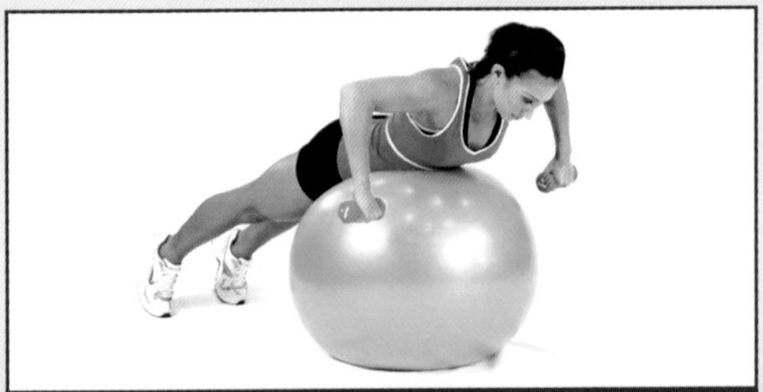

Prone shoulder external rotation, start

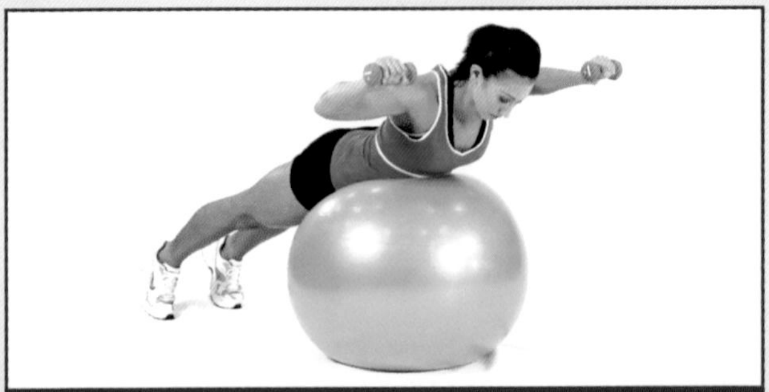

Prone shoulder external rotation, finish

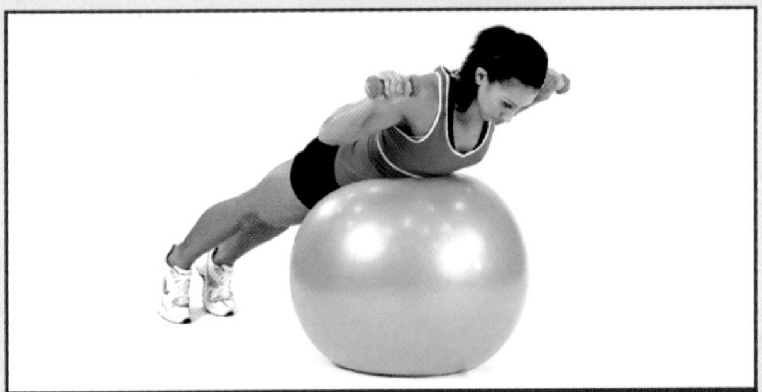

Prone military press, start

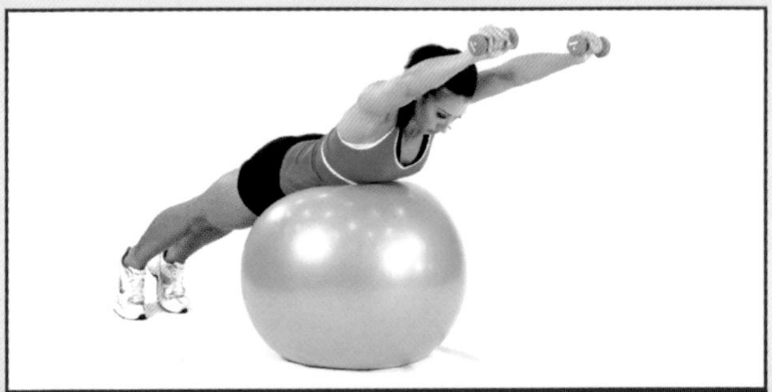

Prone military press, finish

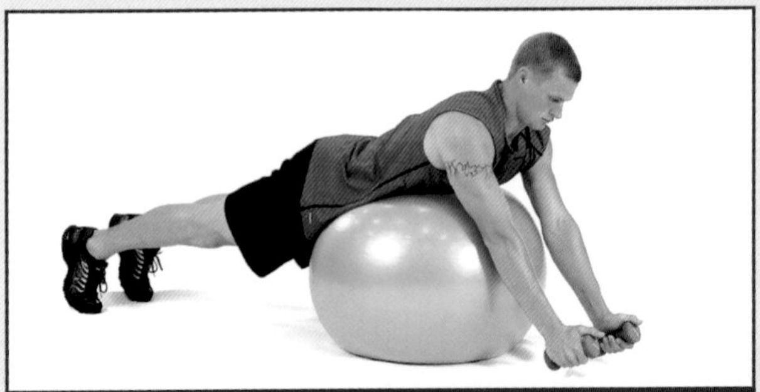

Ball combo I, start

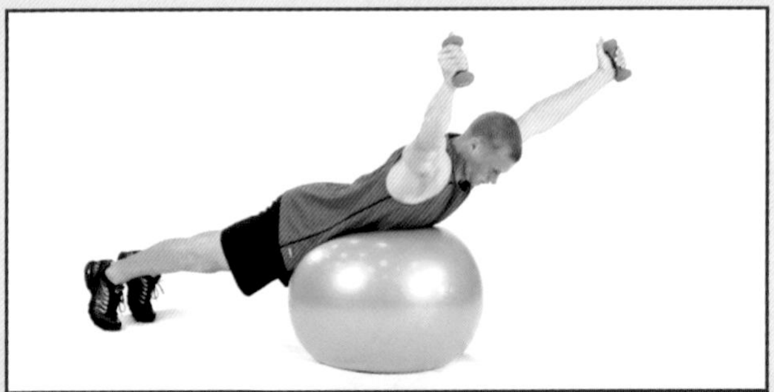

Ball combo I, scaption

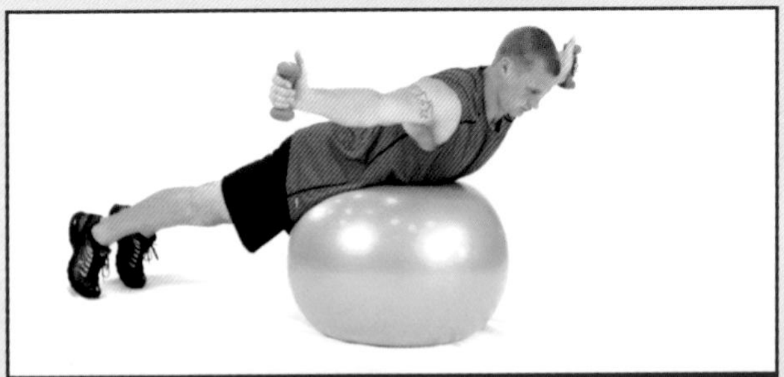

Ball combo I, T

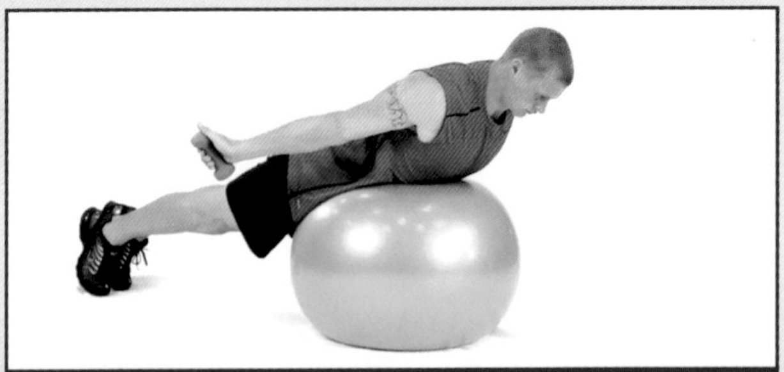

Ball combo I, Cobra (finish)

Example Isolated Strengthening Exercises: Shoulder

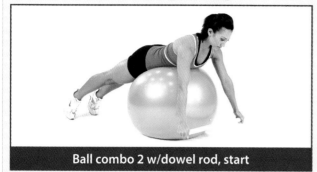

Ball combo 2 w/dowel rod, start

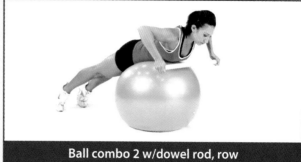

Ball combo 2 w/dowel rod, row

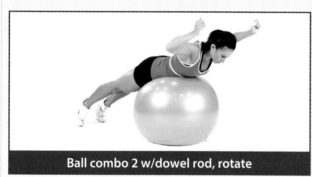

Ball combo 2 w/dowel rod, rotate

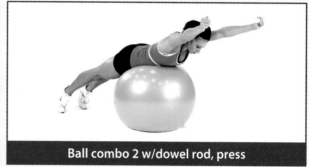

Ball combo 2 w/dowel rod, press

Example Isolated Strengthening Exercises: Elbow and Wrist

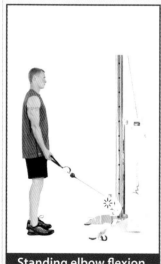

Standing elbow flexion, start

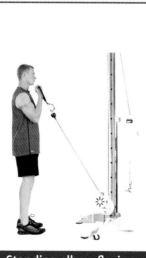

Standing elbow flexion, finish

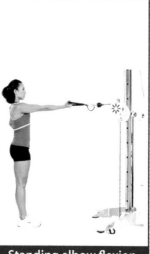

Standing elbow flexion with shoulder flexed, start

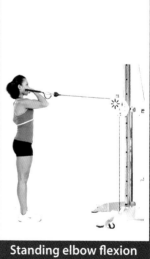

Standing elbow flexion with shoulder flexed, finish

Continued on page 240

Example Isolated Strengthening Exercises: Elbow and Wrist

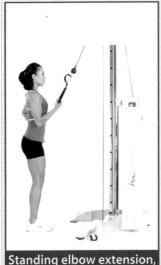

Standing elbow extension, start

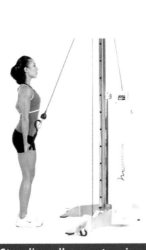

Standing elbow extension, finish

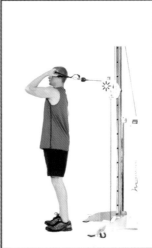

Standing elbow extension with shoulder flexed, start

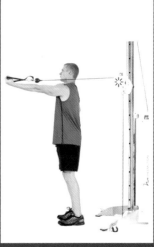

Standing elbow extension with shoulder flexed, finish

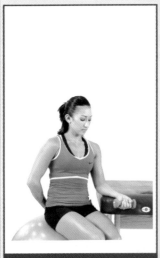

Wrist flexion, start

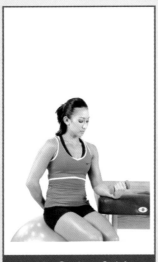

Wrist flexion, finish

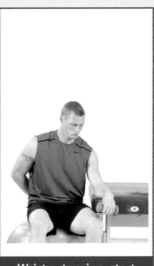

Wrist extension, start

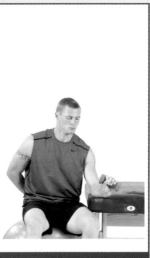

Wrist extension, finish

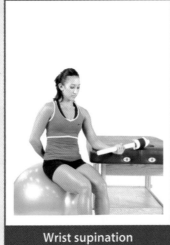

Wrist supination

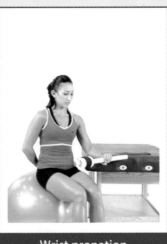

Wrist pronation

Example Isolated Strengthening Exercises: Cervical Spine

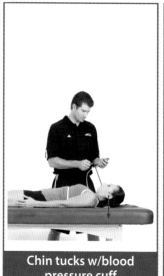

Chin tucks w/blood pressure cuff

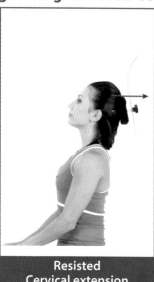

Resisted Cervical extension

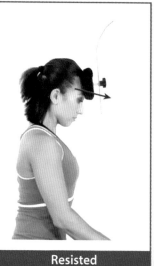

Resisted Cervical flexion

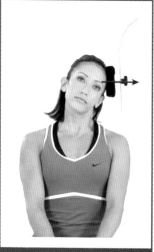

Resisted Cervical lateral flexion

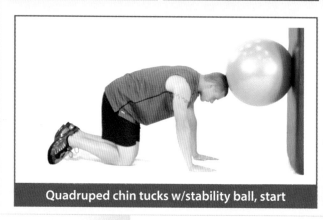

Quadruped chin tucks w/stability ball, start

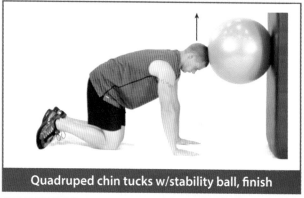

Quadruped chin tucks w/stability ball, finish

Positional Isometrics

A second activation technique that can be used is positional isometrics. Positional isometrics incorporates isometric contractions performed at the end ROM of a joint. It is a static technique meaning that there is no active motion. This technique would be more appropriate for a person with adequate core strength and neuromuscular control as it will involve higher intensity contractions or force. Like isolated strengthening techniques, the purpose of this technique is to increase the intramuscular coordination of specific muscles necessary to heighten the activation levels before integrating them back into their functional synergies. It should be noted that one must be a qualified health and fitness professional (i.e., a licensed professional) to apply positional isometric techniques on clients.

SCIENTIFIC RATIONALE FOR POSITIONAL ISOMETRICS

As previously mentioned, positional isometrics is used to heighten the activation of underactive muscle(s) of a joint. This is based on the premise that isometric muscle contractions generate higher levels of tension than concentric muscle contractions and provide functional strength at approximately 10 degrees on either side of the joint angle of contraction (10,11). Therefore, the use of isometric contractions may provide a better initial stimulus necessary for increased activation of specific muscles while still promoting some functional carryover of strength in a slightly greater joint ROM.

GETTING YOUR FACTS STRAIGHT

Clinical Scenario: The Use of Positional Isometrics

Whenever improvements are made with range of motion of a joint, there will be associated weakness of the muscles that facilitate movement at that joint. Positional isometrics provides an appropriate form of treatment to address this weakness and should be considered.

(Text continues on page 245)

APPLICATION GUIDELINES FOR POSITIONAL ISOMETRICS

➤ PRECAUTIONS AND CONTRAINDICATIONS

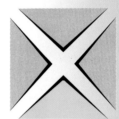

Precautions for positional isometrics follow those for most forms of training and can be seen in the accompanying table.

PRECAUTIONS AND CONTRAINDICATIONS FOR POSITIONAL ISOMETRICS	
Precautions	**Contraindications**
Special populations Neuromuscular disorders	Acute injury or muscle strain or tear of the muscle being worked Acute rheumatoid arthritis of the effected joint Hypertension Coronary heart disease (CHD) Poor core stabilization strength Early postoperative muscle or tendon repair where circulatory compromise or force exertion should be avoided

ACUTE VARIABLES

The acute variables for positional isometrics can be seen in the following table. Positional isometrics can be used as needed and consists of one set of four repetitions. Each repetition increases in intensity from 25% up to 100% of maximal voluntary contraction (MVC).

ACUTE VARIABLES FOR POSITIONAL ISOMETRICS			
Frequency	**Sets**	**Repetitions**	**Duration of Rep**
As needed	1	4	4-second isometric holds at 25%, 50%, 75%, and 100% MVC (2 seconds' rest between contractions)

MVC = maximal voluntary contraction.

Example Positional Isometric Techniques

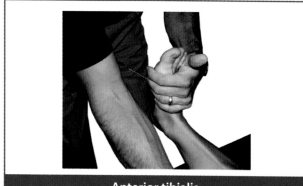

Anterior tibialis

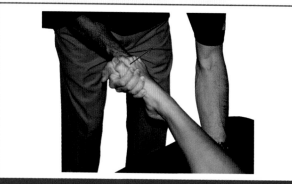

Posterior tibialis

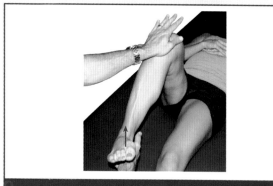

Medial hamstring

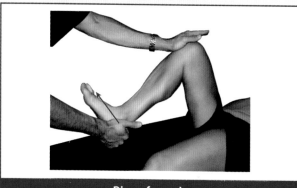

Bicep femoris

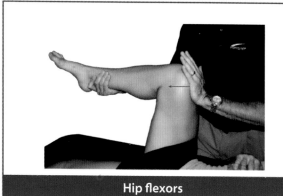

Hip flexors

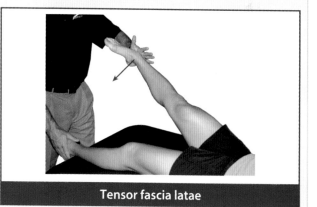

Tensor fascia latae

Continued on page 244

Example Positional Isometric Techniques

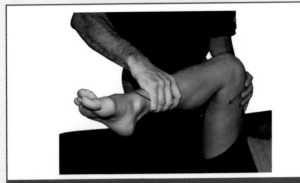

Sartorius

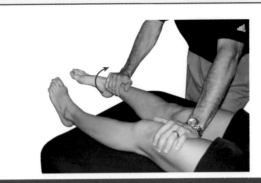

Gracilis

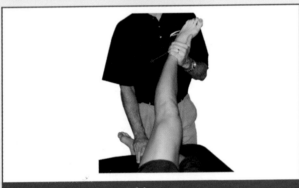

Adductors

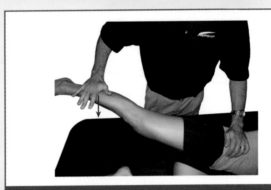

Gluteus medius

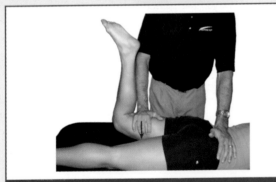

Gluteus maximus

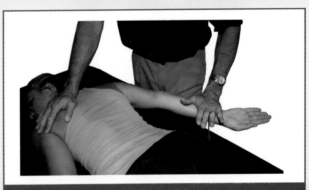

Latissimus dorsi

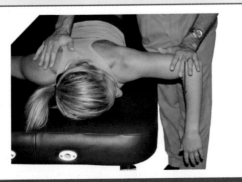

Rhomboids

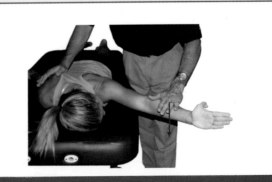

Lower trapezius

INTEGRATION TECHNIQUES

Integrated Dynamic Movement

Once the appropriate muscles have been activated, the last component of the Corrective Exercise Continuum, integration techniques (Figure 11.1) through the use of integrated dynamic movement, can be performed. Integrated dynamic movement involves the use of dynamic total body exercises. Collectively, integrated dynamic movement enhances the functional capacity of the human movement system by increasing multiplanar neuromuscular control. This is achieved by using exercises that focus on the synergistic function of the stabilization and mobilization muscles of the body. The remainder of this chapter will review the scientific rationale for integrated dynamic movement and provide application guidelines for integrated dynamic movement exercises.

SCIENTIFIC RATIONALE FOR INTEGRATED DYNAMIC MOVEMENT

It is suggested that many injuries occur during eccentric deceleration in the frontal and transverse planes as a result of the inability to control postural alignment (12–15). Furthermore, it is known that multijoint motions promote and require greater **intermuscular coordination** to achieve the desired outcome and is often the reason for their use (1). Research has shown that the short-term use of both unilateral and bilateral exercises is effective at increasing performance measures and that unilateral exercise has a greater influence on unilateral performance (16). Also, the use of overhead movements, often used in integrated dynamic movements, help to place increased stress on the core musculature (17).

This alludes to the importance of using multijoint exercises in all planes of motion from both bilateral and unilateral stances to help increase intermuscular coordination and reeducate the neuromuscular system to maintain proper postural alignment during functional activity. Thus, the premise with integrated dynamic movements is to promote high levels of intermuscular coordination (neuromuscular efficiency) in a progressive manner to simulate functional activities. By doing this, we help to reestablish postural control and decrease the risk of injury.

Integrated dynamic movement involves low load and controlled movement in ideal posture. This helps to ensure that joints start and remain in proper alignment, muscles function in their proper length-tension relationships, and synergistic muscle recruitment is optimal. An example of integrated dynamic movement may include a ball squat with an overhead press (Figure 11-3).

The importance of integrated dynamic movement lies not just in the movement patterns themselves, but in the progression of the movement patterns as well. For example, a base exercise would consist of a two-legged exercise with minimal challenge to stability (i.e., ball wall squat). Progression from here would be to an alternating or staggered stance exercise (i.e., step-up) and then progress to a lunge and then

> Intermuscular coordination: the ability of the neuromuscular system to allow all muscles to work together with proper activation and timing between them.

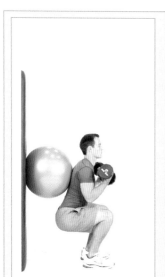
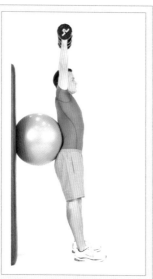

Figure 11.3A Ball Squat with Overhead Press, start.

Figure 11.3B Ball Squat with Overhead Press, finish.

to a single-leg base of support exercise (i.e., single-leg squat) to more dynamic movements on one leg (such as hopping) (Figure 11-4). This progression can be performed first in the sagittal plane, then progress to the frontal (side to side) and transverse planes (rotation). The incorporation of upper body movement, plane of motion, and challenge to stability can also be added (18,19).

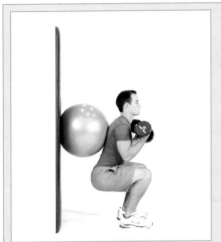

Figure 11.4A Sample Integrated Dynamic Movement Progression, two-leg.

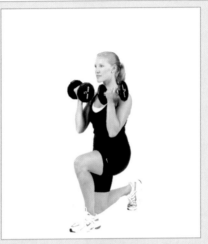

Figure 11.4B Sample Integrated Dynamic Movement Progression, alternating leg.

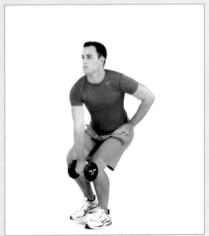

Figure 11.4C Sample Integrated Dynamic Movement Progression, single leg.

GETTING YOUR FACTS STRAIGHT

The Use of Resistance Training Exercises in Unstable Environments

Resistance training performed on unstable surfaces could be considered to assist in improvements in movement. Although research has shown the benefits to performing exercises in more stable environments (1–5), new research is showing the benefits of performing resistance training exercises in more unstable environments (6–8). Behm and Anderson found both increased trunk and limb muscle activity when performing exercises in more unstable versus stable environments (6). Carter and associates found that stability ball training may provide improvements in spinal stability in the sedentary population (7). Marshall and Murphy found increased deltoid and abdominal activity when performing a bench press on a stability ball in comparison to performing it on a stable bench (8). However, more research into this form of training still needs to done.

1. American College of Sports Medicine. Position stand: progression models in resistance training for healthy adults. Med Sci Sports Exerc 2009;41(3):687–708.
2. Kraemer WJ, Bush JA. Factors affecting the acute neuromuscular responses to resistance exercise. In: Roitman JL, ed. ACSM Resource Manual for Guidelines for Exercise Testing and Prescription. 3rd ed. Baltimore, MD: Lippincott Williams & Wilkins; 1998. p 164–173.
3. Sale D, MacDougall D. Specificity in strength training: a review for the coach and athlete. Can J Appl Sport Sci 1981;6(2):87–92.
4. Willardson J. The effectiveness of resistance exercises performed on unstable equipment. J Strength Cond Res 2004;26(5):70–4.
5. Cressey EM, West CA, Tiberio DP, Kraemer WJ, Maresh CM. The effects of ten weeks of lower body unstable surface training on markers of athletic performance. J Strength Cond Res 2007;21(2):561–7.
6. Behm DG, Anderson KG. The role of instability with resistance training. J Strength Cond Res 2006;20(3):716–22.
7. Carter JM, Beam WC, McMahan SG, Barr ML, Brown LE. The effects of stability ball training on spinal stability in sedentary individuals. J Strength Cond Res 2006;20(2):429–35.
8. Marshall PWM, Murphy BA. Increased deltoid and abdominal muscle activity during Swiss ball bench press. J Strength Cond Res 2006;20(4):745–50.

APPLICATION GUIDELINES FOR INTEGRATION TECHNIQUES

➤ PRECAUTIONS AND CONTRAINDICATIONS

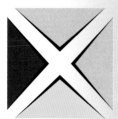

Precautions and contraindications for integrated dynamic movement exercises follow the same general guidelines for all exercise and can be seen in the accompanying table. Again, it is important to perform an assessment for each client before utilizing integrated dynamic movement exercises to ensure that the exercises selected are appropriate and safe.

PRECAUTIONS AND CONTRAINDICATIONS FOR INTEGRATED DYNAMIC MOVEMENT	
Precautions	**Contraindications**
Special populations Neuromuscular disorders	Acute injury or muscle strain or tear of the muscle being worked Acute rheumatoid arthritis of the effected joint Position of exercise (prone, supine, decline position) relative to the client's condition (pregnancy, CHD, etc.) Acute injury to joint involved during movement

CHD = coronary heart disease.

Acute Variables

Acute variables for integrated dynamic movement can be seen in the table here (19). These exercises can be safely performed anywhere from three to five days per week depending on the intensity and volume used. Generally, only one integrated dynamic movement is necessary to use, although others can be incorporated if desired. The individual's physical capabilities should also be taken into consideration when selecting an integrated dynamic movement. See Figure 11-7 for more examples of integrated dynamic movements.

ACUTE VARIABLES FOR INTEGRATED DYNAMIC MOVEMENT			
Frequency	**Sets**	**Repetitions**	**Duration of Rep**
3–5 days per week	1–3	10–15	Slow and controlled

Example Integrated Dynamic Movement Exercises

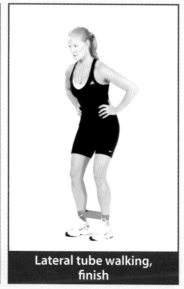

Lateral tube walking, start

Lateral tube walking, finish

Continued on page 248

Example Integrated Dynamic Movement Exercises

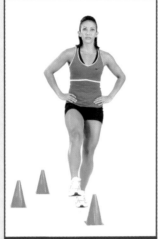

Single-leg balance w/multi-planar reach, sagittal

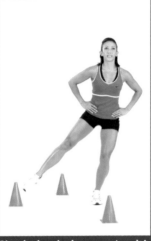

Single-leg balance w/multi-planar reach, frontal

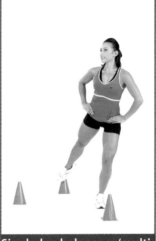

Single-leg balance w/multi-planar reach, transverse

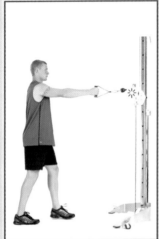

Single-arm row to arrow position, start

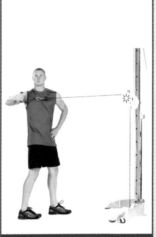

Single-arm row to arrow position, finish

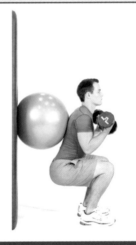

Ball squat to overhead press, start

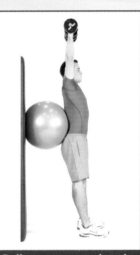

Ball squat to overhead press, finish

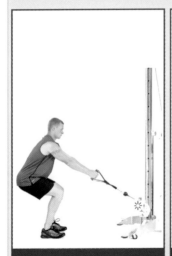

Squat to row, start

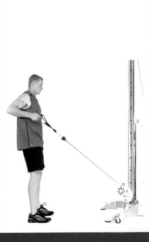

Squat to row, finish

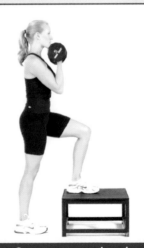

Step up to overhead press, start

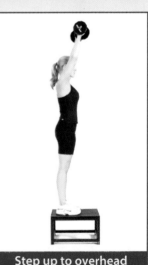

Step up to overhead press, finish

Example Integrated Dynamic Movement Exercises

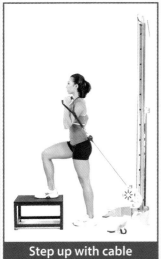

Step up with cable press, start

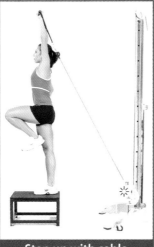

Step up with cable press, finish

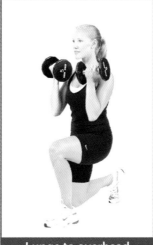

Lunge to overhead press, start

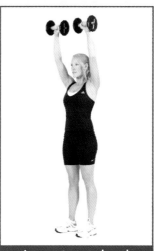

Lunge to overhead press, finish

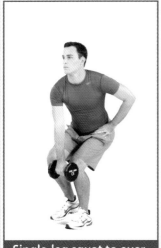

Single-leg squat to overhead press, start

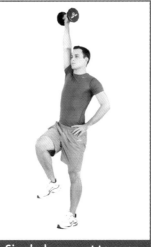

Single-leg squat to overhead press, finish

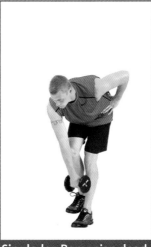

Single-leg Romanian deadlift to PNF pattern, start

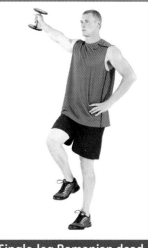

Single-leg Romanian deadlift to PNF pattern, finish

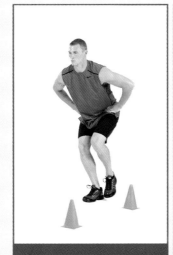

Hop w/stabilization, start

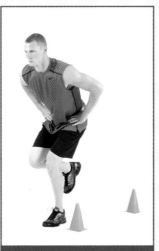

Hop w/stabilization, finish

SUMMARY • The activation and integration phases complete the Corrective Exercise Continuum as introduced previously in this text. This chapter offers the rationale and description of various techniques to address the reeducation of underactive myofascial tissue. The application of these principles to localized muscle components followed by integration into synergistic and functional movement patterns completes a comprehensive program for both training and rehabilitation.

References

1. Enoka RM. Neuromechanics of Human Movement. 3rd ed. Champaign, IL: Human Kinetics; 2002.
2. Bruhn S, Kullmann N, Gollhofer A. The effects of a sensorimotor training and a strength training on postural stabilisation, maximum isometric contraction and jump performance. *Int J Sports Med* 2004;25(1):56–60.
3. Roos EM, Engström M, Lagerquist A, Söderberg B. Clinical improvement after 6 weeks of eccentric exercise in patients with mid-portion Achilles tendinopathy: a randomized trial with 1 year follow-up, *Scand J Med Sci Sports* 2004;14(5):286–95.
4. Ohberg L, Lorentzon R, Alfredson H. Eccentric training in patients with chronic Achilles tendinosis: normalised tendon structure and decreased thickness at follow up. *Br J Sports Med* 2004;38(1):8–11.
5. Kaminski TW, Wabbersen CV, Murphy RM. Concentric versus enhanced eccentric hamstring strength training: clinical implications. *J Athl Train* 1998;33(3):216–21.
6. Ellenbecker TS, Davies GJ, Rowinski MJ. Concentric versus eccentric strengthening of the rotator cuff. *Am J Sports Med* 1988;16:64–9.
7. Colliander EB, Tesch PA. Effects of eccentric and concentric muscle actions in resistance training. *Acta Physiol Scand* 1990;140(1):31–9.
8. Roig M, O'Brien K, Kirk G, et al. The effects of eccentric versus concentric resistance training on muscle strength and mass in healthy adults: a systematic review with meta-analysis. *Br J Sports Med* 2009;43:556–68.
9. American College of Sports Medicine. Progression models in resistance training for healthy adults. *Med Sci Sports Exerc* 2009;41(3):687–708.
10. Alter MJ. Science of Flexibility. 3rd ed. Champaign, IL: Human Kinetics; 2004.
11. Kitai TA, Sale DG. Specificity of joint angle in isometric training. *Eur J Appl Physiol Occup Physiol* 1989;58(7):744–8.
12. Ford KR, Myer GD, Hewett TE. Valgus knee motion during landing in high school female and male basketball players. *Med Sci Sports Exerc* 2003;35(10):1745–50.
13. Ireland ML, Wilson JD, Ballantyne BT, McClay I. Hip strength in females with and without patellofemoral pain. *J Orthop Sports Phys Ther* 2003;33(11):671–6.
14. Nyland J, Smith S, Beickman K, et al. Frontal plane knee angles affects dynamic postural control strategy during unilateral stance. *Med Sci Sports Exerc* 2002;34(7):1150–7.
15. Powers CM. The influence of altered lower-extremity kinematics on patellofemoral joint dysfunction: a theoretical perspective. *J Orthop Sports Phys Ther* 2003;33(11):639–46.
16. McCurdy KW, Langford GA, Doscher MW, Wiley LP, Mallard KG. The effects of short-term unilateral and bilateral lower-body resistance training on measures of strength and power. *J Strength Cond Res* 2005;19(1): 9–15.
17. Richardson C, Hodges P, Hides J. Therapeutic Exercise for Lumbopelvic Stabilization. A Motor Control Approach for the Treatment and Prevention of Low Back Pain. London: Churchill Livingstone; 2004.
18. Clark MA, Lucett SC, Corn RJ. NASM Essentials of Personal Fitness Training. 3rd ed. Baltimore, MD: Lippincott Williams & Wilkins; 2008.
19. Voight ML, Cook G. Impaired Neuromuscular Control: Reactive Neuromuscular Training. In: Voight ML, Hoogenboom BJ, Prentice WE, eds. Musculoskeletal Interventions: Techniques for Therapeutic Exercise. Boston, MA: McGraw Hill; 2007. p 181–214.

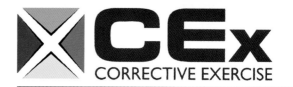

SECTION 4

CORRECTIVE EXERCISE STRATEGIES

CHAPTER 12

Corrective Strategies for Foot and Ankle Impairments

OBJECTIVES *Upon completing this chapter, you will be able to:*

➤ Understand basic functional anatomy for the foot and ankle complex.

➤ Understand the mechanisms for common foot and ankle injuries.

➤ Determine common risk factors that can lead to foot and ankle injury.

➤ Incorporate a systematic assessment and corrective exercise strategy for foot and ankle impairments.

INTRODUCTION

THE human body is susceptible to movement dysfunctions and neuromusculo-skeletal imbalances. Some causes may include repetitive movements, overuse, sedentary living, and improper movement techniques. These dysfunctions in turn lead to many of the common injuries seen in an active population. The foot and ankle complex may greatly influence the entire HMS. This region represents the platform from which our base of support is derived and is the main contact point between the ground and the body. As such, it must withstand a high amount of contact force (ground reaction force) with each step taken because it is closest to the impact site (foot strike). As the body is an interconnected chain (kinetic chain), compensation or dysfunction in one region such as the foot and ankle may lead to dysfunctions in other areas of the body (1,2). This chapter will review basic functional anatomy of the foot and ankle complex, its relationship with other segments of the body during movement, and corrective strategies to help improve foot and ankle movement dysfunction.

REVIEW OF FOOT AND ANKLE FUNCTIONAL ANATOMY

The foot and ankle is a complex structure with great potential for influence on the rest of the human movement system. There are a number of bones, joints, and muscles that may be affected by dysfunction in the foot and ankle; however, this section seeks only to provide a general review of the most pertinent structures. This is not intended to be an exhaustive and detailed review.

Bones and Joints

Examining the foot and ankle region specifically (Figure 12-1), the phalanges, metatarsals, and tarsals make up the metatarsophalangeal (MTP) and tarsometatarsal joints. The tarsal bones consist of the cuboid; medial, intermediate, and lateral cuneiforms; navicular; talus; and calcaneus. The transverse arch consists of the cuboid and cuneiforms (Figure 12-2). The medial longitudinal arch is composed of the calcaneus, talus, navicular, medial cuneiform, and first metatarsal (Figure 12-2). Additional articulations include the subtalar joint (talus and calcaneus), talonavicular and calcaneocuboid joints.

Moving to the lower leg, the tibia and fibula bones form the proximal and distal tibiofibular joints as well as the talocrural joint (tibia, fibula, and talus), commonly called the "ankle" joint.

More proximally (Figure 12-3), the patella, femur, and the pelvis, in conjunction with the tibia, constitute the tibiofemoral, patellofemoral, and

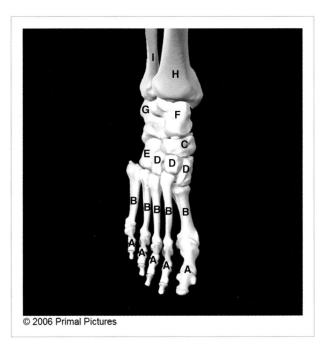

© 2006 Primal Pictures

Figure 12.1 Bones of the foot, ankle and lower leg.
(A) phalanges. (B) metatarsals. (C) navicular. (D) medial, intermediate, and lateral cuneiform. (E) cuboid. (F) talus.
(G) calcaneus. (H) tibia. (I) fibula.

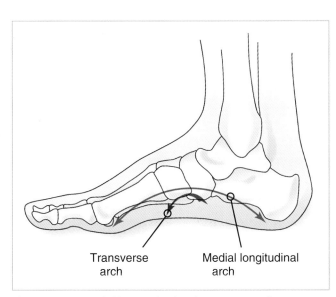

Transverse arch   Medial longitudinal arch

Figure 12.2 Medial longitudinal and transverse arches of the foot.

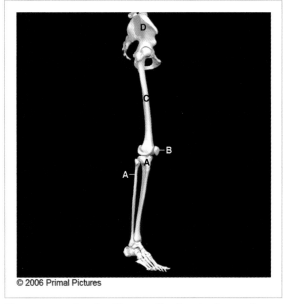

© 2006 Primal Pictures

Figure 12.3 Proximal bones affecting the foot and ankle. (A) tibia and fibula. (B) patella. (C) femur. (D) pelvis.

Table 12.1 KEY MUSCLES ASSOCIATED WITH THE FOOT AND ANKLE COMPLEX	
• Flexor hallucis longus • Gastrocnemius • Soleus • Peroneals	• Posterior tibialis • Anterior tibialis • Medial hamstrings • Gluteus medius and maximus

iliofemoral joints that anchor proximal myofascial tissues. These structures are important in terms of corrective exercise because dysfunction at one joint may influence behavior at a distant joint and the musculature controlling it (3–5).

Muscles

There are a number of muscles in the lower leg and lumbo-pelvic-hip complex whose function may be related to the foot and ankle complex (Table 12-1) (3–5). It is important to restore and maintain normal range of motion and strength, and to eliminate any muscle inhibition, to ensure joints are operating optimally (3–5). See chapter two for a detailed review of the location and function of these muscles.

COMMON FOOT AND ANKLE INJURIES AND ASSOCIATED MOVEMENT DEFICIENCIES

Plantar fasciitis: irritation and swelling of the thick tissue on the bottom of the foot. The most common complaint is pain in the bottom of the heel.

Plantar Fasciitis

The plantar fascia is a thick, fibrous band of tissue that runs from the calcaneus and fans out to insert on the metatarsal heads to support the medial longitudinal arch of the foot. An inflamed and irritated plantar fascia can be very painful (Figure 12-4). **Plantar fasciitis** is a common cause of heel pain, and most patients report pain in the heel region, particularly after getting out of bed in the morning or after sitting for extended periods (6). Lack of ankle dorsiflexion has been associated with plantar fasciitis (6,7), as has a pronated foot type (8). Increased body mass index in a nonathletic population has also been indicated as a predisposing factor (7). However, there is not strong evidence to associate foot type or first metatarsophalangeal joint motion with plantar fasciitis (6,7). Stretching of the calf or plantar fascia appears to provide short-term pain relief and improvements in dorsiflexion range of motion (7).

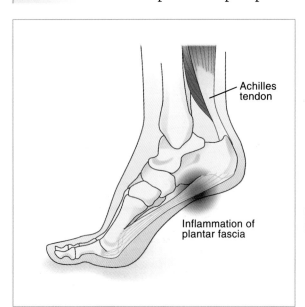

Achilles tendon

Inflammation of plantar fascia

Figure 12.4   Plantar fasciitis.

Achilles' Tendinopathy

The gastrocnemius complex, which consists of the gastrocnemius and soleus muscles, share a common Achilles' tendon that inserts on the base of the calcaneus. Tendonitis, or inflammation of this tendon, is a

Tendinopathy: a combination of pain, swelling, and impaired performance commonly associated with the Achilles' tendon.

Tendinosis: damage to a tendon at a cellular level, but does not present to inflammation.

common sports-related injury (Figure 12-5). Alternately, if inflammation is not present, but **tendinopathy** and tissue degeneration are present, it is termed **tendinosis** (9). Jumping and running are common causes of Achilles' tendinopathy (10). Signs and symptoms may include pain during physical activities or at rest, inflammation, swelling, and thickening of the tendon. A tight Achilles' tendon (lack of dorsiflexion) (9) and increased rearfoot inversion has been associated with Achilles' tendinopathy (11). Additionally, runners with Achilles' tendinopathy demonstrated decreased knee range of motion, and decreased activity in the tibialis anterior, rectus femoris, and gluteus medius muscles in the time before and after heel strike (12). Eccentric exercise of the tendons appears to treat the condition, but care must be taken to not worsen the injury (9).

Medial Tibial Stress Syndrome

Medial tibial stress syndrome (shin splints): pain in the front of the tibia caused by an overload to the tibia and the associated musculature.

Periosteum: a membrane that lines the outer surface of all bones.

Medial tibial stress syndrome (Figure 12-6), which has also been called shin splints (13), is an overuse injury thought to be caused by excessive running or training, poor shoes, type of training surface, or biomechanical factors (13). Individuals with medial tibial stress syndrome complain of pain and tenderness along the medial tibia, usually in the distal one third. Pain is often worst during or after activity (14). Pain is attributed to either irritation of the **periosteum** or bone stress reaction in the tibia (13,15). Increased plantar flexion range of motion, or differences in ankle joint range of motion, and the use of orthotics have been associated with medial tibial stress syndrome (13,14,16). Overpronation has also been linked as a risk factor, as has increased passive inversion and eversion range of motion at the ankle, internal and external rotation at the hip, and lack of muscular endurance in the calf (13). Women and individuals with decreased running or activity experience seem to be more at risk for this injury (13). There is not evidence to support intensity, distance, training surface, change in shoes, or age of shoes as risk factors (13).

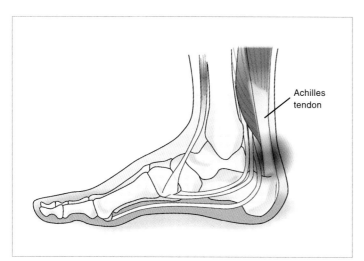

Figure 12.5   Achilles' tendonitis.

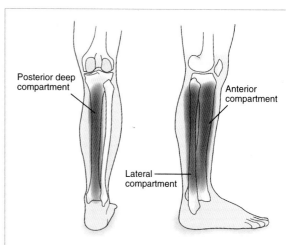

Figure 12.6   Medial tibial stress syndrome.

Ankle Sprains and Chronic Ankle Instability

Ankle sprain: an injury to the ankle ligaments in which small tears occur in the ligaments.

Chronic ankle instability: repetitive episodes of giving way at the ankle, coupled with feelings of instability.

Ankle sprains are reported to be the most common sports-related injury (17). Lateral ankle sprains are the most common type of sprain, and affect the lateral ankle ligaments, including the anterior talofibular ligament, calcaneofibular ligament, and posterior talofibular ligament (Figure 12-7) (18). Individuals who experience a lateral ankle sprain are at risk for developing chronic ankle instability (18). **Chronic ankle instability** is defined as repetitive episodes of giving way at the ankle, coupled with feelings of instability (18). Several risk factors for ankle sprain have been identified, including previous sprain (19) and decreased ankle dorsiflexion range of motion (20,21). Individuals with increased arch height and women with increased calcaneal eversion range of motion are also at increased risk for ankle sprain (22). Foot width and type, anatomic alignment, sex, and generalized joint laxity have been proposed as risk factors for ankle sprain, but there is little evidence to support these (19,22). Although strength is an important consideration in the prevention of ankle sprains, there is also limited conclusive evidence to link muscular weakness to ankle sprain (19,21,23,24). Evertor muscle weakness does not appear to be a factor in ankle sprain (23). However, invertor strength deficits may be present in those with chronic ankle instability (23,25). It has also been shown that individuals may experience hip weakness after an ankle sprain (26). Additionally, individuals with ankle instability may demonstrate arthrogenic muscle inhibition of the soleus and peroneals (27).

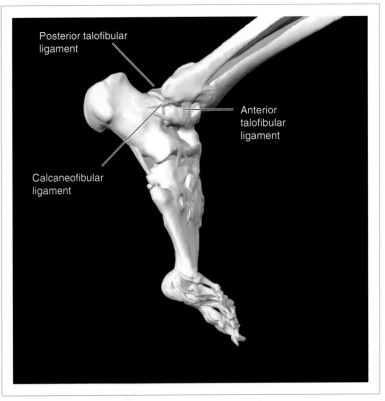

Figure 12.7 Lateral ankle ligaments.

FOOT AND ANKLE DYSFUNCTION AND THE HUMAN MOVEMENT SYSTEM CHAIN REACTION

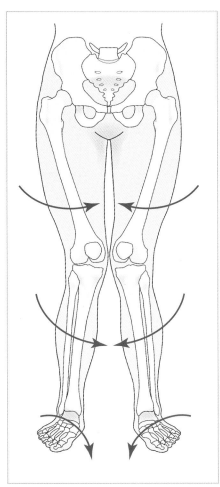

Figure 12.8 Effects of excessive foot and ankle pronation.

If the foot excessively externally rotates and/or everts (excessive pronation) during movement, the foot and ankle complex and lower leg will alter motion accordingly as components of the kinetic chain. From a mechanical perspective, foot pronation can lead to tibial rotation and femoral adduction and internal rotation (or knee valgus) (Figure 12-8) (3,28). Musculature imbalance and tightness is theorized to contribute to this position (3). Specifically, tightness of the lateral ankle musculature (lateral gastrocnemius, soleus, and peroneals) may influence tibial abduction and rotation, which can influence femoral adduction and internal rotation. If antagonistic muscles (medial gastrocnemius, anterior tibialis, and posterior tibialis) are weak, they may be unable to overcome the valgus joint positioning. This constant valgus position could potentially lead to additional tightness of the short head of the biceps femoris (tibial abduction with concomitant femoral adduction) as well as tightness in the tensor fascia latae (TFL; femoral internal rotation). The medial gastrocnemius has been identified as a dynamic stabilizer of the knee and counteracts a knee valgus moment (29). An electromyography (EMG) study of muscle electrical activity indicated that individuals with pronated feet demonstrated increased EMG amplitude in the tibialis anterior, lateral gastrocnemius, and soleus in some phases of gait, and decreased EMG for the soleus, medial gastrocnemius, and lateral gastrocnemius in others (30). When arch height was increased via an orthotic insert, increased EMG activity was noted in the vastus medialis and gluteus medius during a single-leg squat and a lateral step-down (31). It appears that pronation may have an effect on lower extremity muscle activity, and that increasing arch height (decreasing pronation) can alter that muscle activity (30).

(Text continues on page 265)

ASSESSMENT AND CORRECTIVE EXERCISES FOR FOOT AND ANKLE IMPAIRMENTS

➤ SYSTEMATIC PROCESS TO DETERMINE FOOT AND ANKLE IMPAIRMENTS

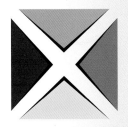

Identification of dysfunction is achieved through an integrated assessment process, which includes static posture, transitional movement assessments, dynamic movement assessments, goniometric (range of motion) measurements, and manual muscle testing (for those licensed to do so). The integrated assessment process allows the health and fitness professional to identify range of motion restrictions, muscle weakness or imbalance, and poor movement patterns. Once these deficits are identified, the corrective exercise strategy can be developed. A summary of the assessment process and common findings indicating potential dysfunction is listed below.

Continued on page 258

SAMPLE FOOT AND ANKLE ASSESSMENT PROCESS AND OBSERVATIONS	
Assessment	**Observation**
Static posture	Feet excessively pronated
Overhead squat	Feet turn out (externally rotate) or flatten (evert)
Single-leg squat	Feet flatten
Gait	Excessive lower extremity pronation
Goniometric measurement	Decreased dorsiflexion (less than 15 degrees) and/or secondary decrease in the knee extension 90/90 position (hamstring—short head of biceps femoris) and/or hip extension (TFL)
Manual muscle testing	One or more of the following muscles tested "weak": Anterior tibialis, posterior tibialis, medial gastrocnemius and/or medial hamstring; Proximally, the gluteus medius and/or gluteus maximus

STATIC POSTURE

As mentioned in chapter five, the first step in developing a corrective exercise strategy is a static postural assessment, which should be performed with the individual barefoot and in shorts. There are several methods to determine foot type and foot posture, which are beyond the scope of this book. For a general identification, feet may be divided into three categories: normal arch, **pes planus**, and **pes cavus**. Pes planus is characterized by a flattened medial longitudinal arch during weight-bearing, and pes cavus by a high medial longitudinal arch when weight-bearing. Individuals with pes planus or less than normal arch height often display increased pronation of the foot and ankle complex. Increased pronation is characterized by flattening, externally rotating, and everting of the feet, coupled with tibial internal rotation, knee valgus, and femur internal rotation (32). Hyperpronation has been associated with lower leg dysfunction and lower limb pathology. Increased hyperpronation may also cause an increased anterior pelvic tilt (hip flexion) (32), potentially leading to tightness of the hip flexor complex (iliopsoas, TFL). This malalignment may be minimized by rotating the individual's feet out of hyperpronation into a more neutral alignment.

Pes planus: a flattened medial arch during weight-bearing.

Pes cavus: a high medial arch when weight-bearing.

Hyperpronation

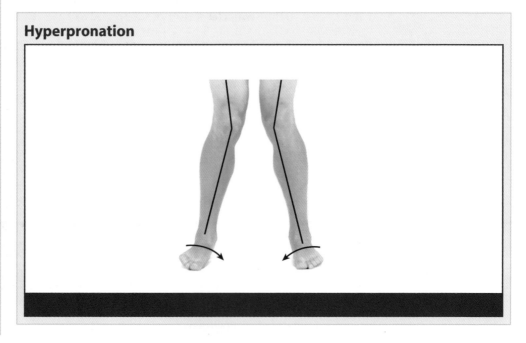

> **ORTHOTICS**
> *Some foot postures and types may benefit from an orthotic, or shoe insert, designed to cushion or realign the foot-ankle complex into neutral. Orthotics may be soft, semirigid, or rigid, depending on the foot type.*

TRANSITIONAL MOVEMENT ASSESSMENT

The second step in developing a corrective exercise strategy is a transitional movement assessment such as the overhead squat (chapter six). Health and fitness professionals should be assessing the feet to determine whether they turn out and/or flatten. This may mimic the observations from the static assessment or may be more excessive. If the knees come together during the squat (knee valgus), the individual may have decreased calf flexibility, greater hip external range of motion, and decreased plantar flexion strength (3). Based on the collective information obtained from the assessment, the health and fitness professional can begin to identify potential muscle imbalances and joint range of motion deficiencies to address. It is likely that poor performance on the transitional movement assessment is attributable to multiple factors, at multiple joints. Several structures, as well as underlying mechanical malalignment, may need to be addressed.

Transitional Movement Compensations

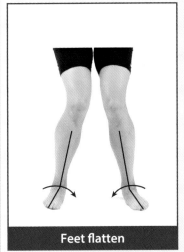

Feet flatten

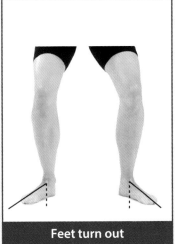

Feet turn out

DYNAMIC MOVEMENT ASSESSMENT

Dynamic movement assessments (chapter six) can also help to determine whether foot and ankle movement deficiencies exist while performing more dynamic movements such as gait. When performing a gait assessment, observe the individual's feet for flattening and/or external rotation. This may be accompanied by knee valgus. These compensations may mimic the observations from the static and transitional movement assessments or may be more excessive. This can be viewed from either an anterior or posterior view.

RANGE OF MOTION ASSESSMENTS

Once static and movement assessments are completed, range of motion assessments (chapter seven) can be performed to help identify the specific areas that need to be addressed through inhibitory and lengthening techniques. Key goniometric assessments to determine range of motion deficiencies that may be contributing to foot and ankle dysfunction include the first MTP joint (flexor hallucis longus), ankle dorsiflexion (gastrocnemius and soleus), and/or hip extension (hip flexors). Hamstring flexibility (biceps femoris, semitendinosus, and semimembranosus) may also be assessed by extending the knee when the individual is supine and the hip is flexed to 90 degrees. See chapter seven to view proper execution of these assessments and average range of motion values. Decreased range of motion at these joints may be caused by tightness of any of these muscles, which could affect the arthrokinematics of the lower extremity. Deficits and side-to-side differences in range of motion should be determined, and a stretching program provided (inhibitory and lengthening techniques) to decrease those deficits and bilateral differences.

Continued on page 260

STRENGTH ASSESSMENTS

Lastly, manual muscle tests (chapter eight) will be used to determine possible strength deficits and will help identify specific muscles that need to be activated in the corrective exercise process. Key muscles to test include the anterior and posterior tibialis, medial gastrocnemius, medial hamstring, gluteus medius, and gluteus maximus. Weakness of any of these muscles could contribute to foot and ankle dysfunction. See chapter eight to view proper execution of these assessments.

➤ SYSTEMATIC CORRECTIVE EXERCISE STRATEGIES FOR FOOT AND ANKLE IMPAIRMENTS

Once muscle weakness and range of motion deficiencies have been identified, the corrective exercise strategy can be developed using NASM's Corrective Exercise Continuum. Prevention and rehabilitation programs have proved effective at decreasing the incidence of foot and ankle injuries in physically active individuals and improving ankle function (33). Most programs also incorporate proprioceptive or balance training with or without functional movements on a daily or multiple times per week schedule. Several studies used single-leg stance exercises on a wobble board, in either a home exercise program with sport-specific balance training (34,35), or with eyes open or closed on different surfaces (36). Similarly, foam pads have been used to provide unstable surfaces to improve balance (37). Other general foot and ankle injury prevention and rehabilitation programs include restoring range of motion at the ankle, particularly in closed kinetic chain dorsiflexion using gastrocnemius and soleus muscle stretching. Strengthening of the foot and ankle musculature is also incorporated, either using resistance bands, weights, or body weight, as are functional activities like hopping, lateral movements, and cutting maneuvers (33). Programs typically progress in number of repetitions, speed, and direction over the course of several weeks (33).

The table below provides a sample programming strategy using the Corrective Exercise Continuum for foot and ankle impairment. Following are exercises that can be done for each component of the continuum to help address the issue of foot and ankle impairments. Which exercises are used will be dependent on the findings of the assessments and the individual's physical capabilities (integration exercises).

SAMPLE CORRECTIVE EXERCISE PROGRAM FOR FOOT AND ANKLE IMPAIRMENT			
Phase	**Modality**	**Muscle(s)/Exercise**	**Acute Variables**
Inhibit	SMR	Lateral gastrocnemius and peroneals Biceps femoris (short head)	Hold on tender area for 30 seconds
Lengthen	Static stretching OR **NMS**	Gastrocnemius/soleus Biceps femoris (short head)	30-second hold **OR** 7- to 10-second isometric contraction, 30-second hold
Activate	**Positional isometrics** AND/OR **isolated strengthening**	Posterior tibialis Anterior tibialis Medial hamstrings	4 reps of increasing intensity 25, 50, 75, 100% **OR** 10–15 reps with 2-second isometric hold and 4-second eccentric
Integrate*	**Integrated dynamic movement**	Step-up to balance Single-leg balance reach	10–15 reps under control

*NOTE: If client is not initially capable of performing the integrated dynamic movement exercise listed, he or she may need to be regressed to a more suitable exercise.

Step 1: Inhibit Key regions to inhibit via foam rolling include the soleus and lateral gastrocnemius, peroneals, biceps femoris, and tensor fascia latae.

Self-Myofascial Release

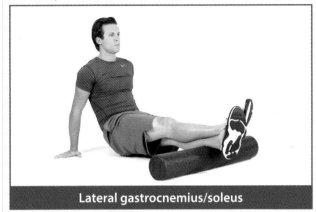

Lateral gastrocnemius/soleus

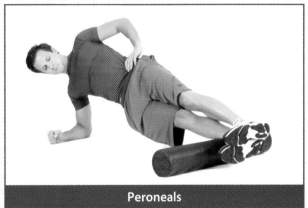

Peroneals

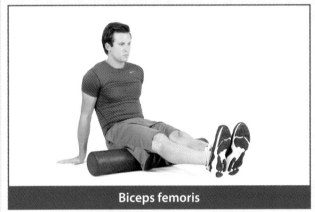

Biceps femoris

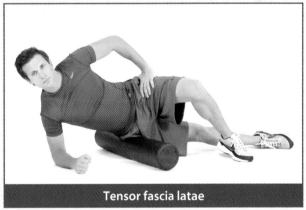

Tensor fascia latae

Step 2: Lengthen Key lengthening exercises via static or neuromuscular stretches would include the soleus and gastrocnemius, biceps femoris, and tensor fascia latae.

Static Stretches

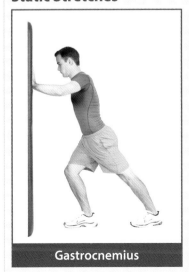

Gastrocnemius

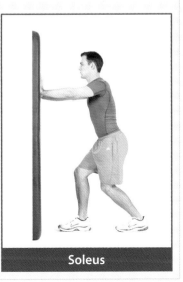

Soleus

Continued on page 262

Static Stretches

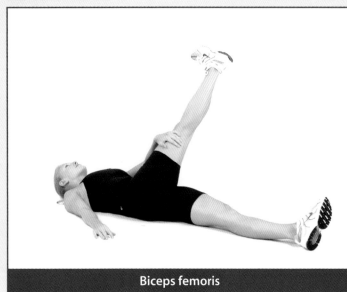

Biceps femoris

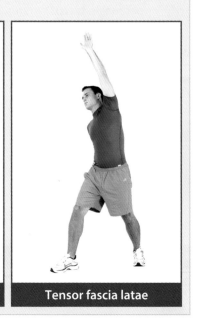

Tensor fascia latae

Neuromuscular Stretches

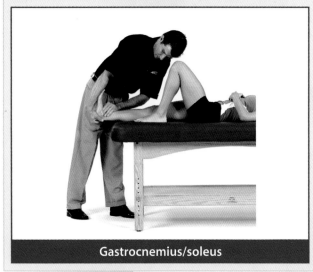

Gastrocnemius/soleus

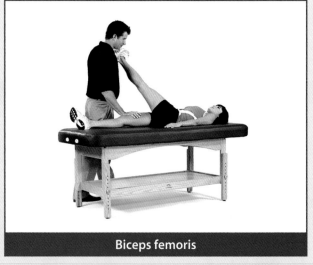

Biceps femoris

Step 3: Activate Key activation exercises via isolated strengthening exercises or positional isometrics include the toe flexors and intrinsic foot muscles, medial gastrocnemius, medial hamstrings, anterior tibialis, and posterior tibialis.

Isolated Strengthening Exercises

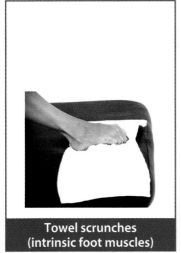

Towel scrunches (intrinsic foot muscles)

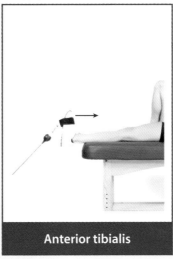

Anterior tibialis

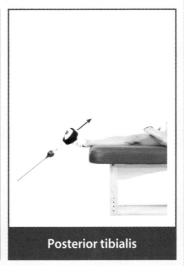

Posterior tibialis

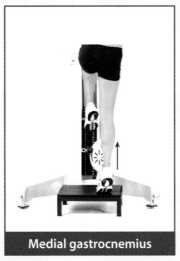

Medial gastrocnemius

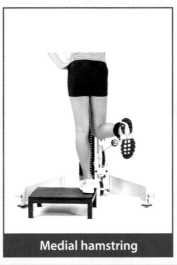

Medial hamstring

Positional Isometric Techniques

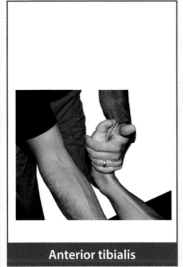

Anterior tibialis

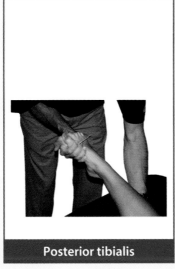

Posterior tibialis

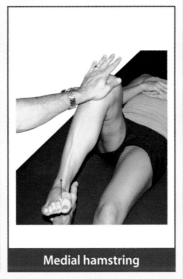

Medial hamstring

Continued on page 264

Step 4: Integration Progression

An integration progression process could first include uniplanar exercises (sagittal plane) and then progress to multiplanar exercises (frontal and transverse). Exercises can begin as more transitional (moving with no change in the base of support, such as a single-leg balance reach) to more dynamic exercises (movement with a change in the base of support, such as a step-up to balance, to a lunge to balance, to a single-leg squat).

Integrated Dynamic Movements

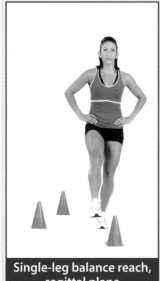

Single-leg balance reach, sagittal plane

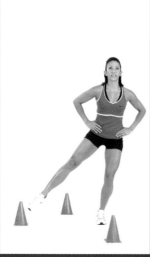

Single-leg balance reach, frontal plane

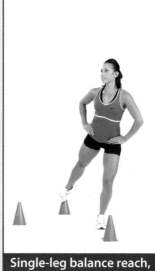

Single-leg balance reach, transverse plane

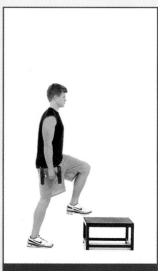

Step up to balance, start

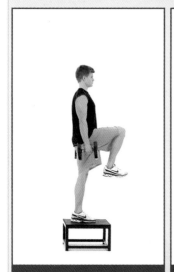

Step up to balance, finish

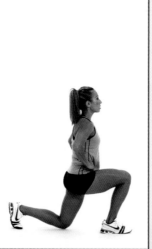

Lunge to balance, start

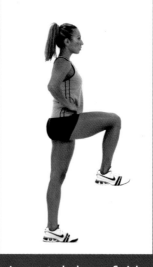

Lunge to balance, finish

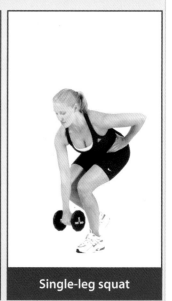

Single-leg squat

SUMMARY • The foot and ankle complex may greatly influence the entire human movement system. It must withstand a high amount of contact force through ground reactive forces, momentum, and gravity. As the body is an interconnected chain, compensation or dysfunction in one region such as the foot and ankle may lead to dysfunctions in other areas of the body. For this reason, it becomes a crucial region to assess. Symptoms that are being felt in other regions of the body could potentially be caused by dysfunction at the foot and ankle complex. If not assessed, the symptoms may be addressed, but the cause of those symptoms is not, with reoccurring injury being the result.

References

1. Powers CM. The influence of altered lower-extremity kinematics on patellofemoral joint dysfunction: a theoretical perspective. *J Orthop Sports Phys Ther* 2003;33:639–46.
2. Sahrmann S. Diagnosis and Treatment of Movement Impairment Syndromes. St. Louis. MO: Mosby; 2002.
3. Bell DR, Padua DA, Clark MA. Muscle strength and flexibility characteristics of people displaying excessive medial knee displacement. *Arch Physical Med Rehabil* 2008;89:1323–8.
4. Geraci MC, Brown W. Evidence-based treatment of hip and pelvic injuries in runners. *Phys Med Rehabil Clin N Am* 2005;16:711–47.
5. Beckman SM, Buchanan TS. Ankle inversion injury and hypermobility: effect on hip and ankle muscle electromyography onset latency. *Arch Physical Med Rehabil* 1995;76:1138–43.
6. Irving DB, Cook JL, Menz HB. Factors associated with chronic plantar heel pain: a systematic review. *J Sci Med Sport* 2006;9:11–22.
7. McPoil TG, Martin RL, Cornwall MW, Wukich DK, Irrgang JJ, Godges JJ. Heel pain-plantar fasciitis: clinical practice guidelines linked to the international classification of function, disability, and health from the orthopaedic section of the American Physical Therapy Association. *J Orthop Sports Phys Ther* 2008;38:A1–18.
8. Irving DB, Cook JL, Young MA, Menz HB. Obesity and pronated foot type may increase the risk of chronic plantar heel pain: a matched case-control study. *BMC Musculoskelet Disord* 2007;8:41.
9. Rees JD, Maffulli N, Cook J. Management of tendinopathy. *Am J Sports Med* 2009;37:1855–67.
10. Krivickas LS. Anatomical factors associated with overuse sports injuries. *Sports Med* 1997;24:132–46.
11. Kaufman KR, Brodine SK, Shaffer RA, Johnson CW, Cullison TR. The effect of foot structure and range of motion on musculoskeletal overuse injuries. *Am J Sports Med* 1999;27:585–93.
12. Azevedo LB, Lambert MI, Vaughan CL, O'Connor CM, Schwellnus MP. Biomechanical variables associated with Achilles tendinopathy in runners. *Br J Sports Med* 2008;43:288–92.
13. Moen MH, Tol JL, Weir A, Steunebrink M, De Winter TC. Medial tibial stress syndrome: a critical review. *Sports Med* 2009;39:523–46.
14. Hubbard TJ, Carpenter EM, Cordova ML. Contributing factors to medial tibial stress syndrome: a prospective investigation. *Med Sci Sports Exerc* 2009;41:490–6.
15. Tweed JL, Avil SJ, Campbell JA, Barnes MR. Etiologic factors in the development of medial tibial stress syndrome: a review of the literature. *J Am Podiatr Med Assoc* 2008;98:107–11.
16. Tweed JL, Campbell JA, Avil SJ. Biomechanical risk factors in the development of medial tibial stress syndrome in distance runners. *J Am Podiatr Med Assoc* 2008;98:436–44.
17. Fong DT, Hong Y, Chan LK, Yung PS, Chan KM. A systematic review on ankle injury and ankle sprain in sports. *Sports Med* 2007;37:73–94.
18. Hertel J. Functional anatomy, pathomechanics, and pathophysiology of lateral ankle instability. *J Athl Train* 2002;37:364–75.
19. Fong DT, Chan YY, Mok KM, Yung P, Chan KM. Understanding acute ankle ligamentous sprain injury in sports. *Sports Med Arthrosc Rehabil Ther Technol* 2009;1:14.
20. Drewes LK, McKeon PO, Casey Kerrigan D, Hertel J. Dorsiflexion deficit during jogging with chronic ankle instability. *J Sci Med Sport* 2009;12(6):685-7.
21. de Noronha M, Refshauge KM, Herbert RD, Kilbreath SL, Hertel J. Do voluntary strength, proprioception, range of motion, or postural sway predict occurrence of lateral ankle sprain? *Br J Sports Med* 2006;40:824–8.
22. Morrison KE, Kaminski TW. Foot characteristics in association with inversion ankle injury. *J Athl Train* 2007;42:135–42.
23. Holmes A, Delahunt E. Treatment of common deficits associated with chronic ankle instability. *Sports Med* 2009;39(3):207–24.
24. Kaminski TW, Hartsell HD. Factors contributing to chronic ankle instability: a strength perspective. *J Athl Train* 2002;37:394–405.
25. Sekir U, Yildiz Y, Hazneci B, Ors F, Aydin T. Effect of isokinetic training on strength, functionality and proprioception in athletes with functional ankle instability. *Knee Surg Sports Traumatol Arthrosc* 2007;15(5):654–64.
26. Friel K, McLean N, Myers C, Caceres M. Ipsilateral hip abductor weakness after inversion ankle sprain. *J Athl Train* 2006;41(1):74–8.
27. McVey ED, Palmieri RM, Docherty CL, Zinder SM, Ingersoll CD. Arthrogenic muscle inhibition in the leg

muscles of subjects exhibiting functional ankle instability. *Foot Ankle Int* 2005;26:1055–61.

28. Gross MT. Lower quarter screening for skeletal malalignment: suggestions for orthotics and shoewear. *J Orthop Sports Phys Ther* 1995;21:389–405.

29. Lloyd DG, Buchanan TS. Strategies of muscular support of varus and valgus isometric loads at the human knee. *J Biomech* 2001;34:1257–67.

30. Murley GS, Landorf KB, Menz HB, Bird AR. Effect of foot posture, foot orthoses and footwear on lower limb muscle activity during walking and running: a systematic review. *Gait Posture* 2009;29(2):172–87.

31. Hertel J, Sloss BR, Earl JE. Effect of foot orthotics on quadriceps and gluteus medius electromyographic activity during selected exercises. *Arch Physical Med Rehabil* 2005;86:26–30.

32. Khamis S, Yizhar Z. Effect of feet hyperpronation on pelvic alignment in a standing position. *Gait Posture* 2007;25:127–34.

33. Hale SA, Hertel J, Olmsted-Kramer LC. The effect of a 4-week comprehensive rehabilitation program on postural control and lower extremity function in individuals with chronic ankle instability. *J Orthop Sports Phys Ther* 2007;37:303–11.

34. Emery CA, Rose MS, McAllister JR, et al. A prevention strategy to reduce the incidence of injury in high school basketball: a cluster randomized controlled trial. *Clin J Sports Med* 2007;17:17–24.

35. McGuine TA, Keene JS. The effect of a balance training program on the risk of ankle sprains in high school athletes. *Am J Sports Med* 2006;34:1103–11.

36. Mohammadi F. Comparison of 3 preventive methods to reduce the recurrence of ankle inversion sprains in male soccer players. *Am J Sports Med* 2007;35:922–6.

37. McHugh MP, Tyler TF, Mirabella MR, et al. The effectiveness of a balance training intervention in reducing the incidence of noncontact ankle sprains in high school football players. *Am J Sports Med* 2007;35:1289–94.

Corrective Strategies for Knee Impairments

INTRODUCTION

LOWER-EXTREMITY injuries account for more than 50% of injuries in college (1) and high school athletes (2), and among lower-extremity injuries, the knee is one of the most commonly injured regions of the body. Researchers have estimated health-care costs to be approximately $2.5 billion annually for anterior cruciate ligament (ACL) injuries (3). To prevent these injuries from occurring and allow for individuals to maintain healthy and physically active lifestyles, it is important to understand the anatomy, causes, and most appropriate corrective exercise strategies for prevention and management. This chapter will review each of these components as they relate to the knee.

REVIEW OF KNEE FUNCTIONAL ANATOMY

The knee is a part of a kinetic chain that is greatly affected by the linked segments from the proximal and distal joints. The foot and ankle and the lumbo-pelvic-hip complex (LPHC) play a major role in knee impairment, as the structures that help to form the ankle and hip joints make up the knee joint. This region is a prime example of how alterations in other joints within the human movement system can dramatically affect the movement and increase the stress and injury capacity of another joint, which leads to knee impairments.

Bones and Joints

Looking at the knee region specifically (Figure 13-1), the tibia and femur make up the tibiofemoral joint, and the patella and femur make up the patellofemoral joint. The fibula is also noted as it is the attachment site of the biceps femoris, which crosses and affects the knee.

Proximally, the femur and the pelvis make up the iliofemoral joint, and the sacrum and pelvis make up the sacroiliac joint (Figure 13-2). Collectively, these structures anchor the proximal myofascial tissues. These bones and joints are of importance in corrective exercise because they will also have a functional impact on the arthrokinematics of the knee.

Distally, the tibia and fibula help form the talocrural (ankle) joint (Figure 13-3). Collectively, these structures anchor the distal myofascial tissues of the knee. These bones and joints are of importance in corrective exercise because they will also have a functional impact on the arthrokinematics of the knee.

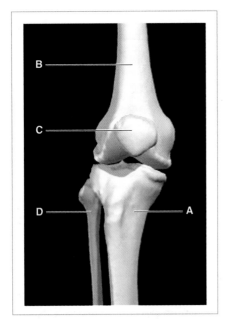

Figure 13.1 Bones of the knee. (A) Tibia. (B) Femur. (C) Patella. (D) Fibula.

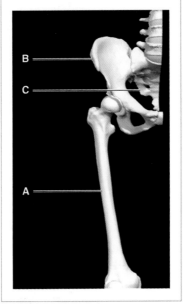

Figure 13.2 Proximal bones affecting the knee. (A) Femur. (B) Pelvis. (C) Sacrum.

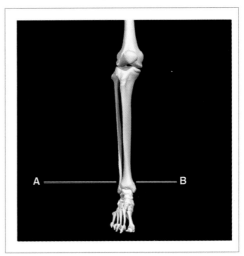

Figure 13.3 Distal bones affecting the knee. (A) Distal fibula. (B) Distal tibia.

Muscles

There are a number of muscles in the lower leg and lumbo-pelvic-hip complex whose function may be related to the knee (Table 13-1). It is important to restore and maintain normal range of motion and strength, and eliminate any muscle inhibition, to ensure joints are operating optimally. See chapter two for a detailed review of the location and function of these muscles.

Table 13.1 KEY MUSCLES ASSOCIATED WITH THE KNEE	
• Gastrocnemius/soleus	• Tensor fascia latae/IT-band
• Adductor complex	• Quadriceps
• Medial and lateral hamstring complex	• Gluteus medius and maximus

COMMON KNEE INJURIES AND ASSOCIATED MOVEMENT DEFICIENCIES

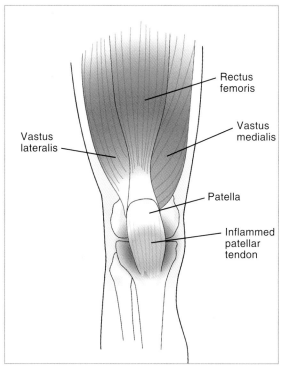

Figure 13.4 Patellar tendinopathy.

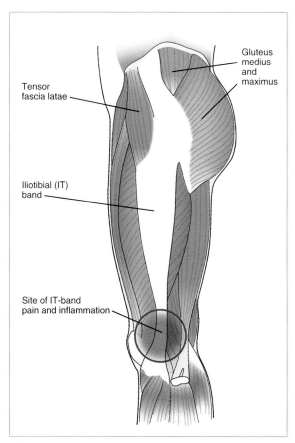

Figure 13.5 IT-band syndrome.

Patellar Tendinopathy (Jumper's Knee)

Patellar tendinopathy is a common overuse injury (Figure 13-4). It occurs when an individual places repeated stress on the patellar tendon. The stress results in tiny tears in the tendon, which may cause necrotic degenerative change or inflammation in the tendon and pain.

Patellar tendinopathy is an injury common with, but not limited to, athletes, particularly those participating in jumping sports such as basketball (4–8), volleyball (7–10), or long jumping (7,10). Risk factors for patellar tendinopathy include the following (4,10–12):

- Knee valgus and varus
- An increased Q-angle
- Poor quadriceps and hamstring complex flexibility
- Poor eccentric deceleration capabilities
- Overtraining and playing on hard surfaces

Iliotibial Band (IT-Band) Syndrome (Runner's Knee)

Iliotibial band syndrome (ITBS) is the result of inflammation and irritation of the distal portion of the iliotibial tendon as it rubs against the lateral femoral condyle (Figure 13-5), or less commonly, the greater trochanter of the hip, causing a greater trochanteric bursitis. Inflammation and irritation of the iliotibial band (ITB) may occur because of a lack of flexibility of the tensor fascia latae (TFL), which can result in an increase in tension on the ITB during the stance phase of running.

Iliotibial band syndrome (ITBS) typically is caused by overuse. The injury is most commonly reported in runners as a result of abnormal gait or running biomechanics (13–17), although other athletes (e.g., cyclists, tennis players) also may be affected. Weakness of muscle groups in the kinetic chain may also result in the development of ITBS. Weakness in the hip abductor muscles, such as the gluteus medius, may result in synergistic dominance of the TFL (increasing frontal plane instability). This in turn may lead to increased tension of the ITB and thus increased friction on the tissue, with inflammation being the end result.

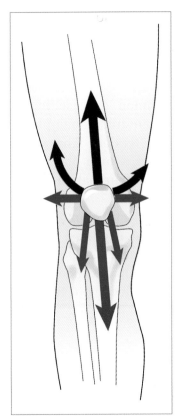

Figure 13.6 Patellofemoral syndrome.

Patellofemoral Syndrome

One of the most commonly accepted causes of patellofemoral syndrome (PFS) is abnormal tracking of the patella within the femoral trochlea (Figure 13-6). When the patella is not properly aligned within the femoral trochlea, the stress per unit area on the patellar cartilage increases owing to a smaller contact area between the patella and the trochlea (4). Abnormal tracking of the patella may be attributable to static (i.e., increased Q-angle) or dynamic lower-extremity malalignment (i.e., increased femoral rotation, adduction, and knee valgus), altered muscle activation of surrounding knee musculature, decreased strength of the hip musculature, or various combinations (5–8).

Anterior Cruciate Ligament (ACL) Injury

Beyond the common injuries indicated that are more chronic in onset, recent studies also indicate that altered lower-extremity neuromusculoskeletal control imbalances can increase the risk of acute injures such as ACL ruptures (Figure 13-7) (9–12). Specifically, peak landing forces were significantly predicted by valgus torques at the knee, women demonstrated decreased relative knee flexor torque during landing compared with men, and women had greater side-to-side differences in normalized hamstring complex peak torque (13). Insufficient neuromusculoskeletal control of lower limb biomechanics, particularly frontal plane control of the knee joint, leads to high-risk patterns in female athletes during execution of common, albeit potentially hazardous, movements (12). These sex differences are evident during landing and cutting in soccer and basketball athletes (14,15). Female athletes also have significant differences between their dominant and nondominant sides in maximum valgus knee angle (14,15).

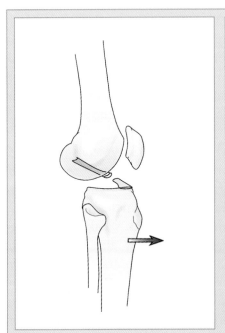

Figure 13.7A Anterior force.

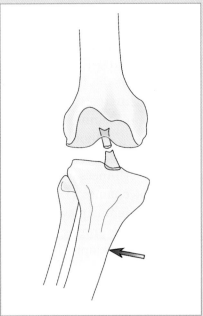

Figure 13.7B Lateral force.

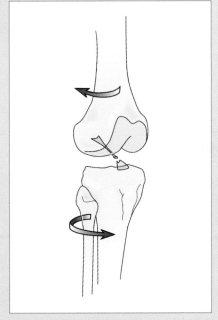

Figure 13.7C Rotational force.

These differences in valgus measures (ligament dominance) and limb-to-limb asymmetries (leg dominance) reflect neuromusculoskeletal control deficits that may be indicative of decreased dynamic knee joint control in female athletes (14).

Subsequent studies systematically evaluated more proximal neuromusculoskeletal control deficits at the hip and trunk to help determine potential contributing mechanisms to high-risk knee mechanics during landing (16,17). When performing single-leg landing tasks, female athletes demonstrated increased trunk flexion and lateral tilt range of motion. In addition to greater knee abduction angles, female athletes had increased hip frontal plane excursion compared with men during both types of landings (18). The increased hip adduction motion seen in the frontal plane during athletic activities likely contributes to the dynamic valgus knee position that may place the athlete at increased risk of knee injury (17–20).

(Text continues on page 288)

ASSESSMENT AND CORRECTIVE EXERCISE STRATEGIES FOR KNEE IMPAIRMENTS

➤ SYSTEMATIC PROCESS TO DETERMINE KNEE IMPAIRMENTS

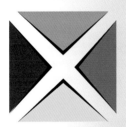

The first step in developing a corrective exercise strategy for knee impairments is an integrated assessment process. On the basis of the information obtained from these assessments collectively, the neuromusculoskeletal control deficits can be identified for targeted treatments. A summary of the assessment process for knee impairments and common findings indicating potential dysfunction are listed below.

SAMPLE KNEE ASSESSMENT PROCESS AND OBSERVATIONS	
Assessment	**Observation**
Static Posture	Pronation distortion syndrome (tibial and femoral adduction and internal rotation)
Overhead Squat	Knees move inward (adduct and internally rotate) Knees move outward (abduct and externally rotate)
Single-leg Squat	Knee moves inward (adduct and internally rotate)
Tuck Jump Assessment	Knee and thigh deficits (i.e., excessive knee valgus on landing)
	Foot placement deficits and poor landing technique
Goniometric Measurement	Decreased dorsiflexion (less than 15°) Decreased knee extension in 90/90 position (hamstring complex–biceps femoris) Decreased hip extension (TFL) Decreased hip internal rotation (biceps femoris, piriformis, and/or adductor magnus)
Manual Muscle Testing	One or more of the following muscles tested "weak": Anterior/posterior tibialis, gluteus medius and/or maximus, medial hamstring complex, adductors (knees move outward during overhead squat)

Continued on page 272

STATIC POSTURE

A key static postural distortion syndrome to look for to determine potential movement dysfunction at the knee is the pronation distortion syndrome. As mentioned in chapter five, this is characterized as possessing flat feet with knee valgus (tibial and femoral adduction and internal rotation). This position of the knee can place excessive stress on the muscles and connective tissue associated with the joint during dynamic movement.

Pronation Distortion Syndrome

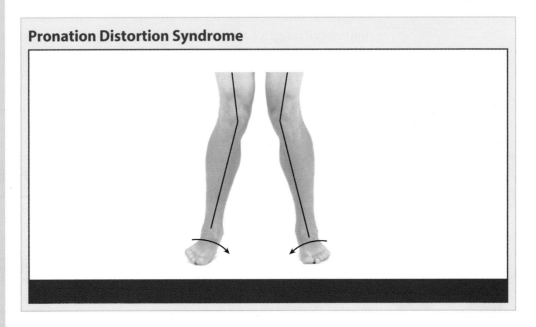

TRANSITIONAL MOVEMENT ASSESSMENTS

When performing the overhead squat, the key movement compensations to look for with knee dysfunction includes the knee moving inward (knee valgus) or outward (knee varus).

Compensations During Overhead Squat

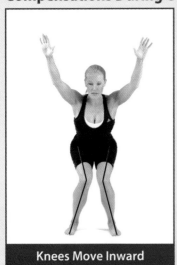
Knees Move Inward

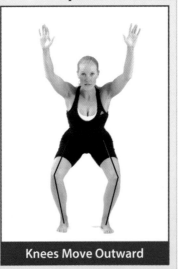
Knees Move Outward

The knee moving inward during the overhead squat (excessive compensatory pronation) may be indicative of calf, TFL/IT-band, and adductor tightness as well as anterior tibialis, posterior tibialis, and/or gluteus medius and gluteus maximus weakness. Because this compensation could be a result of lower leg and/or hip dysfunction, using the modified version of the overhead squat with the heels elevated would be warranted to determine whether the primary cause is coming from the lower leg or from the hip. As described in chapter six, if the compensation improves with the heels elevated (putting the gastrocnemius and soleus in "slack"), then the primary focus may be at the hip (weakness). If the compensation does not improve with the heels elevated, then the primary area to address may be the foot and ankle complex or the foot and ankle complex and hip in combination. Performing further assessments can help isolate the target area(s).

If the knees move outward during an overhead squat assessment, this may be indicative of tightness in the lateral gastrocnemius/soleus, piriformis, and biceps femoris (externally rotates the tibia and femur) and weakness of the adductors and medial hamstring complex (adducts and internally rotates the femur and tibia).

The single-leg squat is also an important transitional assessment to perform to assess potential injury risks at the knee joint. Having to squat on one leg may show dysfunction not evident when squatting on two feet. Like the overhead squat, the key compensation to look for when performing the single-leg squat is whether the knee moves inward.

Compensation During Single-Leg Squat, Knee Moves Inward

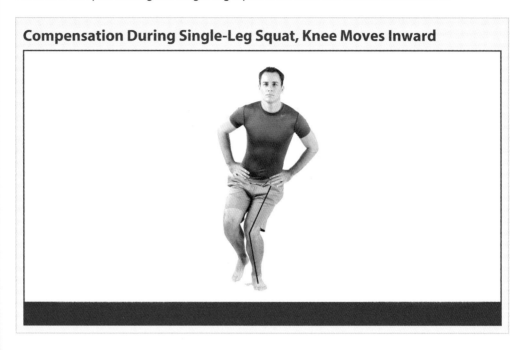

DYNAMIC MOVEMENT ASSESSMENTS

The tuck jump exercise may be useful to the health and fitness professional for the identification of lower-extremity technical flaws during a plyometric activity (19,21). The tuck jump requires a high level of effort from the individual, which may allow a health and fitness professional to readily identify potential deficits, especially during the first few repetitions when the individual places most of his or her cognitive efforts solely on the performance of this difficult jump (19,21). In addition, the tuck jump exercise may be used to assess improvement in lower-extremity biomechanics as the individual progresses through training (19,21).

Tuck Jump Assessment

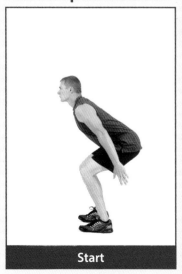

Start

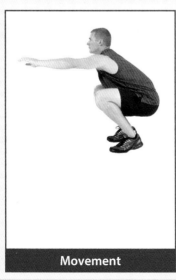

Movement

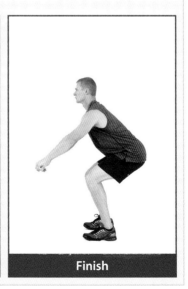

Finish

Continued on page 274

The below figure provides the "health and fitness professional friendly" landing assessment tool that the health and fitness professional may use to monitor an individual's technical performance of the tuck jump before, during, and after training. As reviewed in chapter six, the individual is instructed to perform repeated tuck jumps for 10 seconds, while the health and fitness professional visually grades the outlined criteria (19). To improve the ease of the assessment, a standard two-dimensional camera in the frontal and sagittal planes may be used to assist the health and fitness professional. The individual's technique should be subjectively graded as either having an apparent deficit (checked) or not. Indicators of flawed techniques should be noted for each individual and should be the focus of feedback during subsequent training sessions (19). The individual's baseline performance can be compared with repeated assessments performed at the midpoint and conclusion of training protocols to objectively track improvement with jumping and landing technique. Empiric laboratory evidence suggests that individuals who do not improve their scores, or who demonstrate six or more flawed techniques, should be targeted for further technique training (19).

Tuck Jump Assessment Chart

Tuck Jump Assessment	Pre	Mid	Post	Comments
Knee and Thigh Motion				
(1) Lower extremity valgus at landing	☐	☐	☐	
(2) Thighs do not reach parallel (peak of jump)	☐	☐	☐	
(3) Thighs do not equal side-to-side (during flight)	☐	☐	☐	
Foot Position During Landing				
(4) Foot placement not shoulder width apart	☐	☐	☐	
(5) Foot placement not parallel (front to back)	☐	☐	☐	
(6) Foot contact timing not equal	☐	☐	☐	
(7) Excessive landing contact noise	☐	☐	☐	
Plyometric Technique				
(8) Pause between jumps	☐	☐	☐	
(9) Technique declines prior to 10 seconds	☐	☐	☐	
(10) Does not land in same footprint (excessive in-flight motion)	☐	☐	☐	
	Total _____	Total _____	Total _____	

One specific area that the health and fitness professional should focus on when training to prevent ACL injury risk is the correction of lower-extremity valgus at landing and improvement of side-to-side differences in lower-extremity movements, which are both target deficits to be assessed with the tuck jump assessment tool (12,19). The tuck jump assessment tool can be used to improve these high-risk techniques during an exercise that requires a high effort level from the individual (19). If individuals can improve their neuromusculoskeletal control and biomechanics during this difficult jump and landing sequence, they may gain dynamic neuromusculoskeletal control of the lower extremity and create a learned skill that can be transferred to competitive play (if performing with an athlete) and ultimately reduces their injury risk (12,19).

If an individual does not have the capabilities to perform the tuck jump assessment, a basic gait analysis can also be performed as a dynamic movement assessment, looking for overpronation of the foot and excessive knee valgus.

RANGE OF MOTION ASSESSMENTS

Once static and movement assessments are completed, range of motion assessments (chapter seven) can be performed to help identify the specific areas that need to be addressed through inhibitory and lengthening techniques. Key goniometric assessments to determine range of motion deficiencies that may be contributing to knee dysfunction include ankle dorsiflexion (gastrocnemius/soleus) and hip extension (TFL). Hamstring complex flexibility (biceps femoris, semitendinosus, and semimembranosus) may also be assessed by extending the knee when the individual is supine and the hip flexed to 90°. Lastly, hip internal rotation can also be assessed to determine transverse plane extensibility of the biceps femoris, adductor magnus, and piriformis, particularly if the knees move outward during an overhead squat assessment. See chapter seven to view proper execution of these assessments and average range of motion values.

STRENGTH ASSESSMENTS

Lastly, manual muscle tests (chapter eight) are suggested to be used to determine possible strength deficits and will help identify specific muscles that need to be activated in the corrective exercise process. Key muscles to test include the medial gastrocnemius, medial hamstring complex, gluteus medius, and gluteus maximus. Medial hamstring complex and adductor weakness may also need to be assessed if the knees move outward during the overhead squat assessment. Weakness of any of these muscles could contribute to knee dysfunction. See chapter eight to view proper execution of these assessments.

➤ SYSTEMATIC CORRECTIVE EXERCISE STRATEGIES FOR KNEE IMPAIRMENTS

Neuromusculoskeletal control imbalances are often evident in adolescent female athletes, which include ligament dominance (decreased lower-extremity frontal plane stability), quadriceps dominance (decreased relative strength or recruitment of the posterior chain musculature), and leg dominance (limb-to-limb asymmetries in neuromusculoskeletal control or muscle recruitment) (21). To target ligament dominance deficits, the health and fitness professional should instruct the individual to use the knee as a single-plane (sagittal) hinge joint allowing flexion and extension, not valgus and varus motion at the knee (21). The health and fitness professional should also use training movements that will facilitate both identification and correction of unwanted knee motions in the frontal plane. Teaching dynamic control of knee motion in the sagittal plane may be achieved through progressive exercises that challenge the neuromusculoskeletal system (21). To target the deficits described as ligament dominance, the health and fitness professional must first make the individual aware of proper form and technique as well as undesirable and potentially dangerous positions. To achieve this awareness, individuals can be videotaped or placed in front of a mirror to improve their awareness of undesirable medial knee alignments during movement (21). Second, the health and fitness professional must be diligent in providing adequate feedback of correct technical performance to facilitate the desirable neuromusculoskeletal alterations. If inadequate or inappropriate feedback is provided, then the individual may be reinforcing improper techniques with the neuromusculoskeletal training (21).

Continued on page 276

Before teaching the dynamic movement exercises, individuals should be shown the proper athletic position. The athletic position is a functionally stable position with the knees comfortably flexed, shoulders back, eyes up, feet approximately shoulder-width apart, and the body mass balanced over the balls of the feet. The knees should be over the balls of the feet, and the chest should be over the knees (13,21). This is the individual's ready position and should be the starting and finishing position for most of the training exercises.

Athletic Position

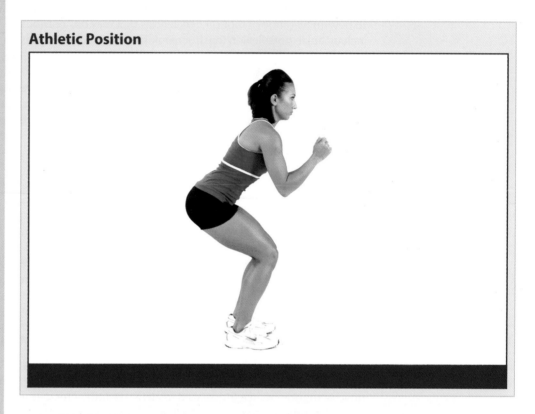

Wall jumps are an example of an integrated dynamic movement exercise that could be used to target ligament dominance deficits. This low-to-moderate intensity jump movement allows the health and fitness professional to begin analysis of the athlete's degree of valgus or varus motion in the knee (21). During wall jumps, the individual does not go through deep knee flexion angles, with most of the vertical movement provided by active ankle plantar flexion (21). The relatively straight knee makes even slight amounts of medial knee motion easy to identify visually. When medial knee motion is observed, the health and fitness professional should begin to give verbal feedback cues to the individual during this low-to-moderate intensity exercise (21). This feedback allows the athlete to cognitively process the proper knee motion required to perform the exercise. Neuromusculoskeletal control of medial knee motion is critical when landing with knee angles close to full extension, as this is a commonly reported mechanism of injury (22).

Wall Jumps

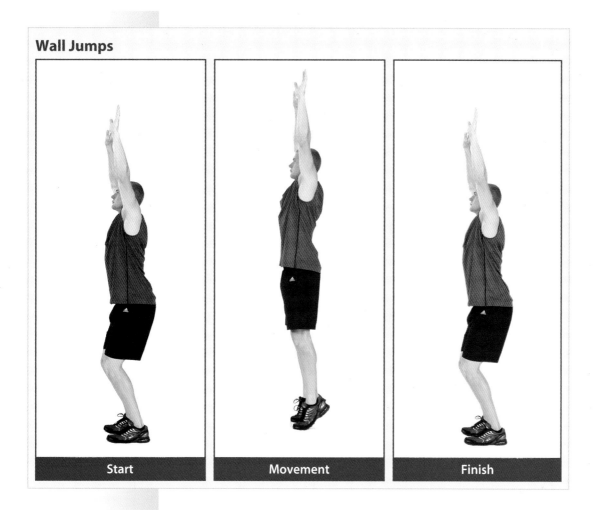

| Start | Movement | Finish |

Another useful exercise to target the ligament-dominant individual is the tuck jump (as shown earlier in the chapter). Although used as an assessment, the tuck jump can also be used as an exercise that is on the opposite end of the intensity spectrum from the wall jump and requires a high level of effort from the individual. During the tuck jump exercise, the health and fitness professional can quickly identify an individual who may demonstrate abnormal levels of frontal plane knee displacement during jumping and landing because the individual usually devotes minimal attention to technique on the first few repetitions (21). As mentioned earlier, tuck jumps can also be used to assess improvements in lower-extremity biomechanics (19).

The long jump and hold exercise allows the health and fitness professional to assess the individual's knee motion while he or she progresses through movements in the sagittal plane (21). The achievement of dynamic knee control during tasks performed in all planes of movement is critical to address deficits that may transfer into competitive sports participation or everyday activities. During competition, athletes may display "active valgus," a position of hip adduction and knee abduction that is the result of muscular contraction rather than ground reaction forces (21). The long jump is a moderate-intensity integrated dynamic movement exercise that can provide another opportunity for the health and fitness professional to assess active valgus and provide feedback on more desirable techniques, which can assist the individual's cognitive recognition during each jump to perfect technique. When performing the long jump exercise, individuals may demonstrate active valgus when taking off from a jump rather than landing. This movement deficit should be identified and corrected during training. In addition, individuals should

Continued on page 278

Long Jump and Hold

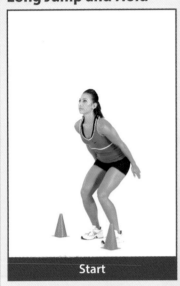

Start | Finish

be instructed to hold the landing (stabilize) for 5 seconds, which forces the individual to gain and maintain dynamic knee control for a more prolonged period (21). The prolonged deep hold may facilitate feedback-driven lower-extremity alignment adjustments and ultimately improved frontal plane alignment of the knee.

The 180° jump is an integrated dynamic movement exercise that is incorporated into dynamic movement training to teach dynamic body and lower-extremity control while the body is rotating in the transverse plane. The rotational forces created by the 180° jump must be quickly absorbed and redirected in the opposite direction (21). This movement is important to teach the individual to recognize and control dangerous rotational forces that can improve body awareness and control that will reduce injury risk and also improve measures of performance (13,21,23).

180° Jump

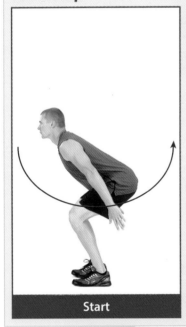
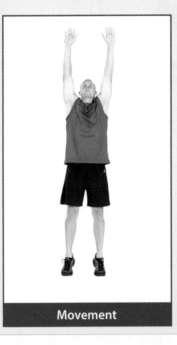
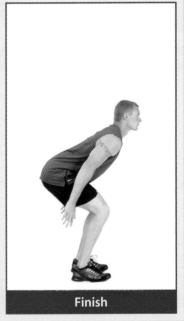

Start | Movement | Finish

Once the individual has been trained to maintain appropriate knee alignment during the jump, land, and hold of the long jump exercise with double-leg stance, the single-leg hop and hold exercise can be incorporated into the training (21). Most noncontact ACL injuries occur when landing or decelerating on a single limb (24). The single-leg hop and hold exercise roughly mimics a mechanism of an ACL injury during competitive play (21). When initiating the single-leg hop and hold exercise, the individual should be instructed to jump only a few inches and land with deep knee flexion. As he or she masters the low-intensity jumps, the distance can be progressively increased, as long as he or she can

Single-Leg Hop and Hold

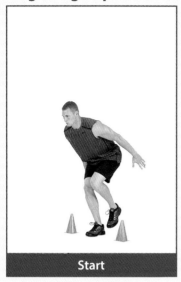
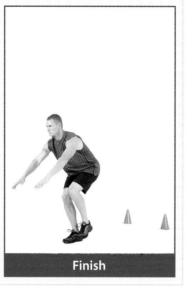

| Start | Finish |

continue to maintain deep knee flexion when landing and control unwanted frontal plane motion at the knee (21). Proper progression into the single-leg hop and hold is critical to ensure individual safety during training (21). This point is salient for the health and fitness professional, as ACL injury prevention techniques should not introduce inappropriate risk of injury during training.

The end stages of training targeted toward ligament-dominance deficits is achieved through the use of unanticipated cutting movements. Before teaching unanticipated cutting, individuals should first be able to attain proper athletic position proficiently (21). This ready position is the goal position to achieve before initiating a directional cut. Adding the directional cues to the unanticipated part of training can be as simple as pointing or as sports-specific as using partner mimic or ball retrieval drills (21).

Cutting Maneuvers

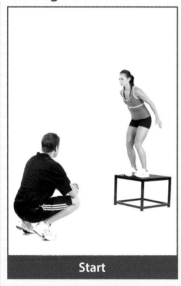
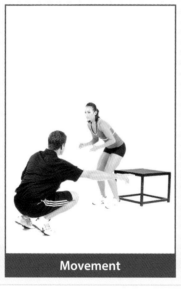
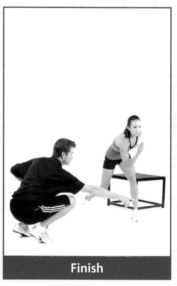

| Start | Movement | Finish |

Single-faceted sagittal plane training and conditioning protocols that do not incorporate cutting maneuvers will not provide similar levels of external varus or valgus or rotational loads that are seen during sport-specific cutting maneuvers (21,25). Training programs that incorporate safe levels of varus or valgus stress may induce more muscle-dominant neuromusculoskeletal adaptations (26). Such adaptations may prepare the individual for the multidirectional movement demands that occur during sport competition, which can improve performance and reduce risk of lower-extremity injury (12,13,21,23,27,28). Research has shown that female athletes perform cutting techniques with decreased knee flexion and increased valgus angles (15,21,29). Knee valgus loads can double when performing unanticipated cutting maneuvers similar to those used in sport (21,30). Thus the end point of training designed to reduce ACL loading via valgus torques can be gained through training the athlete to use movement techniques that produce low frontal plane knee loads (26). Recent evidence demonstrates that training which

Continued on page 280

incorporates unanticipated movements can reduce knee joint loads and lower-extremity injury risk (12,23,31). Additionally, training individuals to preactivate their musculature before ground contact may facilitate kinematic adjustments, reducing the potential for increased knee loads (21,30,32,33). Training the individual to use safe cutting techniques in unanticipated sport situations or everyday activities may also help impart technique adaptations that will integrate into the athlete's competitive movements during sport competition or during activities of daily living. If naturally ligament-dominant individuals achieve muscular (sagittal) -dominant movement strategies, their future risk of ACL and other knee injuries will likely be reduced (13,21,28).

It is important to note that not all individuals will have the physical capabilities to perform many of the aforementioned jump task progressions. In this situation, a basic functional movement progression that incorporates total body integration in multiple planes can be used as integrated dynamic movements. This progression could begin with ball squats, then to step-ups, then to lunges, then to single-leg squats (from more stable/less dynamic to more unstable/more dynamic). For each exercise, it will be important to cue the individual to keep the knee(s) in line with the toes and to not allow the knee to move inside or outside of the foot to ensure proper arthrokinematics and neuromuscular control.

Functional Movement Progressions

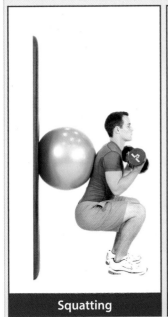

Squatting

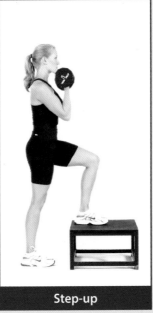

Step-up

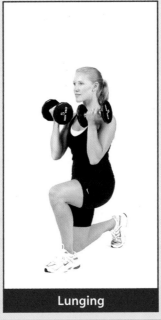

Lunging

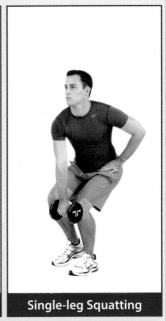

Single-leg Squatting

The following table provides a sample programming strategy using the Corrective Exercise Continuum for knee impairments. The photos illustrate the exercises that can be done for each component of the continuum to help address the issue of knee impairments (knees move inward and knees move outward). Which exercises are used will be dependent on the findings of the assessments and the individual's physical capabilities (integration exercises).

SAMPLE CORRECTIVE EXERCISE PROGRAM FOR KNEE IMPAIRMENT

Phase	Modality	Muscle(s)/Exercise	Acute Variables
Inhibit	SMR	Gastrocnemius/soleus, adductors, TFL/IT-band, biceps femoris (short head) Piriformis (knee moves out during overhead squat)	Hold on tender area for 30 seconds
Lengthen	**Static stretching** OR **NMS**	Gastrocnemius/soleus, adductors, TFL, biceps femoris Piriformis (knee moves out during overhand squat)	30-second hold **OR** 7–10-second isometric contraction, 30-second hold
Activate	**Positional isometrics** AND/ OR **isolated strengthening**	Anterior/posterior tibialis, gluteus medius, gluteus maximus Adductors and medial hamstring complex (knee moves out during overhead squat)	4 reps of increasing intensity 25, 50, 75, 100% **OR** 10–15 reps with 2-second isometric hold and 4-second eccentric contraction
Integrate	**Integrated dynamic movement**	Jumping progression* Functional movement progression: • Ball squats • Step-ups • Lunges • Single-leg squat	10–15 reps under control

***NOTE:** Use the functional movement progression if the individual cannot perform jumping progressions.

KNEE IMPAIRMENT: KNEE MOVES INWARD

Step 1: Inhibit Key regions to inhibit via foam rolling include the gastrocnemius/soleus, adductors, TFL/IT-band, and the short head of the biceps femoris.

Self-Myofascial Release

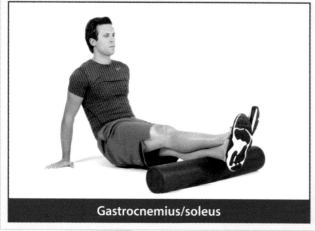

Gastrocnemius/soleus

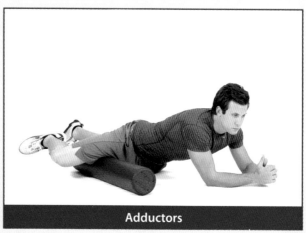

Adductors

Continued on page 282

Self-Myofascial Release

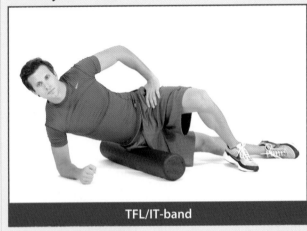

TFL/IT-band

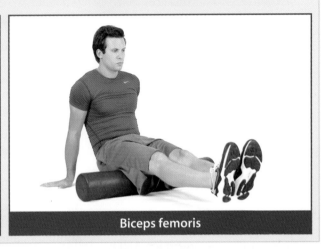

Biceps femoris

Step 2: Lengthen Key lengthening exercises via static and/or neuromuscular stretches would include the gastrocnemius/soleus, adductors, TFL, and biceps femoris (short head).

Static Stretches

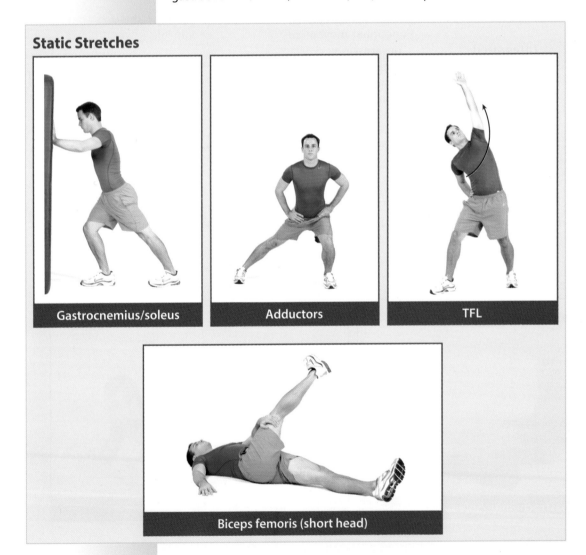

Gastrocnemius/soleus

Adductors

TFL

Biceps femoris (short head)

Neuromuscular Stretches

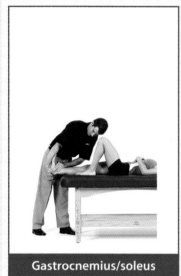

Gastrocnemius/soleus

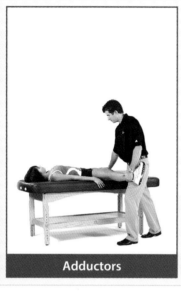

Adductors

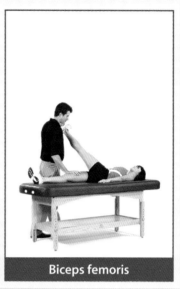

Biceps femoris

Step 3: Activate   Key activation exercises via isolated strengthening exercises and/or positional isometrics include the anterior tibialis, posterior tibialis, gluteus medius, and gluteus maximus.

Isolated Strengthening Exercises

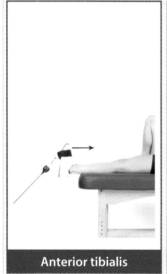

Anterior tibialis

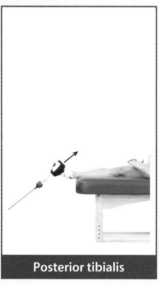

Posterior tibialis

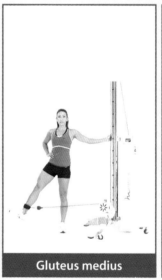

Gluteus medius

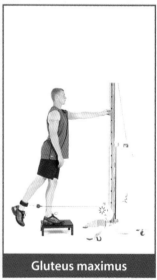

Gluteus maximus

Continued on page 284

Positional Isometric Techniques

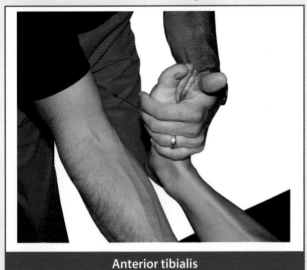

Anterior tibialis

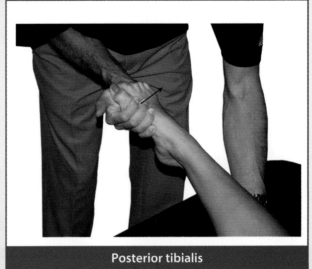

Posterior tibialis

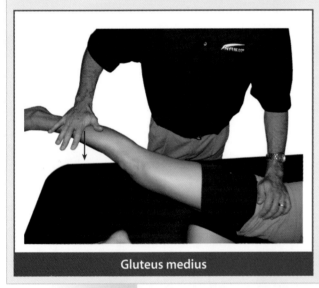

Gluteus medius

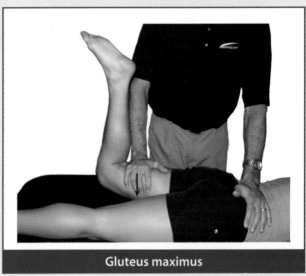

Gluteus maximus

Step 4: Integration Progression

An integration progression could progress by starting with wall jumps, then progress to tuck jumps, then to long jumps with two feet, then to 180° jumps, then to single-leg hops, then to cutting maneuvers (as shown earlier in the chapter). If the individual cannot perform these tasks, use the functional movement progression also shown earlier in the chapter.

Step 1: Inhibit Key regions to inhibit via foam rolling include the gastrocnemius/soleus, piriformis, and biceps femoris (long head).

Self-Myofascial Release

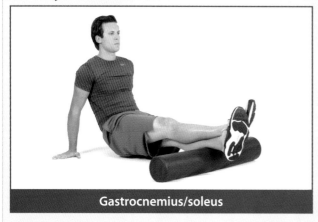

Gastrocnemius/soleus

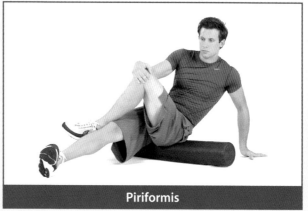

Piriformis

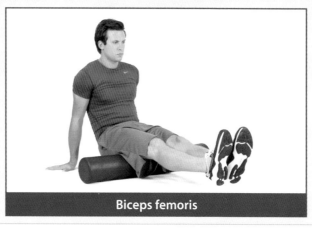

Biceps femoris

Step 2: Lengthen Key lengthening exercises via static and/or neuromuscular stretches would include the gastrocnemius/soleus, piriformis, and biceps femoris (long head).

Continued on page 286

Static Stretches

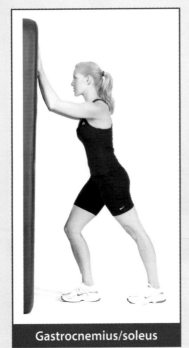

Gastrocnemius/soleus

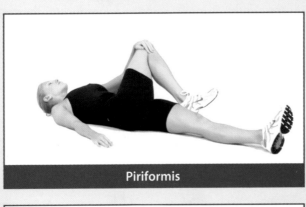

Piriformis

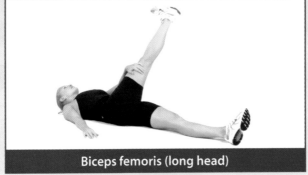

Biceps femoris (long head)

Neuromuscular Stretches

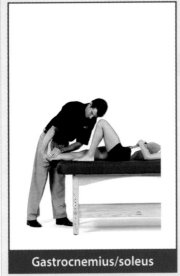

Gastrocnemius/soleus

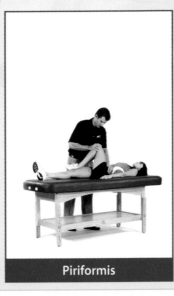

Piriformis

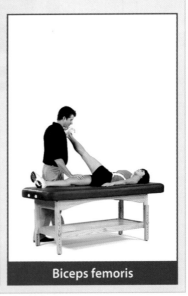

Biceps femoris

Step 3: Activate Key activation exercises via isolated strengthening exercises and/or positional isometrics include the adductors, medial hamstring complex, and gluteus maximus.

Isolated Strengthening Exercises

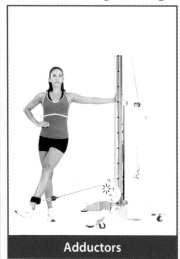
Adductors

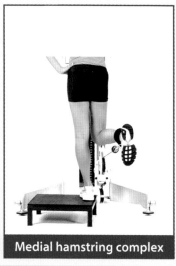
Medial hamstring complex

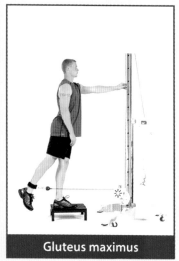
Gluteus maximus

Positional Isometric Techniques

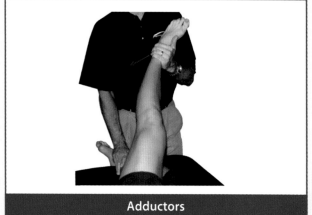

Adductors

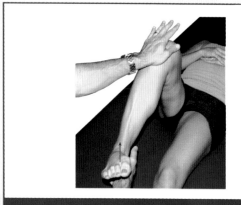
Medial hamstring complex

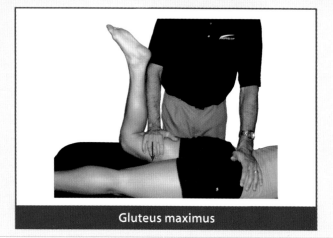
Gluteus maximus

Step 4: Integration Progression An integration progression used for this compensation could be the same progression used for the compensation of the knee moving inward.

SUMMARY • Lower-extremity injuries account for a majority of the total injuries in both college and high school athletes. Among lower-extremity injuries, the knee is one of the most commonly injured regions of the body. The knee is a part of a kinetic chain that is impacted by the linked segments from the proximal and distal joints. The described integrated assessment process uses four primary assessments of the linked segments from the proximal and distal joints, which include static posture, movement assessments, goniometric measurements, and manual muscle testing. On the basis of the collective information obtained from these assessments, neuromusculoskeletal control deficits are identified for targeted treatments. Use of the outlined corrective exercise strategies for knee impairments provide health and fitness professionals with a systematic approach that can ultimately reduce the risk of knee and lower-extremity injuries while improving performance measures.

References

1. Hootman JM, Dick R, Agel J. Epidemiology of collegiate injuries for 15 sports: summary and recommendations for injury prevention initiatives. *J Athl Train* 2007;42(2):311–9.
2. Fernandez WG, Yard EE, Comstock RD. Epidemiology of lower extremity injuries among U.S. high school athletes. *Acad Emerg Med* 2007;14(7):641–5.
3. Garrick JG, Requa RK. ACL injuries in men and women—How common are they? In: Griffin LY, ed. *Prevention of Noncontact ACL Injuries.* Rosemont, IL: American Academy of Orthopaedic Surgeons; 2001.
4. Greslamer RP, Klein JR. The biomechanics of the patellofemoral joint. *J Orthop Sports Phys Ther* 1998;28(5):286–98.
5. Fulkerson JP. Diagnosis and treatment of patients with patellofemoral pain. *Am J Sports Med* 2002;30(3):447–56.
6. Ireland ML, Willson JD, Ballantyne BT, Davis IM. Hip strength in females with and without patellofemoral pain. *J Orthop Sports Phys Ther* 2003;33(11):671–6.
7. Thomee R, Augustsson J, Karlsson J. Patellofemoral pain syndrome: a review of current issues. *Sports Med* 1999;28:245–62.
8. Myer GD, Ford KR, Foss KD, et al. Incidence and potential pathomechanics of patellofemoral pain in female athletes. Paper presented at National Strength and Conditioning Association National Meeting, 2009; Las Vegas, NV.
9. Baumhauer J, Alosa D, Renstrom A, Trevino S, Beynnon B. A prospective study of ankle injury risk factors. *Am J Sport Med* 1995;23(5):564–70.
10. Knapik JJ, Bauman CL, Jones BH, Harris JM, Vaughan L. Preseason strength and flexibility imbalances associated with athletic injuries in female collegiate athletes. *Am J Sports Med* 1991;19(1):76–81.
11. Uhorchak JM, Scoville CR, Williams GN, Arciero RA, St Pierre P, Taylor DC. Risk factors associated with noncontact injury of the anterior cruciate ligament: a prospective four-year evaluation of 859 West Point cadets. *Am J Sports Med* Nov-Dec 2003;31(6):831–42.
12. Hewett TE, Myer GD, Ford KR, Heidt RS Jr, Colosimo AJ, McLean SG, van den Bogert AJ, Paterno MV, Succop P. Biomechanical measures of neuromuscular control and valgus loading of the knee predict anterior cruciate ligament injury risk in female athletes: a prospective study. *Am J Sports Med* Feb 8 2005;33(4):492–501.
13. Hewett TE, Stroupe AL, Nance TA, Noyes FR. Plyometric training in female athletes: decreased impact forces and increased hamstring torques. *Am J Sports Med* 1996;24(6):765–73.
14. Ford KR, Myer GD, Hewett TE. Valgus knee motion during landing in high school female and male basketball players. *Med Sci Sports Exerc* Oct 2003;35(10):1745–50.
15. Ford KR, Myer GD, Toms HE, Hewett TE. Gender differences in the kinematics of unanticipated cutting in young athletes. *Med Sci Sports* Jan 2005;37(1):124–9.
16. Zazulak BT, Ponce PL, Straub SJ, Medvecky MJ, Avedisian L, Hewett TE. Gender comparison of hip muscle activity during single-leg landing. *J Orthop Sports Phys Ther* May 2005;35(5):292–9.
17. Hewett TE, Ford KR, Myer GD, Wanstrath K, Scheper M. Gender differences in hip adduction motion and torque during a single leg agility maneuver. *J Orthop Res* 2006;24(3):416–21.
18. Ford KR, Myer GD, Smith RL, Vianello RM, Seiwert SL, Hewett TE. A comparison of dynamic coronal plane excursion between matched male and female athletes when performing single leg landings. *Clin Biomech (Bristol, Avon)* 2006;21(1):33–40.
19. Myer GD, Ford KR, Hewett TE. Tuck jump assessment for reducing anterior cruciate ligament injury risk. *Athl Ther Today* 2008;13(5):39–44.
20. Zazulak BT, Hewett TE, Reeves NP, Goldberg B, Cholewicki J. The effects of core proprioception on knee ligament injury: a prospective biomechanical-epidemiological study. Accepted AOSSM Specialty Day, San Diego, CA; 2007.
21. Myer GD, Ford KR, Hewett TE. Rationale and clinical techniques for anterior cruciate ligament injury prevention among female athletes. *J Athl Train* Dec 2004;39(4):352–64.
22. Olsen OE, Myklebust G, Engebretsen L, Bahr R. Injury mechanisms for anterior cruciate ligament injuries in team handball: a systematic video analysis. *Am J Sports Med* Jun 2004;32(4):1002–12.

23. Myer GD, Ford KR, Palumbo JP, Hewett TE. Neuromuscular training improves performance and lower-extremity biomechanics in female athletes. *J Strength Cond Res* Feb 2005;19(1):51–60.

24. Boden BP, Dean GS, Feagin JA, Garrett WE. Mechanisms of anterior cruciate ligament injury. *Orthopedics* 2000;23(6):573–8.

25. Lloyd DG, Buchanan TS. Strategies of muscular support of varus and valgus isometric loads at the human knee. *J Biomech* 2001;34(10):1257–67.

26. Lloyd DG. Rationale for training programs to reduce anterior cruciate ligament injuries in Australian football. *J Orthop Sports Phys Ther* Nov 2001;31(11):645–54; discussion 661.

27. Cahill BR, Griffith EH. Effect of preseason conditioning on the incidence and severity of high school football knee injuries. *Am J Sports Med* Jul-Aug 1978;6(4):180–4.

28. Hewett TE, Lindenfeld TN, Riccobene JV, Noyes FR. The effect of neuromuscular training on the incidence of knee injury in female athletes: a prospective study. *Am J Sports Med* 1999;27(6):699–706.

29. Malinzak RA, Colby SM, Kirkendall DT, Yu B, Garrett WE. A comparison of knee joint motion patterns between men and women in selected athletic tasks. *Clin Biomech (Bristol, Avon)* Jun 2001;16(5):438–45.

30. Besier TF, Lloyd DG, Ackland TR, Cochrane JL. Anticipatory effects on knee joint loading during running and cutting maneuvers. *Med Sci Sports Exerc* 2001;33(7):1176–81.

31. Myer GD, Ford KR, Brent JL, Hewett TE. Differential neuromuscular training effects on ACL injury risk factors in "high-risk" versus "low-risk" athletes. *BMC Musculoskel Disord* 2007;8(39):1–7.

32. Neptune RR, Wright IC, van den Bogert AJ. Muscle coordination and function during cutting movements. *Med Sci Sports Exerc* Feb 1999;31(2):294–302.

33. Myer GD, Ford KR, Khoury J, Succop P, Hewett TE. A laboratory based prediction tool for identification of female athletes with high ACL injury risk knee loads during landing. *Br J Sports Med* 2010. In press.

CHAPTER 14

Corrective Strategies for Lumbo-Pelvic-Hip Impairments

OBJECTIVES   *Upon completion of this chapter, you will be able to:*

➤ Understand basic functional anatomy for the lumbo-pelvic-hip complex.

➤ Understand the mechanisms for common lumbo-pelvic-hip complex injuries.

➤ Determine common risk factors that can lead to lumbo-pelvic-hip complex injuries.

➤ Incorporate a systematic assessment and corrective exercise strategy for lumbo-pelvic-hip complex impairments.

INTRODUCTION

THE lumbo-pelvic-hip complex (LPHC) is a region of the body that has a massive influence on the structures above and below it. The LPHC has between 29 and 35 muscles that attach to the lumbar spine or pelvis (1,2). The LPHC is directly associated with both the lower extremities and upper extremities of the body. Because of this, dysfunction of both the lower extremities and upper extremities can lead to dysfunction of the LPHC and vice versa.

REVIEW OF LPHC FUNCTIONAL ANATOMY

As previously stated, the LPHC has a great influence on the rest of the kinetic chain. There are many bones, joints, and muscles involved in the dysfunction of the LPHC; however, the purpose of this section is to provide a general review of the most pertinent structures. This is not intended to be an exhaustive and detailed review.

Bones and Joints

In the LPHC region specifically, the femur and the pelvis make up the iliofemoral joint and the pelvis and sacrum make up the sacroiliac joint (Figure 14-1). The lumbar spine and sacrum form the lumbosacral junction (Figure 14-1). Collectively, these structures anchor many of the major myofascial tissues that have a functional impact on the arthrokinematics of the structures above and below them.

Above the LPHC are the thoracic and cervical spine, rib cage, scapula, humerus, and clavicle. These structures make up the thoracolumbar and cervicothoracic junctions of the spine, the scapulothoracic, glenohumeral, acromioclavicular (AC), and sternoclavicular (SC) joints (Figure 14-2).

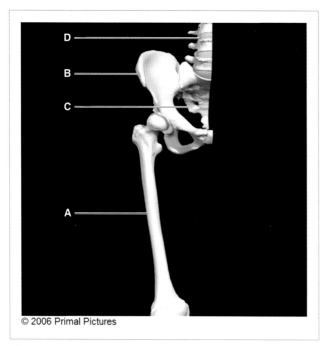

© 2006 Primal Pictures

Figure 14.1 Bones of the LPHC. (A) Femur. (B) Pelvis. (C) Sacrum. (D) Lumbar spine.

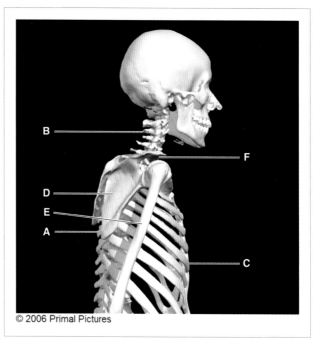

© 2006 Primal Pictures

Figure 14.2 Bones above the LPHC. (A) Thoracic spine. (B) Cervical spine. (C) Rib cage. (D) Scapula. (E) Humerus. (F) Clavicle.

As mentioned in earlier chapters, below the LPHC, the tibia and femur make up the tibiofemoral joint, and the patella and femur make up the patellofemoral joint (Figure 14-3). The fibula is also noted as it is the attachment site of the biceps femoris, which originates from the pelvis.

Also mentioned in previous chapters, the tibia, fibula, and talus help to form the talocrural (ankle) joint (Figure 14-4). Collectively, these structures anchor the myofascial tissues of the LPHC such as the biceps femoris, medial hamstring comoplex, and rectus femoris. These bones and joints are of importance in corrective exercise because they will also have a functional impact on the arthrokinematics of the LPHC.

Muscles

There are a number of muscles in the upper and lower extremities whose function may be related and have an effect on the LPHC (Table 14-1). As with

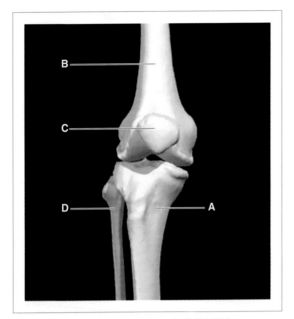

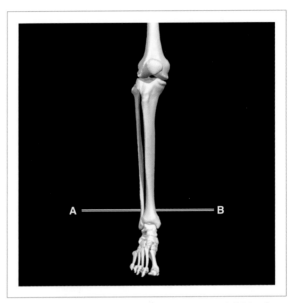

Figure 14.3 Bones below the LPHC. (A) Tibia. (B) Femur. (C) Patella. (D) Fibula.

Figure 14.4 Bones below the LPHC (con't). (A) Distal Fibula. (B) Distal Tibia.

all muscles, it is important to restore and maintain normal range of motion and strength as well as eliminate any muscle inhibition to ensure joints are operating optimally (3–5). See chapter two for a detailed review of the location and function of these muscles.

Table 14.1	KEY MUSCLES ASSOCIATED WITH THE LPHC
• Gastrocnemius/soleus • Adductor complex • Hamstring complex • Hip flexors • Abdominal complex	• Erector spinae • Intrinsic core stabilizers • Latissimus dorsi • Tensor fascia latae/IT-band • Gluteus medius and maximus

COMMON LPHC INJURIES AND ASSOCIATED MOVEMENT DEFICIENCIES

Many of the common injuries associated with the LPHC include low-back pain, sacroiliac joint dysfunction, and hamstring complex, quadriceps, and groin strains (Table 14-2). However, the body is an interconnected chain, and compensation or dysfunction in the LPHC region can lead to dysfunctions in other areas of the body (3–8). Moving above the LPHC, common injuries are often seen in the cervical-thoracic spine, ribs (9–11), and shoulder (12–14), which can stem from dysfunction in the LPHC. Moving below the LPHC toward the knee, common injuries include patellar tendinosis (jumper's knee) and iliotibial band (IT-band) tendonitis (runner's knee) (15–17) as well as anterior cruciate ligament (ACL) tears (18,19). At the foot and ankle, common injuries that can stem from LPHC dysfunction include plantar fasciitis, Achilles tendinopathy, and medial tibial stress syndrome (20,21).

Table 14.2   COMMON INJURIES ASSOCIATED WITH LPHC IMPAIRMENT

Local Injuries	Injuries Above LPHC	Injuries Below LPHC
Low-back pain Sacroiliac joint dysfunction Hamstring complex, quadriceps, and groin strains	Shoulder and upper-extremity injuries Cervical-thoracic spine Rib cage	Patellar tendonitis (jumper's knee) IT-band tendonitis (runner's knee) Medial, lateral, and anterior knee pain Chondromalacia patellae Plantar fasciitis Achilles tendonitis Posterior tibialis tendonitis (shin splints)

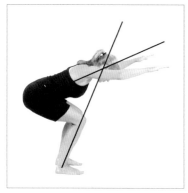

Figure 14.5   Excessive forward lean.

Applying this concept practically, if the ankle is restricted and unable to move during the descent of a squat, the hip will be required to move more (relative flexibility) (22). If there is a lack of sagittal plane dorsiflexion at the ankle owing to an overactive or tight gastrocnemius and soleus, the LPHC will be forced to increase forward flexion to alter the body's center of gravity to maintain balance (Figure 14-5). The underactivity of the erector spinae and gluteus maximus to maintain an upright trunk position produces the compensation of an excessive forward lean.

The gluteus maximus and latissimus dorsi along with the thoracolumbar fascia work synergistically to form the posterior oblique subsystem (Figure 14-6) (23,24). As a compensatory mechanism

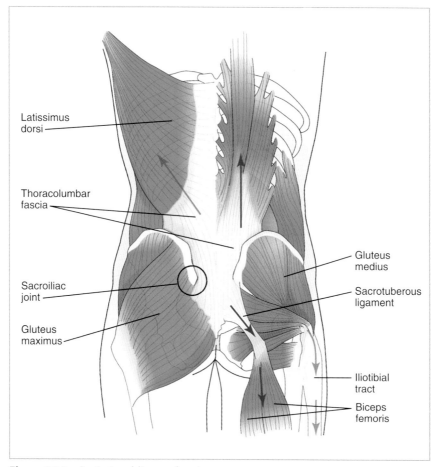

Figure 14.6   Posterior oblique subsystem.

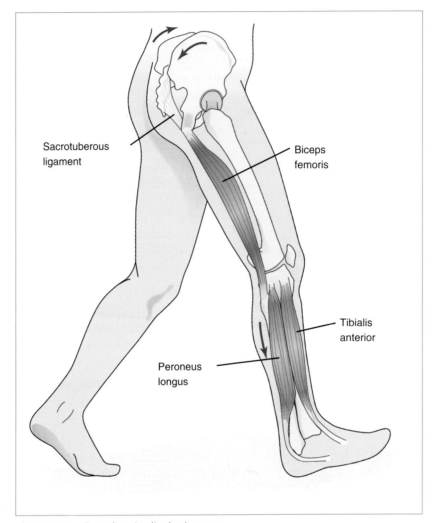

Figure 14.7   Deep longitudinal subsystem.

for the underactivity and inability of the gluteus maximus to maintain an upright trunk position, the latissimus dorsi may become synergistically dominant (overactive or tight) to provide stability through the trunk, core, and pelvis (4). Because the latissimus dorsi crosses the inferior angle of the scapulae and inserts onto the humerus it can alter the rotation of the scapula and instantaneous axis of rotation of the humeral head within the glenoid fossa (4).

The erector spinae, sacrotuberous ligament, biceps femoris, peroneus longus, and anterior tibialis work synergistically to form the deep longitudinal subsystem (Figure 14-7) (23,25,26). With both the anterior tibialis and erector spinae working at a submaximal level, the biceps femoris may become overactive to help maintain stability of the LPHC (4,27). This, however, will alter the position of the pelvis and sacrum and affect the sacroiliac and iliofemoral joints. The latissimus dorsi may also become overactive or tight to provide stability through the pelvis and extension of the spine for the inability of the erector spinae to maintain an upright trunk position. The latissimus dorsi attaches to the pelvis and will anteriorly rotate the pelvis, which causes extension of the lumbar spine (4,27).

From an injury perspective, the increased hip or spinal flexion can lead to excessive stress being placed on the low back, resulting in low-back pain. It can also lead to increased stress in the hamstring complex and adductor magnus, which may be trying to compensate for a weakened gluteus maximus and erector spinae complex to stabilize the LPHC, and result in hamstring complex and groin strains (4). The rectus femoris, being one of the primary hip flexors, tends to be overactive in this scenario. This can decrease its ability to lengthen during functional movements and lead to quadriceps strains as well as knee pain. As mentioned earlier, overactivity or tightness of the latissimus dorsi can affect the shoulder and upper extremities leading to a variety of shoulder and upper-extremity injuries (4,27).

GETTING YOUR FACTS STRAIGHT

Spine Stability Controversy

Exercises to improve spine stability are widely used in rehabilitation and prevention programs. However, there is ongoing debate on which muscles or muscle groups (local or global) to address as well as exercise goals during spine stability training. This is in part because of the assumption that intervertebral stability is automatically achieved and that exercises should focus on improving lumbopelvic stability to achieve spine stability.

There are two primary differences in the approaches toward spine stability training. First, there are differences in the target muscle groups for the prescribed exercises, specifically, exercises for local versus global musculature (1). Second, there are differences in the type of exercises performed in terms of exercises geared toward improving strength and power (abdominal bracing) versus exercises that focus on improving neuromuscular control (abdominal drawing-in maneuver).

The traditional approach to spine stability training uses exercises that focus on the global stabilizers, but not the local stabilizers. This is primarily based on research that suggests that the global muscles are most important for spine stability (2,3). However, this research assumes that intervertebral stability is achieved. As discussed, both local and global muscles contribute to spine stability. Therefore it is critical that exercises for spine stability address both local and global stabilizers. Thus, both bracing and drawing-in can ultimately improve spine stability.

Because drawing-in can influence both intervertebral stability and lumbopelvic stability and because lumbopelvic stability is dependent on intervertebral stability, use of the drawing-in maneuver to train the local muscles and improve intervertebral stability may be considered the starting point for a spine stability training program, then progressing to abdominal bracing.

1. Richardson CA, Jull GA. Muscle control-pain control. What exercises would you prescribe? *Man Ther* 1995;1(1):2–10.
2. Grieve GP. Lumbar instability. *Physiotherapy* 1982;68(1):2–9.
3. McGill SM. Low back stability: from formal description to issues for performance and rehabilitation. *Exerc Sport Sci Rev* 2001;29(1):26–31.

(Text continues on page 314)

ASSESSMENT AND CORRECTIVE EXERCISES FOR LPHC IMPAIRMENTS

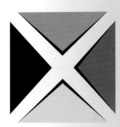

➤ SYSTEMATIC PROCESS TO DETERMINE LPHC IMPAIRMENTS

Because of the freedom of movement at the LPHC and its association with the upper and lower extremities, there are a number of key elements to assess for LPHC dysfunction. This section will review key areas to be assessed when performing an integrated assessment for LPHC impairments.

STATIC POSTURE

A key static postural distortion syndrome to look for to determine potential movement dysfunction at the LPHC is the lower crossed postural distortion syndrome. As mentioned in chapter five, this is characterized by an anterior pelvic tilt (excessive lumbar extension). This position of the pelvis and lumbar spine can place excessive stress on the muscles and connective tissue associated with the LPHC during dynamic movement.

Lower Crossed Syndrome

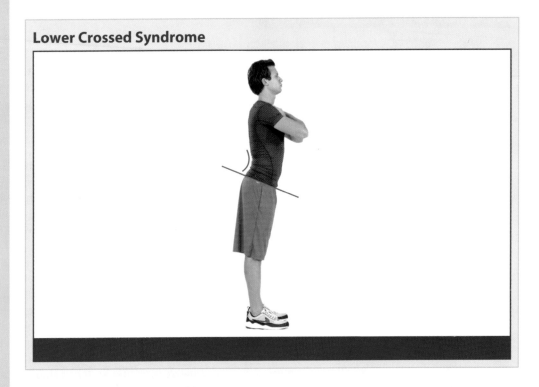

TRANSITIONAL MOVEMENT ASSESSMENTS

There are several LPHC compensations to look for when performing an overhead squat assessment. As outlined in chapter six, these compensations include excessive forward lean, arching of the low back, rounding of the low back, and an asymmetric weight shift. The table below provides a review of the potential overactive and underactive muscles for each compensation.

Overhead Squat LPHC Movement Compensations

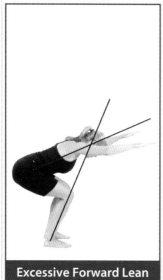

Excessive Forward Lean

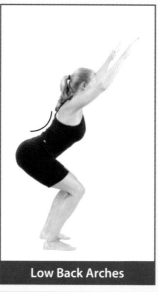

Low Back Arches

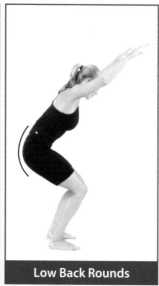

Low Back Rounds

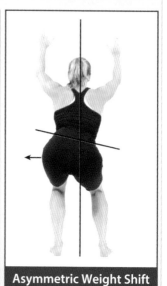

Asymmetric Weight Shift

SUMMARY OF LPHC OVERHEAD SQUAT MOVEMENT COMPENSATIONS

Compensation	Potential Overactive Muscles	Potential Underactive Muscles	Potential Injuries
Excessive forward lean	Soleus Gastrocnemius Hip flexor complex Abdominal Complex	Anterior tibialis Gluteus maximus Erector spinae Intrinsic core stabilizers	Hamstring complex, quadriceps, and groin strain Low-back pain
Low back arches	Hip flexor complex Erector spinae Latissimus dorsi	Gluteus maximus Hamstrings Intrinsic core stabilizers	
Low back rounds	Hamstring complex Adductor magnus Rectus abdominis External obliques	Gluteus maximus Erector spinae Intrinsic core stabilizers Hip flexor complex Latissimus dorsi	
Asymmetrical weight shift	Adductor complex, TFL, (on the side of the shift) Gastrocnemis/soleus, piriformis, biceps femoris, gluteus medius (on side opposite of shift)	Gluteus medius (on side of shift) Anterior tibialis, Adductor complex (on side opposite of shift)	Hamstring complex, quadriceps, and groin strain Low-back pain Sacroiliac joint pain

When performing a single-leg squat, some key compensations to look for would include the knee moving inward and inward or outward trunk rotation as well as the hip hiking and dropping. The table also provides a review of potential overactive and underactive muscles for each compensation.

Continued on page 298

Single-leg Squat LPHC Movement Compensations

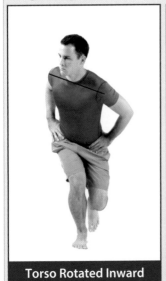
Torso Rotated Inward

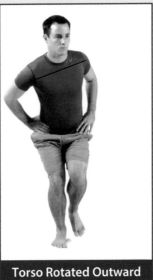
Torso Rotated Outward

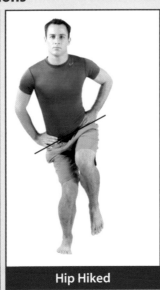
Hip Hiked

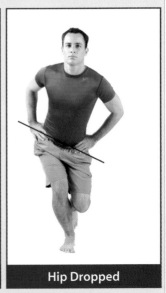
Hip Dropped

SUMMARY OF LPHC SINGLE-LEG SQUAT MOVEMENT COMPENSATIONS

Compensation	Potential Overactive Muscles	Potential Underactive Muscles
Hip hike	Quadratus lumborum (opposite side of stance leg) TFL/gluteus minimus (same side as stance leg)	Adductor complex (same side as stance leg) Gluteus medius (same side as stance leg)
Hip drop	Adductor complex (same side as stance leg)	Gluteus medius (same side as stance leg) Quadratus lumborum (same side as stance leg)
Inward trunk rotation	Internal oblique (same side as stance leg) External oblique (opposite side of stance leg) TFL (same side as stance leg) Adductor complex (same side as stance leg)	Internal oblique (opposite side of stance leg) External oblique (same side as stance leg) Gluteus medius/maximus (same side as stance leg)
Outward trunk rotation	Internal oblique (opposite side of stance leg) External oblique (same side as stance leg) Piriformis (same side as stance leg)	Internal oblique (same side as stance leg) External oblique (opposite side of stance leg) Adductor complex (opposite side as stance leg) Gluteus medius/maximus (same side as stance leg)

DYNAMIC MOVEMENT ASSESSMENTS

Dynamic movement assessments can also help to determine whether LPHC movement deficiencies exist while performing more dynamic movements such as gait (chapter six).

When performing a gait assessment, observe the individual's LPHC for excessive arching and excessive pelvic rotation as well as hip hiking. These compensations could be indicative of poor neuromuscular control of the LPHC and will need to be addressed in the corrective exercise program.

LPHC Compensations During Dynamic Movement Assessment

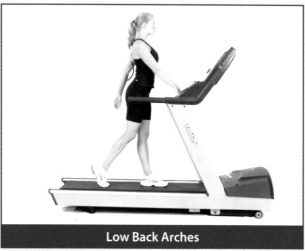

Low Back Arches

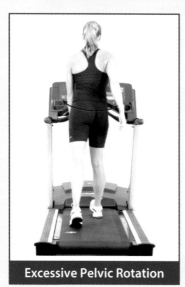

Excessive Pelvic Rotation

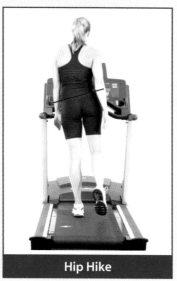

Hip Hike

RANGE OF MOTION ASSESSMENTS

The range of motion (ROM) assessments performed for LPHC impairments will be dependent on the compensations seen during the overhead squat assessment. The table provides a summary of key joints to be measured on potential observations on the basis of the movement compensation(s) seen in the movement assessment. See chapter seven to view proper execution of these assessments and average ROM values.

Continued on page 300

POTENTIAL ROM OBSERVATION	
Compensation	**Potential ROM Observation**
Excessive forward lean	Decreased ankle dorsiflexion Decreased hip extension Decreased hip internal rotation
Low back arches	Decreased hip extension Decreased shoulder flexion Decreased hip internal rotation
Low back rounds	Decrease knee extension Decreased hip internal rotation
Asymmetric weight shift	Decreased hip abduction (same side of shift) Decreased dorsiflexion (opposite side of shift) Decrease knee extension (opposite side of shift) Decreased hip extension (opposite side of shift) Decreased hip internal rotation (opposite side of shift)

STRENGTH ASSESSMENTS

As with the ROM assessments, the manual muscle tests that are selected will also be dependent on the compensations seen during the overhead squat assessment. The table provides a summary of key muscles to be tested on the basis of the movement compensation(s) seen in the movement assessment. See chapter eight to view proper execution of these assessments.

POTENTIAL STRENGTH OBSERVATION	
Compensation	**One or More of the Following Muscles Test "Weak"**
Excessive forward lean	Anterior tibialis or gluteus maximus
Low back arches	Gluteus maximus, hamstring complex, or abdominal complex
Low back rounds	Gluteus maximus or hip flexors
Asymmetric weight shift	Anterior tibialis or adductors (opposite side); gluteus medius (same side)

➤ SYSTEMATIC CORRECTIVE EXERCISE STRATEGIES FOR LPHC IMPAIRMENTS

The following section provides sample programming strategies using the Corrective Exercise Continuum for LPHC impairments. The photos provided illustrate the exercises that can be done for each component of the continuum to help address the issue of LPHC impairments as they relate to the overhead squat assessment (excessive forward lean, low back arches, low back rounds, and asymmetric weight shift). Which exercises are used will be dependent on the findings of the assessments and the individual's physical capabilities (integration exercises).

LPHC IMPAIRMENT: EXCESSIVE FORWARD LEAN

Step 1: Inhibit Key regions to inhibit via foam rolling include the gastrocnemius/soleus and hip flexor complex (rectus femoris).

Self-Myofascial Release

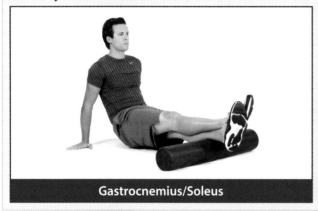

Gastrocnemius/Soleus

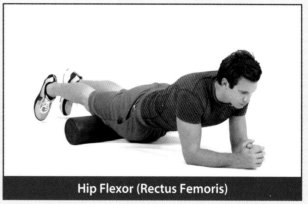

Hip Flexor (Rectus Femoris)

Step 2: Lengthen Key lengthening exercises via static and/or neuromuscular stretches include the gastrocnemius/soleus, hip flexor complex and abdominal complex.

Static Stretches

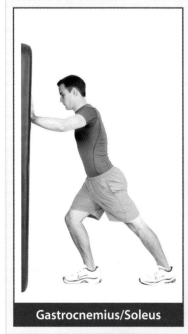

Gastrocnemius/Soleus

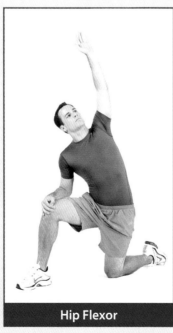

Hip Flexor

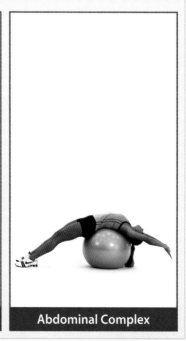

Abdominal Complex

Continued on page 302

Neuromuscular Stretches

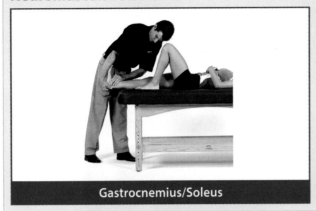
Gastrocnemius/Soleus

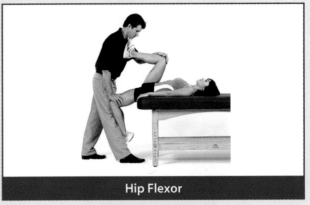
Hip Flexor

Step 3: Activate Key activation exercises via isolated strengthening exercises and/or positional isometrics include the anterior tibialis, gluteus maximus, erector spinae, and intrinsic core stabilizers.

Isolated Strengthening Exercises

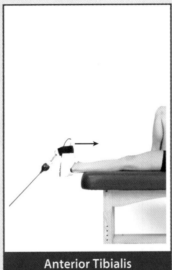
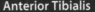
Anterior Tibialis

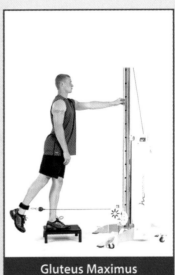
Gluteus Maximus

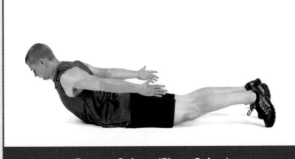
Erector Spinae (Floor Cobra)

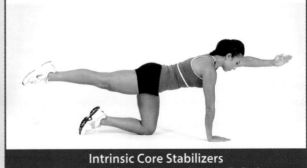
Intrinsic Core Stabilizers
(Quadruped Arm/Opposite Leg Raise)

Positional Isometrics

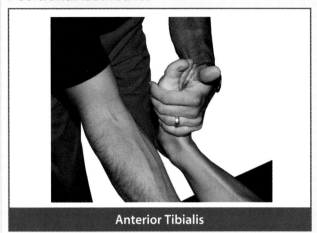

Anterior Tibialis

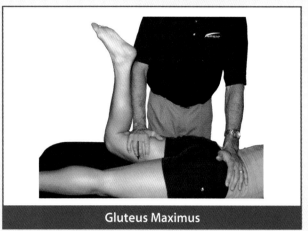

Gluteus Maximus

Step 4: Integration

An integration exercise that could be implemented for this compensation could be a ball squat to overhead press. This exercise will help teach proper hip hinging while maintaining proper lumbo-pelvic control. Adding the overhead press component will place an additional challenge to the core. The individual can then progress to step-ups to overhead presses (sagittal, frontal, and transverse planes), then to lunges to overhead presses (sagittal, frontal, and transverse planes), and then to single-leg squats to overhead presses.

Integrated Dynamic Movement

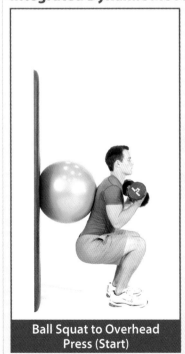

Ball Squat to Overhead Press (Start)

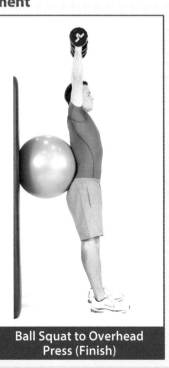

Ball Squat to Overhead Press (Finish)

Continued on page 304

SAMPLE CORRECTIVE EXERCISE PROGRAM FOR LPHC IMPAIRMENT: EXCESSIVE FORWARD LEAN			
Phase	**Modality**	**Muscle(s)**	**Acute Variables**
Inhibit	SMR	Gastrocnemius/soleus Hip flexor complex	Hold on tender area for 30 seconds
Lengthen	**Static stretching** OR **NMS**	Gastrocnemius/soleus Hip flexor complex Abdominal complex	30-second hold **OR** 7–10-second isometric contraction, 30-second hold
Activate	**Positional isometrics** AND/OR **isolated strengthening**	Anterior tibialis Gluteus maximus Erector spinae Core stabilizers	4 reps of increasing intensity 25, 50, 75, 100% **OR** 10–15 reps with 2-second isometric hold and 4-second eccentric contraction
Integrate*	**Integrated dynamic movement**	Ball wall squat with overhead press	10–15 reps under control

***NOTE:** If client is not initially capable of performing the integrated dynamic movement exercise listed he or she may need to be regressed to a more suitable exercise.

LPHC IMPAIRMENT: LOW BACK ARCHES

Step 1: Inhibit   Key regions to inhibit via foam rolling include the hip flexor complex (rectus femoris) and latissimus dorsi.

Self-Myofascial Release

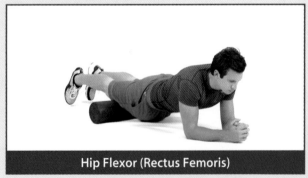

Hip Flexor (Rectus Femoris)

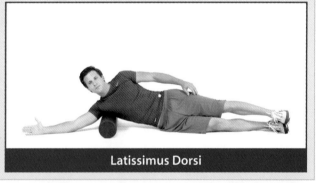

Latissimus Dorsi

Step 2: Lengthen Key lengthening exercises via static and/or neuromuscular stretches include the hip flexor complex, erector spinae, and latissimus dorsi.

Static Stretches

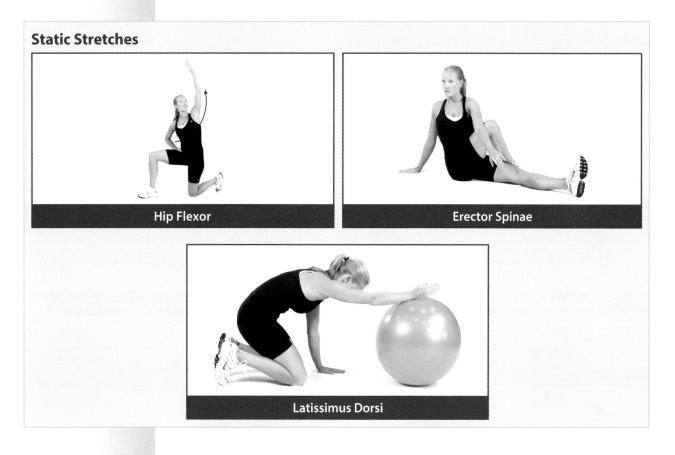

Hip Flexor

Erector Spinae

Latissimus Dorsi

Neuromuscular Stretches

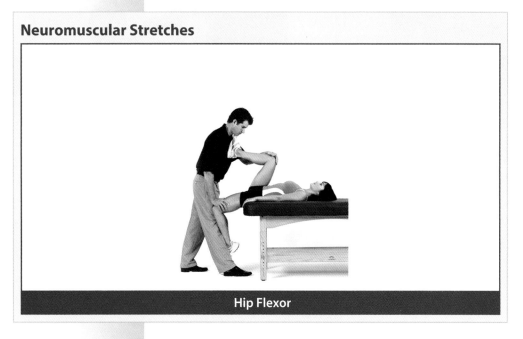

Hip Flexor

Continued on page 306

Step 3: Activate Key activation exercises via isolated strengthening exercises and/or positional isometrics include the gluteus maximus and abdominal complex.

Isolated Strengthening Exercises

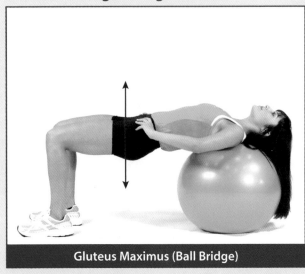

Gluteus Maximus (Ball Bridge)

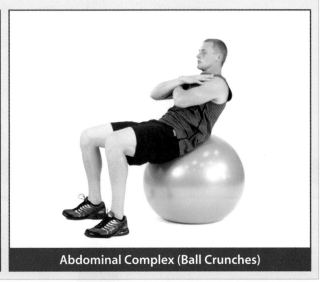

Abdominal Complex (Ball Crunches)

Positional Isometrics

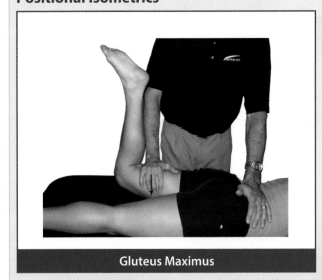

Gluteus Maximus

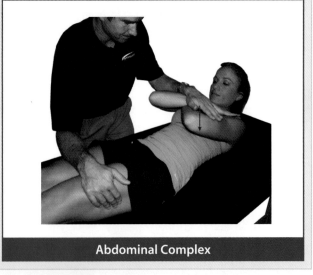

Abdominal Complex

Step 4: Integration   An integration exercise that could also be implemented for this compensation could also be a ball squat to overhead press and use the same integrated progression that was provided for the excessive forward lean programming.

SAMPLE CORRECTIVE EXERCISE PROGRAM FOR LPHC IMPAIRMENT: LOW BACK ARCHES			
Phase	**Modality**	**Muscle(s)**	**Acute Variables**
Inhibit	SMR	Hip flexor complex Latissimus dorsi	Hold on tender area for 30-seconds
Lengthen	Static stretching OR **NMS**	Hip flexor complex Latissimus dorsi Erector spinae	30-second hold **OR** 7–10-second isometric contraction, 30-second hold
Activate	**Positional isometrics** AND/OR **isolated strengthening**	Gluteus maximus Abdominal complex/intrinsic core stabilizers	4 reps of increasing intensity 25, 50, 75, 100% **OR** 10–15 reps with 2-second isometric hold and 4-second eccentric contraction
Integrate*	**Integrated dynamic movement**	Ball wall squat with overhead press	10–15 reps under control

NOTE: If client is not initially capable of performing the integrated dynamic movement exercise listed he or she may need to be regressed to a more suitable exercise.

LPHC IMPAIRMENT: LOW BACK ROUNDS

Step 1: Inhibit   Key regions to inhibit via foam rolling include the hamstring complex and adductor magnus.

Self-Myofascial Release

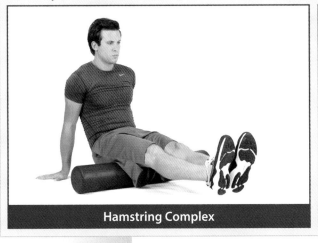

Hamstring Complex

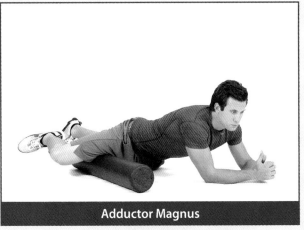

Adductor Magnus

Continued on page 308

Step 2: Lengthen   Key lengthening exercises via static and/or neuromuscular stretches include the hamstring complex and adductor magnus.

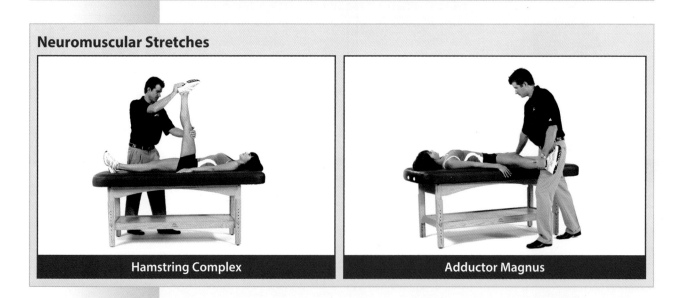

Static Stretches

Hamstring Complex

Adductor Magnus

Abdominal Complex

Neuromuscular Stretches

Hamstring Complex

Adductor Magnus

Step 3: Activate Key activation exercises via isolated strengthening exercises and/or positional isometrics include the gluteus maximus, hip flexors, and erector spinae.

Isolated Strengthening Exercises

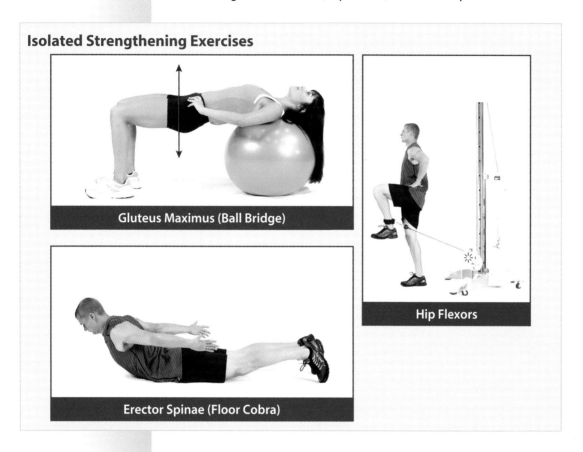

Gluteus Maximus (Ball Bridge)

Hip Flexors

Erector Spinae (Floor Cobra)

Positional Isometrics

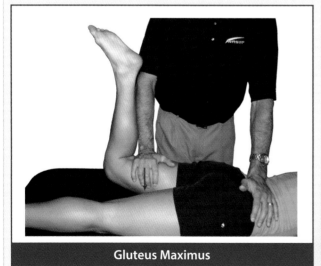

Gluteus Maximus

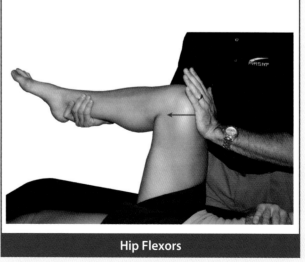

Hip Flexors

Continued on page 310

Step 4: Integration An integration exercise that could also be implemented for this compensation could also be a ball squat to overhead press and use the same integrated progression that was provided for the excessive forward lean programming.

SAMPLE CORRECTIVE EXERCISE PROGRAM FOR LPHC IMPAIRMENT: LOW BACK ROUNDS			
Phase	**Modality**	**Muscle(s)**	**Acute Variables**
Inhibit	SMR	Hamstring complex Adductor magnus	Hold on tender area for 30 seconds
Lengthen	**Static stretching** OR **NMS**	Hamstring complex Adductor magnus	30-second hold **OR** 7–10-second isometric contraction, 30-second hold
Activate	**Positional isometrics** AND/OR **isolated strengthening**	Gluteus maximus Hip flexors Erector spinae	4 reps of increasing intensity 25, 50, 75, 100% **OR** 10–15 reps with 2-second isometric hold and 4-second eccentric contraction
Integrate*	**Integrated dynamic movement**	Ball wall squat with overhead press	10–15 reps under control

*NOTE: If client is not initially capable of performing the integrated dynamic movement exercise listed he or she may need to be regressed to a more suitable exercise.

LPHC IMPAIRMENT: ASYMMETRIC WEIGHT SHIFT

Step 1: Inhibit Key regions to inhibit via foam rolling include the same-side (side toward shift) adductors and TFL/IT-band and the opposite side (side away from shift) piriformis and bicep femoris. The gastrocnemius and soleus can also play a major factor in this compensation as well. As the client descends into the squat, if one of the ankle joints lacks sagittal plane dorsiflexion, this forces the body to shift away from the restricted side and move to the side capable of greater motion. For example, if the left ankle is restricted, it can force the individual to the right to find that ROM.

Self-Myofascial Release

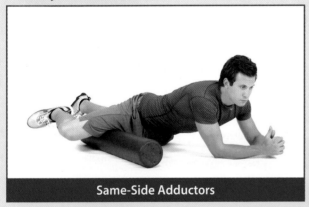

Same-Side Adductors

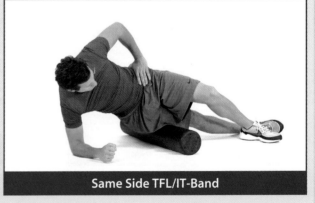

Same Side TFL/IT-Band

Self-Myofascial Release

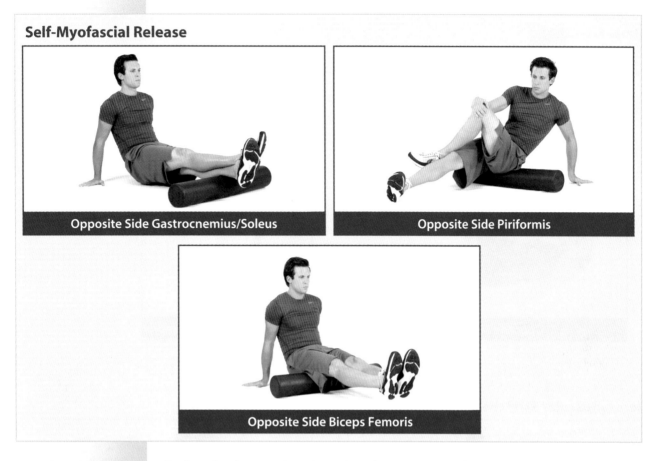

Opposite Side Gastrocnemius/Soleus

Opposite Side Piriformis

Opposite Side Biceps Femoris

Step 2: Lengthen Key lengthening exercises via static and/or neuromuscular stretches include the same-side adductors and the opposite side gastrocnemius/soleus, TFL/IT band, biceps femoris, and piriformis.

Static Stretches

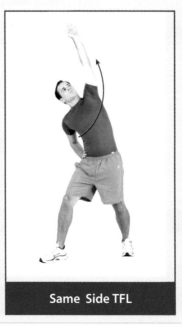

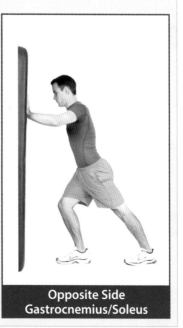

Same-Side Adductors

Same Side TFL

Opposite Side
Gastrocnemius/Soleus

Continued on page 312

Static Stretches

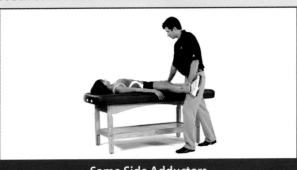

Opposite Side Piriformis

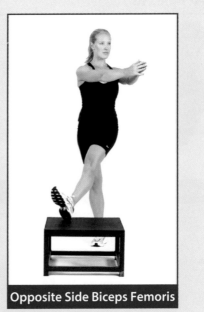

Opposite Side Biceps Femoris

Neuromuscular Stretches

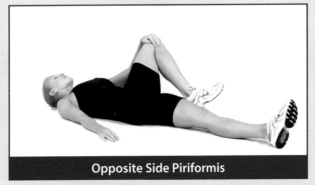

Same Side Adductors

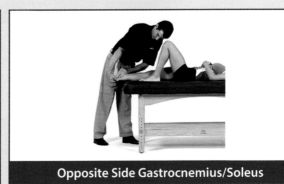

Opposite Side Gastrocnemius/Soleus

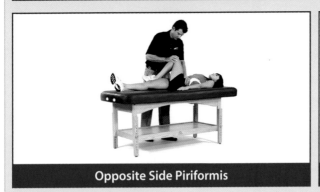

Opposite Side Piriformis

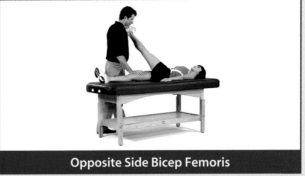

Opposite Side Bicep Femoris

Step 3: Activate Key activation exercises via isolated strengthening exercises and/or positional isometrics include the same-side gluteus medius and the opposite side adductor complex.

Isolated Strengthening Exercises

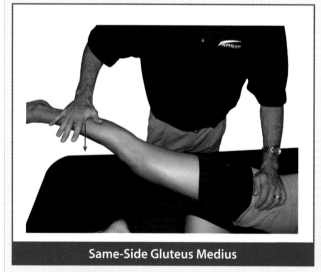

Same Side Gluteus Medius

Opposite Side Adductor Complex

Positional Isometrics

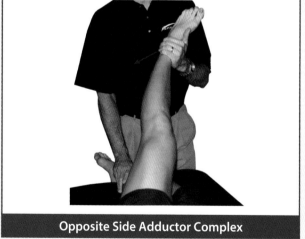

Same-Side Gluteus Medius

Opposite Side Adductor Complex

Continued on page 314

Step 4: Integration An integration exercise that could also be implemented for this compensation could also be a ball squat to overhead press and use the same integrated progression that was provided for the excessive forward lean programming.

SAMPLE CORRECTIVE EXERCISE PROGRAM FOR LPHC IMPAIRMENT: ASYMMETRIC WEIGHT SHIFT			
Phase	**Modality**	**Muscle(s)**	**Acute Variables**
Inhibit	SMR	Adductors and TFL/IT-band (same side) piriformis, bicep femoris and gastrocnemius/soleus (opposite side)	Hold on tender area for 30 seconds
Lengthen	**Static stretching** OR **NMS**	Adductors and TFL (same side) piriformis, gastrocnemius/soleus and biceps femoris (opposite side)	30-second hold **_OR_** 7–10-second isometric contraction, 30-seconds hold
Activate	**Positional isometrics** AND/OR **isolated strengthening**	Gluteus medius (same side) Adductors (opposite side)	4 reps of increasing intensity 25, 50, 75, 100% **_OR_** 10–15 reps with 2-seconds isometric hold and 4-second eccentric contraction
Integrate*	**Integrated dynamic movement**	Ball wall squat to overhead press	10–15 reps under control

*NOTE: If client is not initially capable of performing the integrated dynamic movement exercise listed he or she may need to be regressed to a more suitable exercise.

SUMMARY • The LPHC operates as an integrated functional unit, enabling the entire kinetic chain to work synergistically to produce force, reduce force, and dynamically stabilize against abnormal force. In an efficient state, each structural component distributes weight, absorbs force, and transfers ground reaction forces. This integrated, interdependent system needs to be appropriately trained to enable it to function efficiently during dynamic activities. Because of the many muscles associated with the LPHC, dysfunction in this region can potentially lead to dysfunction in both the upper and lower extremities, and dysfunction in either the upper or lower extremities can lead to LPHC dysfunction. For this reason it becomes a crucial region to assess and will most likely be a region that will need to be addressed in most individuals with movement deficits.

References

1. Porterfield JA, DeRosa C. Mechanical Low Back Pain. 2nd ed. Philadelphia, PA: WB Saunders; 1998.
2. Richardson C, Jull G, Hodges P, Hides J. Therapeutic Exercise for Spinal Segmental Stabilization in Low Back Pain. London: Churchill Livingstone; 1999.
3. Powers CM. The influence of altered lower-extremity kinematics on patellofemoral joint dysfunction: a theoretical perspective. *J Orthop Sports Phys Ther* 2003;33(11):639–46.
4. Sahrmann SA. Diagnosis and Treatment of Movement Impairment Syndromes. St. Louis: Mosby, Inc; 2002.
5. Vesci BJ, Padua DA, Bell DR, Strickland LJ, Guskiewicz KM, Hirth CJ. Influence of hip muscle strength, flexibility of hip and ankle musculature, and hip muscle activation on dynamic knee valgus motion during a double-legged squat. *J Athl Train* 2007;42(Suppl):S-83.

6. Buckley BD, Thigpen CA, Joyce CJ, Bohres SM, Padua DA. Knee and hip kinematics during a double leg squat predict knee and hip kinematics at initial contact of a jump landing task. *J Athl Train* 2007;42(Suppl):S-81.

7. Hollman JH, Kolbeck KE, Hitchcock JL, Koverman JW, Krause DA. Correlations between hip strength and static foot and knee posture. *J Sport Rehab* 2006;15: 12–23.

8. Nadler SF, Malanga GA, DePrince M, Stitik TP, Feinberg JH. The relationship between lower extremity injury, low back pain, and hip muscle strength in male and female collegiate athletes. *Clin J Sport Med* 2000;10:89–97.

9. McLean L. The effect of postural correction on muscle activation amplitudes recorded from the cervicobrachial region. *J Electromyogr Kinesiol* 2002;15:527–35.

10. Thigpen CA, Padua DA, Guskiewicz KM, Michener LA. Three-dimensional shoulder position in individuals with and without forward head and rounded shoulder posture. *J Athl Train* 2006;41(2).

11. Szeto GPY, Straker L, Raine S. A field comparison of neck and shoulder postures in symptomatic and asymptomatic office workers. *Appl Ergo* 2002;33: 75–84.

12. Hirashima M, Kadota H, Sakurai S, Kudo K, Ohtsuki T. Sequential muscle activity and its functional role in the upper extremity and trunk during overarm throwing. *J Sports Sci* 2002;20:301–10.

13. Lewis JS, Green A, Wright C. Subacromial impingement syndrome: the role of posture and muscle imbalance. *J Shoulder Elbow Surg* 2005;14(4):385–92.

14. Bayes MC, Wadsworth LT. Upper extremity injuries in golf. *Phys Sports Med* 2009;37(1):92–6.

15. Fredericson M, Cookingham CL, Chaudhari AM, Dowdell BC, Oestreicher N, Sahrmann SA. Hip abductor weakness in distance runners with iliotibial band syndrome. *Clin J Sport Med* 2000;10:169–75.

16. Ireland ML, Willson JD, Ballantyne BT, Davis IM. Hip strength in females with and without patellofemoral pain. *J Orthop Sports Phys Ther* 2003;33(11): 671–6.

17. Mascal CL, Landel R, Powers C. Management of patellofemoral pain targeting hip, pelvis, and trunk muscle function: 2 case reports. *J Orthop Sports Phys Ther* 2003;33(11):647–60.

18. Myer GD, Ford KR, Hewett TE. Rationale and clinical techniques for anterior cruciate ligament injury prevention among female athletes. *J Athl Train* 2004;39(4):352–64.

19. Hewett TE, Myer GD, Ford KR. Decrease in neuromuscular control about the knee with maturation in female athletes. *J Bone Joint Surg Am* 2004; 86-A(8):1601–8.

20. Hale SA, Hertel J, Olmsted-Kramer LC. The effect of a 4-week comprehensive rehabilitation program on postural control and lower extremity function in individuals with chronic ankle instability. *J Orthop Sports Phys Ther* 2007;37(6):303–11.

21. Riddle DL, Pulisic M, Pidcoe P, Johnson RE. Risk factors for plantar fasciitis: a matched case-control study. *J Bone Joint Surg Am* 2003;85-A(5):872–7.

22. Fry AC, Smith JC, Schilling BK. Effect of knee position on hip and knee torques during the barbell squat. *J Strength Cond Res* 2003;17(4):629–33.

23. Lee D. The Pelvic Girdle. 2nd ed. Edinburgh, UK: Churchill Livingstone; 1999.

24. Mooney V, Pozos R, Vleeming A, Gulick F, Swenski D. Coupled Motion of Contralateral Latissimus Dorsi and Gluteus Maximus: Its Role in Sacroiliac Stabilization. In: Vlemming A, Mooney V, Dorman C, Stoeckart R, eds. Movement, Stability and Low Back Pain. New York: Churchill Livingstone; 1997. p 115–22.

25. Innes K. The Effect of Gait on Extremity Evaluation. In: Hammer W, ed. Functional Soft Tissue Examination and Treatment by Manual Methods. Gaithersburg, MD: Aspen Publishers, Inc; 1999. p 357–68.

26. Vleeming A, Snijders CF, Stoeckart R, Mens FMA. The role of sacroiliac joints in coupling between spine, pelvis, legs and arms. In: Vlemming A, Mooney V, Dorman C, Stoeckart R, eds. Movement, Stability and Low Back Pain. New York: Churchill Livingstone; 1997. p 53–71.

27. Neumann DA. Kinesiology of the Musculoskeletal System: Foundations for Physical Rehabilitation. St. Louis: Mosby; 2002.

CHAPTER 15

Corrective Strategies for Shoulder, Elbow, and Wrist Impairments

Upon completion of this chapter, you will be able to:

➤ Understand basic functional anatomy of the shoulder, elbow, and wrist.

➤ Understand the mechanisms for common shoulder, elbow, and wrist injuries.

➤ Determine common risk factors that can lead to shoulder, elbow, and wrist injuries.

➤ Incorporate a systematic assessment and corrective exercise strategy for shoulder, elbow, and wrist impairments.

SHOULDER

INTRODUCTION

SHOULDER pain is reported to occur in up to 21% of the general population (1,2), with 40% persisting for at least 1 year (3) at an estimated annual cost of $39 billion (4). Shoulder impingement is the most prevalent diagnosis accounting for 40 to 65% of reported shoulder pain (5), whereas traumatic shoulder dislocations account for an additional 15 to 25% of shoulder pain (6–11). The persistent nature of shoulder pain may be the result of degenerative changes to the shoulder's capsuloligamentous structures, articular cartilage, and tendons as the result of altered shoulder mechanics. As many as 70% of individuals with shoulder dislocations experience recurrent instability within 2 years (12,13) and are at risk of developing glenohumeral osteoarthritis secondary to the increased motion at the glenohumeral joint (14,15). Degenerative changes may also affect the rotator cuff by weakening the tendons with time through intrinsic and extrinsic risk factors (5,16–20) such as repetitive overhead use (>60 degrees of shoulder elevation), increased loads raised above shoulder height (21), and forward head and rounded shoulder posture (22), as well as altered scapular kinematics and muscle activity (altered force-couple relationships) (23–26).

These factors are theorized to overload the shoulder muscles, especially the rotator cuff, which can lead to shoulder pain and dysfunction. Given the cost, rate of occurrence, and difficult resolution of shoulder pain, exercise solutions that address these factors are essential in preventing shoulder injuries.

REVIEW OF SHOULDER FUNCTIONAL ANATOMY

Circumduction: the circular movement of a limb.

The unique anatomy of the shoulder girdle enables the joint to balance maximum mobility while maintaining stability through dynamic and static stabilizing structures. Stability is derived primarily from the muscles about the shoulder girdle, and mobility is permitted by the relatively loose capsuloligamentous structures. Stability is maintained by the static and dynamic stabilizers that must work together to create the synchronous motion that allows for the high velocities, large torques, and precise timing such as full **circumduction** during swimming and powerful throwing motions that generate forces at the shoulder in excess of three times one's body weight (27). There are many bones, muscles, and ligaments making up the shoulder girdle, and the reader is invited to review any basic anatomy text for further details.

Bones and Joints

The shoulder girdle has the greatest range of motion of any joint in the body and refers specifically to the articulations between the humerus, scapula, clavicle, rib cage (thorax), and sternum that make up the glenohumeral (GH), acromioclavicular (AC), sternoclavicular (SC), and scapulothoracic joints (Figure 15-1). Below the shoulder are the lumbo-pelvic-hip complex (LPHC; Figure 15-2),

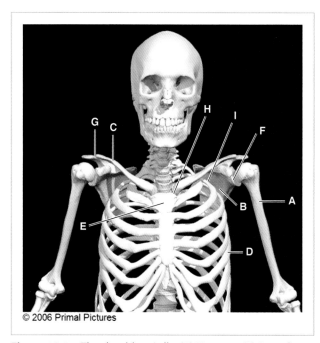

© 2006 Primal Pictures

Figure 15.1   The shoulder girdle. (A) Humerus (B) Scapula (C) Clavicle (D) Ribs (E) Sternum (F) Glenohumeral joint (G) Acromioclavicular joint (H) Sternoclavicular joint (I) Scapulothoracic joint

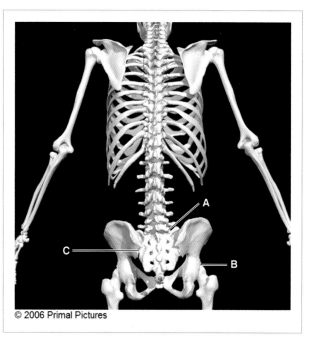

© 2006 Primal Pictures

Figure 15.2   Structures below the shoulder. (A) Lumbosacral joint (B) Iliofemoral joint (C) Sacroiliac joint.

which includes the lumbosacral, sacroiliac, and iliofemoral joints (chapter 14). These structures anchor many of the major myofascial tissues, especially the latissimus dorsi, which functions as a powerful shoulder adductor and internal rotator. Thus, dysfunction at the LPHC can affect proper shoulder function and vice versa.

Glenohumeral Joint

The glenohumeral joint is a ball-and-socket articulation between the head of the humerus and the glenoid of the scapula (Figure 15-3). The joint affords a vast range of motion and great mobility that sacrifices stability (28). The glenoid surface is one third to one fourth the size of the humeral head, producing low contact area and low stability. The joint must rely on the static and dynamic stabilizers for its stability as well as for its motion. The static stabilizers include such structures as the glenoid labrum and the glenohumeral joint capsule consisting of two major ligaments, the middle and inferior glenohumeral ligaments (Figure 15-4). The inferior ligament is divided into three sections: the anterior-inferior, axillary pouch, and posterior-inferior glenohumeral ligaments. Toward the end ranges of glenohumeral motion, these ligaments tighten to limit motion and provide functional stability. These ligaments attach to the glenoid labrum and blend into the humeral head. The complex inferior glenohumeral ligament is the primary stabilizer against anterior translation of the humeral head. The anterior and posterior portions of this ligament help stabilize the joint by becoming taut in extreme ranges of internal and external rotation and often are injured with repetitive use in these positions. However, in midranges of shoulder motion, these ligaments are relatively lax, and the joint must rely heavily on the musculature that surrounds the joint for dynamic stability (29).

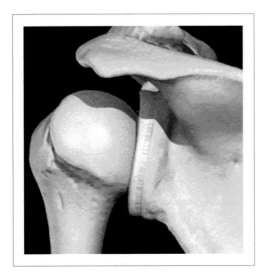

Figure 15.3   Glenohumeral joint.

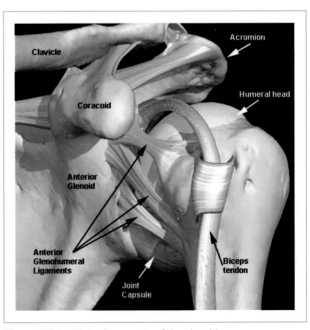

Figure 15.4   Major ligaments of the shoulder.

GETTING YOUR FACTS STRAIGHT

Closed-Packed Position and Behind the Neck Exercises

The closed-packed position is when the shoulder joint surfaces are maximally fit and the capsule and ligaments have the least ability to lengthen. In this position the joint surfaces are compressed and the joint possesses its greatest stability, but least amount of mobility. So to picture this in relative terms, hold a towel at both ends and twist it in opposite directions and notice how as the towel twists your hands move closer together. The joint is compressed by virtue of the fact that the capsule and ligaments are spiralized and tense. In this situation the surface cannot be separated by distractive force, but the position does subject the joint to possible damage because of the compressive and shear stresses.

To be clear, it is not the position that is dangerous, but the direction and amount of external force applied to the joint/limb that will determine the level of risk. To decrease stress on the joint and decrease the risk of injury the joint should be placed in the loose-packed position. This is the position where the joint is least fit and has the most extensibility in the capsule and ligaments. For example, many people try to strengthen their latissimus dorsi and deltoids by performing behind the neck pulldowns or presses. This forces one to place their shoulder into the closed-packed position (shoulder external rotation, abduction, and maximal elevation). However, a simple modification is to pull or press the load in front of the shoulder (front lat pulldowns or front shoulder presses) which avoids the closed-packed position and provides a safer alternative to avoid injuries in the future.

Dynamic Stabilizers

There are a number of muscles associated with the shoulder joint (Table 15-1). The dynamic stability of the glenohumeral joint is dependent on the musculature that surrounds the joint, including the rotator cuff and the scapular stabilizers (29). The rotator cuff is the primary steering mechanism of the glenohumeral joint. The rotator cuff is made up of the supraspinatus and subscapularis anteriorly, with the infraspinatus and teres minor posteriorly (Figure 15-5). The supraspinatus initiates the first 15 degrees of shoulder abduction followed by deltoid activation for the remainder of the arc of motion. The deltoid and supraspinatus work together in a force-couple to control the humeral head in the frontal plane. The main action of the subscapularis is medial rotation of the humerus while also being the primary stabilizer and humeral head depressor (30). The infraspinatus and teres minor externally rotate the glenohumeral joint and decelerate the humerus during internal rotation. The subscapularis and posterior rotator cuff function together in a force-couple controlling the humeral head in the transverse plane (27). See chapter two for a more detailed review of the muscles' location and function.

Table 15.1 KEY MUSCLES ASSOCIATED WITH THE SHOULDER	
• Supraspinatus	• Pectoralis major and minor
• Subscapularis	• Latissimus dorsi
• Infraspinatus	• Rhomboids
• Teres major and minor	• Trapezius
• Deltoid	• Levator scapulae

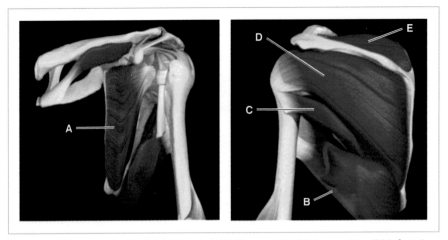

Figure 15.5 Rotator cuff (A) Subscapularis (B) Teres major (C) Teres minor (D) Infraspinatus (E) Supraspinatus.

Function of the Scapula

The scapulothoracic articulation allows shoulder movement beyond the 120 degrees of elevation provided by the glenohumeral joint. It also plays an important role in providing motion and shoulder girdle stability through the 17 muscles that attach to the scapula (29). When these muscles function properly, they provide a stable base for the humerus to glide on and allow for an efficient transfer of force from the lower extremities and trunk. This is accomplished through force-couples of the upper, middle, and lower trapezius as well as the serratus anterior (Figure 15-6). The effectiveness of these force-couples is reliant on the presence of optimal length-tension

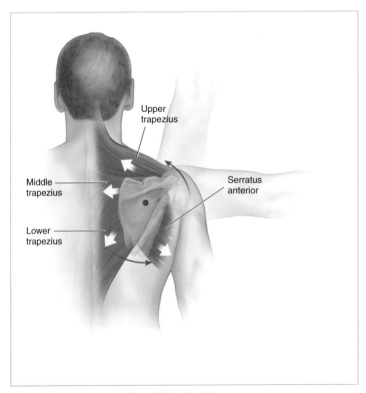

Figure 15.6 Force-couples of the shoulder.

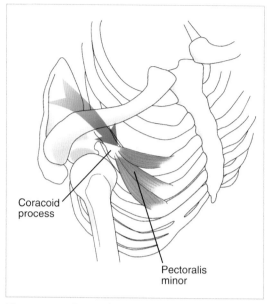

Figure 15.7 Pectoralis minor and scapula malposition.

relationships between opposing muscles. Decreases in force production may lead to disruption in normal muscle synergies and decrease the ability of a force-couple to functionally control joint motion (31). For example, tightness in the pectoralis minor, which inserts on the coracoid process of the scapula, will limit the effectiveness of the serratus anterior to upwardly rotate and posteriorly tilt the scapula. This alters the length-tension relationships of the rotator cuff, decreasing its ability to stabilize the glenohumeral joint (32). Therefore, the pectoralis minor plays an important role in scapula malposition as it can pull the scapula into a more protracted and anteriorly tilted position (33,34) (Figure 15-7).

COMMON SHOULDER INJURIES AND ASSOCIATED MOVEMENT DEFICIENCIES

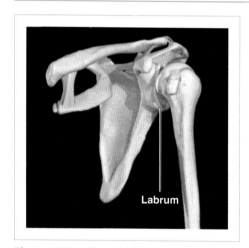

Figure 15.8 Glenoid labrum.

Shoulder injuries can be broadly categorized into those that affect the rotator cuff muscles or those that affect the capsuloligamentous structures of the shoulder (Table 15-2). Rotator cuff conditions such as strains, ruptures, and tendinopathies account for approximately 75 to 80% of shoulder injuries. Rotator cuff strains occur when a muscle group is overexerted, causing microdamage within the muscle belly and tendon, resulting in immediate inflammation and decreased muscle function. In contrast, injuries to the capsuloligamentous structures lead to deficits in the passive stabilizing structures of the shoulder such as the anterior, posterior, or inferior glenohumeral ligaments and the glenoid labrum (Figure 15-8). These injuries are devastating to the ability of the shoulder to facilitate function of the upper extremity in reaching forward or performing overhead tasks.

Table 15.2 COMMON INJURIES ASSOCIATED WITH SHOULDER IMPAIRMENT		
Local Injuries	**Injuries Above Shoulder**	**Injuries Below Shoulder**
Rotator cuff strains	Cervical injuries and	Low-back pain
Rotator cuff ruptures	headaches	Sacroiliac joint dysfunction
Shoulder impingement		Hamstring complex, quadriceps, and groin strains
Biceps tendinopathy		Patellar tendinopathy
Shoulder instability		IT-band syndrome
		Plantar fasciitis
		Achilles tendonitis

Shoulder Impingement

**Subacromial impinge-
ment syndrome (SAIS):
a common diagnosis
broadly defined as
compression of the
structures that run
beneath the cora-
coacromial arch, most
often from a decrease
in the subacromial
space.
Dyskinesis: an altera-
tion in the normal posi-
tion or motion of the
scapula during coupled
scapulohumeral
movements.**

Subacromial impingement syndrome (SAIS) is a common diagnosis broadly defined as compression of the structures that run beneath the coracoacromial arch, most often from a decrease in the subacromial space (Figure 15-9). The impinged structures include the supraspinatus and infraspinatus tendons, the subacromial bursa, and the long head of the biceps tendon. Repetitive compression of these structures with the overhead motions required of many sports and activities of daily living can lead to irritation and inflammation (35). In turn, prolonged inflammation can cause muscular inefficiency, specifically affecting the rotator cuff muscles. SAIS may be the result of bony deformity of the acromion, underlying rotator cuff weakness, shoulder instability, or scapular **dys kinesis** (36). Rotator cuff weakness and shoulder instability results in excessive superior and anterior translation and inadequate external rotation of the humeral head, limiting clearance of the greater tuberosity under the acromion process (36). Decreases in the normal scapular upward rotation and external rotation of the humerus combined with posterior tilting on the thorax cause a decrease in the physiologic space under the coracoacromial arch (35,37–39). Many of these faulty joint motions may be caused by a muscular imbalance or a disruption in force-couple relationships. If these faulty motions are consistently repeated, the resulting decrease in space can lead to impingement of the structures running through the coracoacromial arch. Decreased upward rotation and posterior tilting of the scapula have been shown to occur as the result of forward head posture, forward shoulder posture, or thoracic kyphosis (40–42). With time, this altered initial position is thought to place the serratus anterior, lower trapezius, subscapularis, and posterior rotator cuff at a mechanical disadvantage that can cause weakness and is referred to as the upper crossed syndrome (43) (see chapter five). This altered position of the scapula is thought to result in a decreased subacromial space that could potentially damage the aforementioned structures (35). This impingement or the resulting stresses can damage the rotator cuff, reducing the function of the cuff muscles to suboptimal levels. The resulting alteration in glenohumeral mechanics places the shoulder at an increased risk of injury, especially when combined with overhead activity.

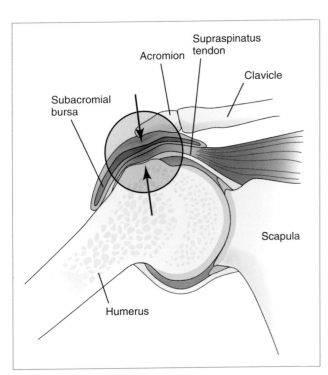

Figure 15.9 Shoulder impingement.

Shoulder Instability

Shoulder instability results from many different mechanisms, but regardless of the mechanism, instability most often manifests itself as anterior or multi-directional. These forms of instability differ greatly in terms of the involved structures and injury mechanisms. Even though the exact injury mechanism may differ, all forms of shoulder instability may occur by means of atraumatic injury mechanisms associated with improper mechanics and poor conditioning (44,45). The most common is traumatic anterior instability as the result of an abducted and externally rotated arm that might occur during a fall on an outstretched arm or reaching behind and to the side to tackle someone (6,7,9–11,46). This results in damage to the anterior/inferior glenohumeral ligament and often the glenoid labrum. The resulting instability usually leads to significant disability with overhead activities that in most cases requires surgical repair (47,48). Shoulder instability may also have an insidious onset as the result of repetitive overhead motion or congenital hypermobility. Repetitive overhead motion of an abducted arm into extreme external or internal rotation results in deformation and failure of the static stabilizers (44). This tissue deformation of the static structures is often termed micro, multidirectional, or atraumatic instability. If overhead motion continues and the previously discussed dynamic stabilizers are not functioning, then rotator cuff fatigue or chronic injury may result. It is generally accepted that tissue deformation occurring from injury causes decreased proprioceptive ability secondary to

> Deafferentation: the elimination or interruption of sensory nerve impulses by destroying or injuring the sensory nerve fibers.

partial **deafferentation** of the joint and its stabilizing structures (49,50). Alteration of the shoulder's neuromuscular control can lead to an asynchronous firing patterns, leading to a maltracking glenohumeral joint, which in and of itself defines shoulder dysfunction. This dysfunction leads to increased distraction forces and tensile stress on the rotator cuff. This process leads to further instability as the static stabilizers are stretched out, the dynamic structures become increasingly weak, and the mechanoreceptors respond slower, thus compromising shoulder performance in the attempt to avoid injury (49,50).

Distal Injuries

As mentioned earlier, because of the connectivity of the structures and tissues of the kinetic chain, shoulder dysfunction can migrate toward or stem from imbalance or injury in the LPHC, knee, and foot and ankle complex, which includes low back pain; sacroiliac joint dysfunction; hamstring complex, quadriceps, and groin strains; patellar tendonitis; iliotibial band (IT-band) tendonitis; plantar fasciitis; Achilles tendonitis; and posterior tibialis tendonitis (shin splints).

(*Text continues on page 337*)

ASSESSMENT AND CORRECTIVE EXERCISE FOR SHOULDER IMPAIRMENTS

➤ SYSTEMATIC PROCESS TO DETERMINE SHOULDER IMPAIRMENTS

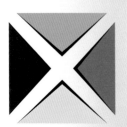

Because of the extreme degrees of freedom of the shoulder joint, its limited contact surface, and its association with the LPHC and cervical spine, there are a number of key elements to assess for shoulder dysfunction. Like the previous chapters, this section will review what to look for when performing static, transitional, and dynamic assessments as well as range of motion and muscle strength tests that will be key to assess when performing an integrated assessment for shoulder impairments. A summary of the assessment process for shoulder impairments and common findings indicating potential dysfunction are listed in the accompanying table.

Continued on page 324

SAMPLE SHOULDER ASSESSMENT PROCESS AND OBSERVATIONS

Assessment	Observation
Static posture	Upper crossed syndrome
Overhead squat	Arms fall forward Low back arches
Horizontal abduction wall test	Elbows flex Shoulders elevate
Rotation wall test	Shoulders elevate Hands away from wall
Shoulder flexion wall test	Shoulders elevate Low back arches
Pushing, pulling, or pressing assessments	Shoulders elevate Forward head Scapular winging (pushing assessment)
Goniometric measurement	Decreased shoulder flexion Decreased glenohumeral internal and/or external rotation
Manual muscle testing	One or more of the following muscle tested "weak": middle, lower trapezius, rhomboids, rotator cuff muscles, serratus anterior

STATIC POSTURE

As mentioned earlier in this chapter, a common static postural distortion syndrome that is associated with shoulder dysfunction is the upper crossed syndrome. As mentioned in chapter five, this is characterized by a rounding of the shoulder and a forward head posture. This position can lead to altered arthrokinematics of the shoulder girdle, increased stress to the shoulder complex, and potential injury. This postural distortion will also be covered further in chapter 16 as it relates to cervical spine dysfunction and injury.

Upper Crossed Syndrome

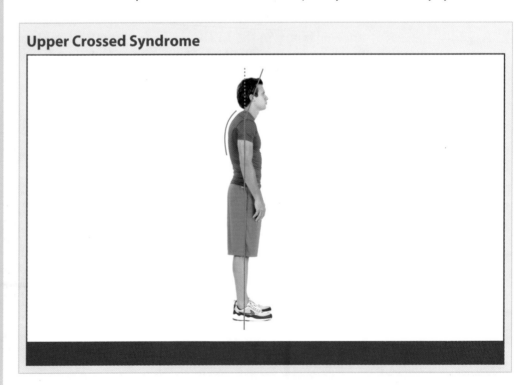

TRANSITIONAL MOVEMENT ASSESSMENTS

The lateral view of the overhead squat test as described in chapter six is most important in the prevention of shoulder injuries. From the lateral view, two main checkpoints, the LPHC and upper body, should be observed for the following compensations: excessive lumbar lordosis (low-back arching) and arms falling forward. The table included here provides a review of the potential overactive and underactive muscles for each compensation.

Overhead Squat Shoulder Compensations

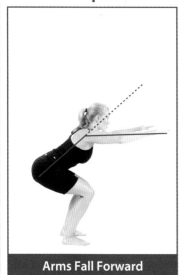

Arms Fall Forward

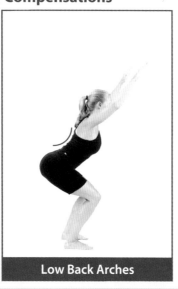

Low Back Arches

SUMMARY OF SHOULDER OVERHEAD SQUAT MOVEMENT COMPENSATIONS			
Compensation	**Potential Overactive Muscles**	**Potential Underactive Muscles**	**Potential Injuries**
Arms fall forward	Latissimus dorsi Pectoralis major/minor Coracobrachialis	Mid/lower trapezius Rhomboids Rotator cuff	Headaches Biceps tendonitis Shoulder impingement Shoulder instability
Low back arches	Latissimus dorsi Erector spinae Hip flexors	Gluteus maximus Hamstrings Core stabilizers	Hamstring, quad and groin strain Low back pain

The horizontal abduction test, rotation test, and shoulder flexion test can be very helpful for the health and fitness professional to determine potential shoulder dysfunction and limited range of motion (chapter six). The three common compensations seen during the upper extremity functional tests include shoulder elevation (shrugging), elbow flexion, and excessive lumbar extension. The accompanying table provides a summary of each and the potential tight and weak musculature that may be contributing to these compensations and may need to be addressed by a corrective exercise program.

Continued on page 326

Examples of Common Upper Extremity Compensations

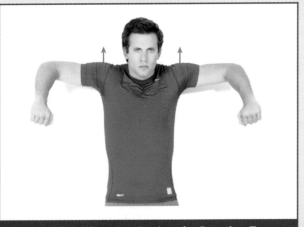

Shoulders Elevating During the Rotation Test

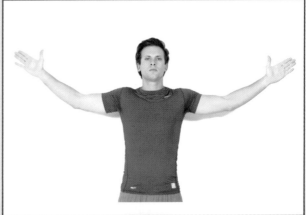

Elbows Flexing During Horizontal Abduction Test

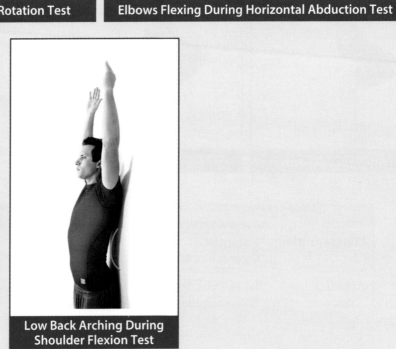

Low Back Arching During
Shoulder Flexion Test

COMMON COMPENSATIONS DURING UPPER EXTREMITY MOVEMENT ASSESSMENTS AND POTENTIAL CAUSES	
Compensation	**Potential Meaning**
Elbows flex	Overactive biceps brachii (long head) Underactive triceps brachii (long head) and rotator cuff
Shoulders elevate	Overactive upper trapezius and levator scapulae Underactive rotator cuff, rhomboids and middle/lower trapezius
Excessive lumbar extension	Overactive erector spinae, pectoralis major/minor, and latissimus dorsi Underactive rotator cuff, rhomboids, middle/lower trapezius, and core stabilizers

Lastly, when performing pushing, pulling, or pressing movements, it will be important to watch for any shoulder elevation, forward migration of the arms (pressing assessment), or scapular winging (push-up assessment). The below table provides a summary of these compensations and the potential tight and weak musculature that may be contributing to these compensations and may need to be addressed by a corrective exercise program.

Example Pushing, Pulling, and Pressing Compensations

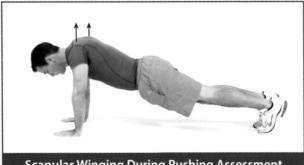

Scapular Winging During Pushing Assessment

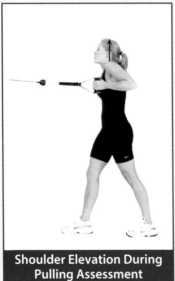

Shoulder Elevation During Pulling Assessment

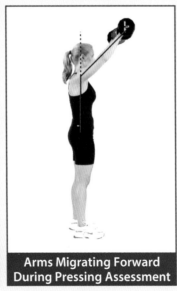

Arms Migrating Forward During Pressing Assessment

COMMON SHOULDER COMPENSATIONS DURING PUSHING, PULLING, AND PRESSING ASSESSMENTS AND POTENTIAL CAUSES

Checkpoint	Compensation	Probable Overactive Muscles	Probable Underactive Muscles
Shoulders	Shoulder elevation	Upper trapezius Levator scapulae	Mid and lower trapezius
	Arms migrate forward	Pectorals Latissimus dorsi	Rotator cuff Mid and lower trapezius
	Scapular winging	Pectoralis Minor	Serratus anterior Mid and lower trapezius

Continued on page 328

DYNAMIC MOVEMENT ASSESSMENTS

The upper extremity Davies test (see photos) is used for dynamic assessment of the upper extremity (UE) as described by Davies et al. (51). This test has been shown to be reliable and is associated with return of rotator cuff strength as well as functional performance of the shoulder (52). Individuals without shoulder dysfunction should be able to complete at least 20 repetitions in 30 seconds. Previous research suggests that closed-chain activities similar to this task are reflective of rotator cuff and scapular muscle function (53–56). Additionally, quality of movement should be assessed during this dynamic assessment. The inability to maintain a neutral LPHC during UE activity may suggest a deficit in core stability. Increased scapular elevation, superior or medial border approximation, or medial border prominence suggests a loss of scapular control and stability. See chapter six to review proper setup and execution of this assessment. If one is not physically capable to perform the Davies Test, you can have them walk on a treadmill as a dynamic movement assessment and from a lateral view, assessment for any rounding of the shoulders and forward head migration.

Upper Extremity Davies Test

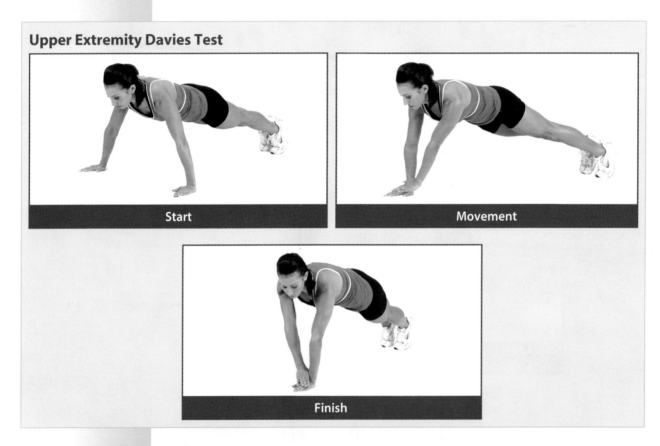

RANGE OF MOTION ASSESSMENTS

The range of motion (ROM) assessments performed for shoulder impairments will be dependent on the compensations seen during the transitional assessments. See the sample shoulder assessment process and observations table on page 324 for a summary of key shoulder joint motions to be measured depending on the movement compensation(s) seen in the movement assessments. See chapter seven to view proper execution of these assessments and average ROM values.

STRENGTH ASSESSMENTS

As with the ROM assessments, the manual muscle tests that are selected will also be dependent on the compensations seen during the transitional movement assessments. The sample shoulder assessment process and observations table seen on page 324 provides a summary of key muscles to be tested on the basis of the compensation(s) seen in the movement assessment. As a reminder, one must be a qualified licensed professional to perform these assessments. See chapter eight to view proper execution of these assessments.

➤ SYSTEMATIC CORRECTIVE EXERCISE STRATEGIES FOR SHOULDER IMPAIRMENTS

The following section will provide sample programming strategies using the Corrective Exercise Continuum for three common shoulder impairments: arms fall forward during the overhead squat; shoulder elevating during upper extremity transitional movement assessments as well as any pushing, pulling, and pressing movements; and scapular winging when performing the push-up assessment. The photos provided illustrate the exercises that can be done for each component of the continuum to help address these common shoulder impairments. Which exercises are used will be dependent on the findings of the assessments and the individual's physical capabilities (integration exercises).

SHOULDER IMPAIRMENT: ARMS FALL FORWARD

Step 1: Inhibit   Key regions to inhibit with foam rolling include the latissimus dorsi and thoracic spine.

Self-Myofascial Release

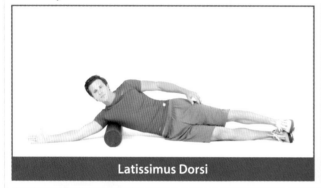
Latissimus Dorsi

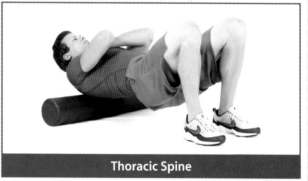
Thoracic Spine

Step 2: Lengthen   Key lengthening exercises with static stretches include the latissimus dorsi and pectorals.

Static Stretches

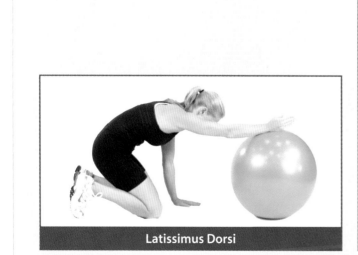
Latissimus Dorsi

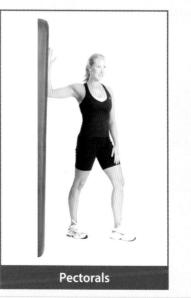
Pectorals

Continued on page 330

Step 3: Activate Key activation exercises with isolated strengthening exercises or positional isometrics include the mid and lower trapezius, rhomboids, and rotator cuff (ball combo II with dowel rod). The ball combo II can also be performed with dumbbells.

Isolated Strengthening Exercises

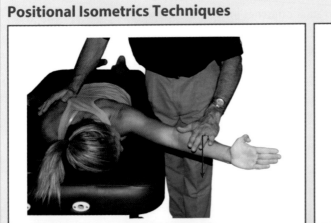

Ball Combo II with Dowel Rod—Start

Ball Combo II with Dowel Rod—Row

Ball Combo II with Dowel Rod—Rotate

Ball Combo II with Dowel Rod—Press (finish)

Positional Isometrics Techniques

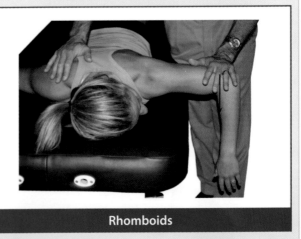

Mid and Lower Trapezius

Rhomboids

Step 4: Integration An integration exercise that could be implemented for this compensation could be a squat to row. This exercise can be progressed by performing it with alternating arms, to one arm, to one arm with trunk rotation, and then going through this same progression on one leg.

Example Integrated Dynamic Movement for Arms Fall Forward

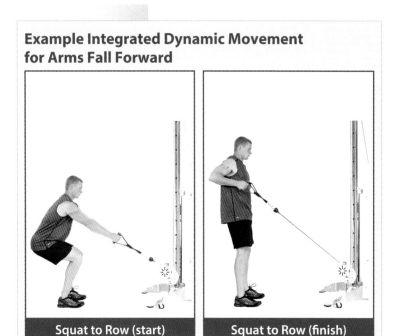

Squat to Row (start)   Squat to Row (finish)

SAMPLE CORRECTIVE EXERCISE PROGRAM FOR SHOULDER IMPAIRMENT: ARMS FALL FORWARD			
Phase	**Modality**	**Muscle(s)**	**Acute Variables**
Inhibit	SMR	Latissimus dorsi Thoracic spine	Hold on tender area for 30 seconds
Lengthen	Static stretching	Latissimus dorsi Pectoralis major	30-seconds hold
Activate	Positional isometrics AND/OR isolated strengthening	Rotator cuff Middle and lower trapezius	4 reps of increasing intensity 25, 50, 75, 100% **OR** 10–15 reps with 2-seconds isometric hold and 4-seconds eccentric
Integrate*	Integrated dynamic movement	Squat to row	10–15 reps under control

*NOTE: If client is not initially capable of performing the integrated dynamic movement exercise listed, he or she may need to be regressed to a more suitable exercise.

SHOULDER IMPAIRMENT: SHOULDER ELEVATION

Step 1: Inhibit Key regions to inhibit with foam rolling and apparatus-assisted modalities include the thoracic spine, upper trapezius, and levator scapulae.

Continued on page 332

Self-Myofascial Release

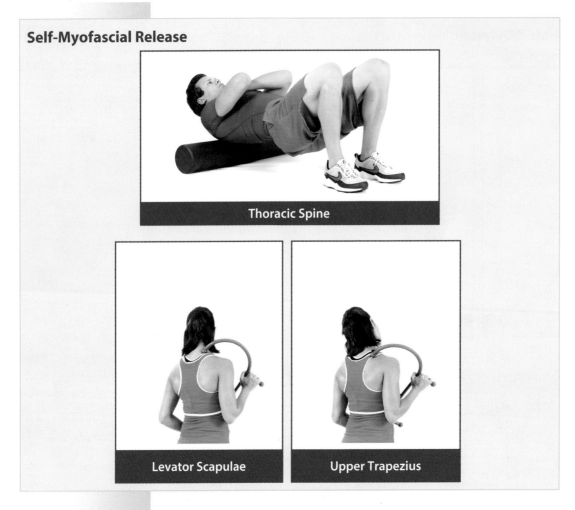

Thoracic Spine

Levator Scapulae

Upper Trapezius

Step 2: Lengthen Key lengthening exercises with static stretches include the pectorals, upper trapezius, and levator scapulae.

Static Stretches

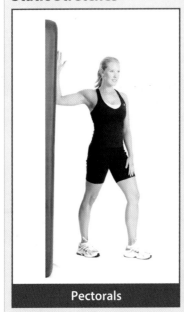

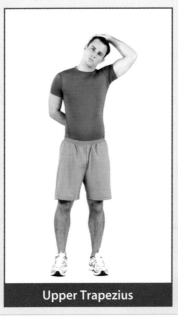

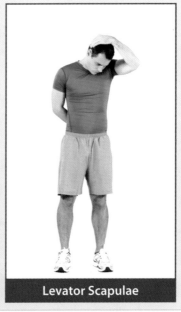

Pectorals

Upper Trapezius

Levator Scapulae

Step 3: Activate   Key activation exercises with isolated strengthening exercises or positional isometrics include the mid and lower trapezius (ball cobra).

Isolated Strengthening Exercises

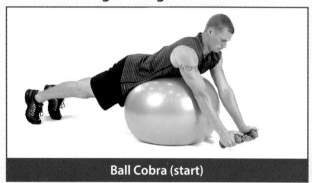

Ball Cobra (start)

Ball Cobra (finish)

Positional Isometrics Techniques

Mid and Lower Trapezius

Step 4: Integration   An integration exercise that could also be implemented for this compensation could be a single-leg Romanian deadlift with PNF (proprioceptive neuromuscular facilitation) pattern.

Continued on page 334

Integrated Dynamic Movement

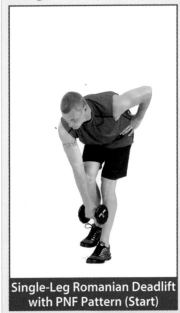

Single-Leg Romanian Deadlift
with PNF Pattern (Start)

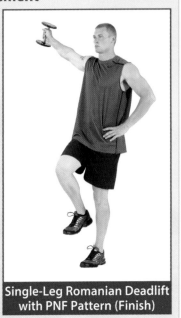

Single-Leg Romanian Deadlift
with PNF Pattern (Finish)

Phase	Modality	Muscle(s)	Acute Variables
SAMPLE CORRECTIVE EXERCISE PROGRAM FOR SHOULDER IMPAIRMENT: SHOULDER ELEVATION			
Inhibit	SMR	Upper trapezius Levator scapulae Thoracic spine	Hold on tender area for 30 seconds
Lengthen	Static stretching	Upper trapezius Levator scapulae Pectorals	30-seconds hold
Activate	Positional isometrics/or isolated strengthening	Middle and lower trapezius	4 reps of increasing intensity 25, 50, 75, 100% **OR** 10–15 reps with 2-seconds isometric hold and 4-seconds eccentric hold
Integrate*	Integrated dynamic movement	Single-leg Romanian deadlift with PNF pattern	10–15 reps under control

***NOTE:** If client is not initially capable of performing the integrated dynamic movement exercise listed he or she may need to be regressed to a more suitable exercise.
PNF, proprioceptive neuromuscular facilitation.

SHOULDER IMPAIRMENT: SCAPULAR WINGING

Step 1: Inhibit Key regions to inhibit with foam rolling include the latissimus dorsi and thoracic spine.

Self-Myofascial Release

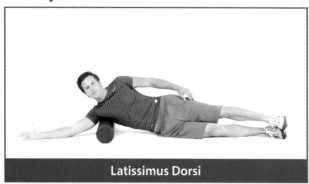

Latissimus Dorsi

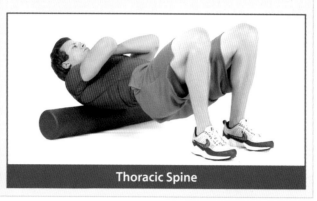

Thoracic Spine

Step 2: Lengthen Key lengthening exercises with static stretches include the latissimus dorsi and pectorals.

Static Stretches

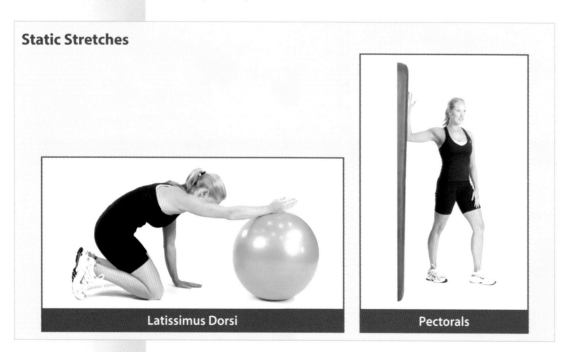

Latissimus Dorsi

Pectorals

Step 3: Activate Key activation exercises with isolated strengthening exercises or positional isometrics include the serratus anterior (push-up with plus) and mid and lower trapezius (ball combo I).

Isolated Strengthening Exercises

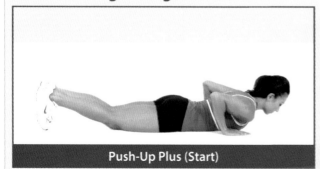

Push-Up Plus (Start)

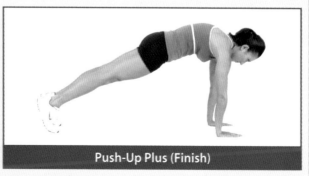

Push-Up Plus (Finish)

Continued on page 336

Key Isolated Strengthening Exercises for Scapular Winging

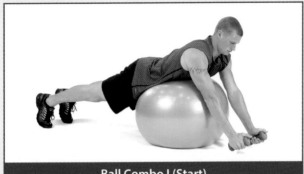

Ball Combo I (Start)

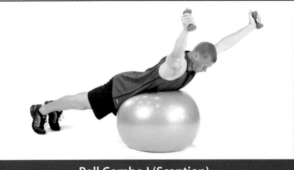

Ball Combo I (Scaption)

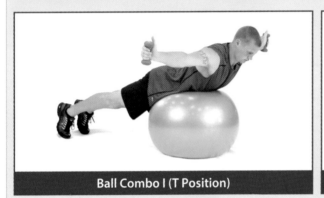

Ball Combo I (T Position)

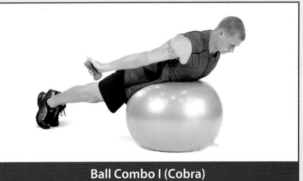

Ball Combo I (Cobra)

Positional Isometrics Techniques

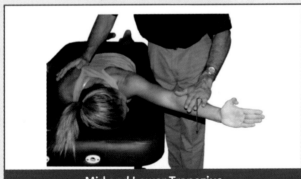

Mid and Lower Trapezius

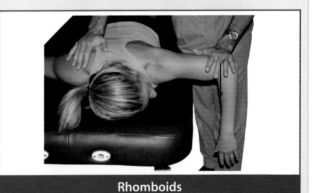

Rhomboids

Serratus Anterior

Step 4: Integration An integration exercise that could also be implemented for this compensation could be a standing one-arm cable chest press.

Integrated Dynamic Movement

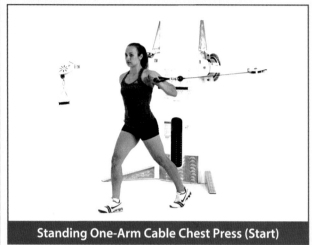

Standing One-Arm Cable Chest Press (Start)

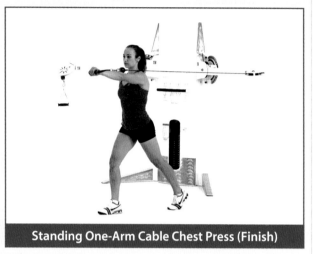

Standing One-Arm Cable Chest Press (Finish)

Phase	Modality	Muscle(s)	Acute Variables
SAMPLE CORRECTIVE EXERCISE PROGRAM FOR SHOULDER IMPAIRMENT: SCAPULAR WINGING			
Inhibit	SMR	Latissimus dorsi Thoracic spine	Hold on tender area for 30 seconds
Lengthen	**Static stretching**	Latissimus dorsi Pectorals Serratus anterior	30-seconds hold
Activate	**Positional isometrics or isolated strengthening**	Middle and lower trapezius	4 reps of increasing intensity 25, 50, 75, 100% **OR** 10–15 reps with 2-seconds isometric hold and 4-seconds eccentric
Integrate*	**Integrated dynamic movement**	Standing 1-arm cable chest press	10–15 reps under control

*****NOTE:** If client is not initially capable of performing the integrated dynamic movement exercise listed he or she may need to be regressed to a more suitable exercise.

ELBOW AND WRIST

INTRODUCTION

MUSCULOSKELETAL injuries to the elbow, forearm, and wrist account for approximately one third of all workday illnesses (57). These injuries are associated with greater loss of productivity and wages than those of other anatomic regions such as the low back. Common diagnoses include tendon-related disorders such as lateral epicondylitis, which occurs in up to 3% of the general population (58). The risk factors for these injuries are similar and include tasks that are repetitive, hand intensive, and forceful (59,60). These factors all increase the stress on the flexor and extensor tendons of the elbow. Therefore, injury prevention and treatment strategies aim to decrease sure to repetitive tasks and limit extremes of elbow and wrist motion.

REVIEW OF ELBOW AND WRIST FUNCTIONAL ANATOMY

Bones and Joints

The elbow's primary function is to transfer energy from the shoulder to the hand, allowing for precise and forceful movements simultaneously. The articulations between the humerus, radius, and ulna form the humeroulnar joint or "true" elbow, humeroradial joint between the capitulum and radial head, and the proximal radioulnar joint. The humeroulnar joint is a hinge joint and is the primary joint responsible for elbow flexion and extension (Figure 15-10). The proximal radioulnar joint is primarily responsible for forearm pronation and supination (Figure 15-10).

The wrist is composed of the distal radioulnar joint and articulations between the proximal (scaphoid, lunate, triquetrum, pisiform) and distal (trapezium, trapezoid, capitate, hamate, or TFCC [triangular fibrocartilage complex]) carpal rows. The proximal wrist is the articulation between the radius, scaphoid and lunate, and TFCC. The distal wrist joint is considered the articulations between the proximal and distal carpal rows. The majority of wrist flexion and extension and radial and ulnar deviation range of motion derives from the proximal wrist joint (Figure 15-11).

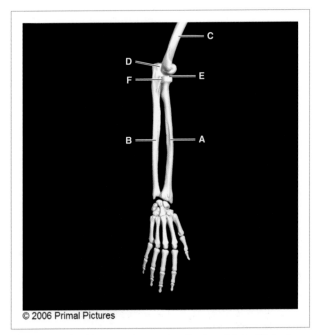

© 2006 Primal Pictures

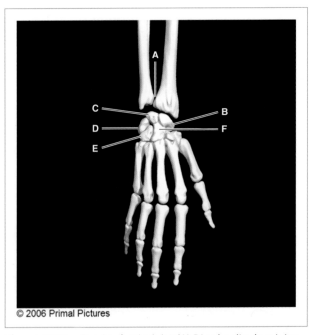

© 2006 Primal Pictures

Figure 15.10   Humeroulnar and radioulnar joints (A) Radius (B) Ulna (C) Humerus (D) Humeroulnar joint (E) Humeroradial joint (F) Proximal radioulnar joint.

Figure 15.11   Proximal wrist joint (A) Distal radioulnar joint (B) Scaphoid (C) Lunate (D) Triquetrum (E) Hamate (F) Capitate.

CORRECTIVE STRATEGIES FOR SHOULDER, ELBOW, AND WRIST IMPAIRMENTS

Muscles

Muscles about the elbow, forearm, and wrist can be simply divided into elbow flexors and extensors and wrist flexors and extensors (Table 15-3). The brachialis is the primary flexor of the elbow and is assisted by the biceps, which is also an important supinator in certain positions. The elbow extensors include the long and short head of the triceps and are an important stabilizer with the brachialis to allow the elbow to maintain a constant position during powerful pronation and supination and wrist motion. See chapter two for a detailed review of the location and integrated function of these muscles.

Table 15.3 KEY MUSCLES ASSOCIATED WITH THE ELBOW AND WRIST	
• Biceps brachii • Triceps brachii • Brachialis • Brachioradialis • Pronator quadratus	• Pronator teres • Supinator • Wrist flexors • Wrist extensors

The wrist is unique in that the majority of muscles that control the joint do not actually attach to the wrist. Instead, the wrist flexors attach to the medial epicondyle of the humerus by means of the common flexor tendon, and the wrist extensors attach to the lateral epicondyle by means of the common extensor tendon. These muscles have relatively short muscle bellies and long tendons that flex and extend not only the wrist, but also the fingers (Figure 15-12). All of the muscles described function concentrically to create motion about a given joint. But more importantly, they control motion (eccentrically) to allow for powerful wrist and hand motions such as turning a wrench or swinging a

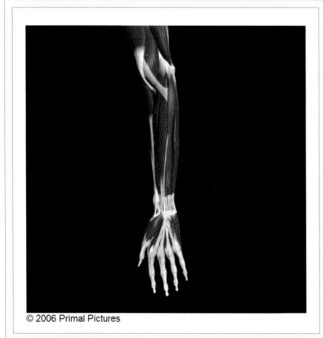
© 2006 Primal Pictures

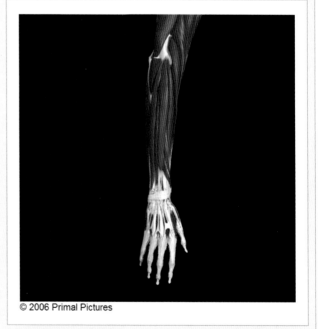
© 2006 Primal Pictures

Figure 15.12A Structure of wrist musculature. Wrist flexors.

Figure 15.12B Structure of wrist musculature. Wrist extensors.

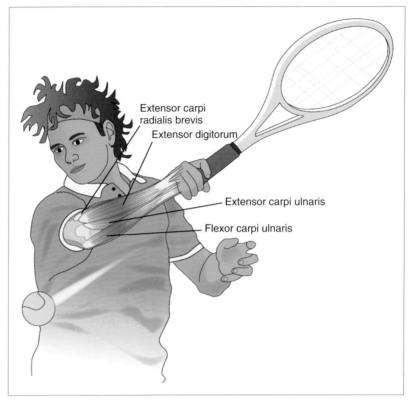

Figure 15.13 Example of eccentric control of the wrist.

tennis racquet (Figure 15-13). Therefore, optimal corrective exercise programs will work to maximize flexibility, thereby limiting resistance to power production and stabilization ability. Additionally, these muscles must be trained to function eccentrically to allow for adequate stabilization of the elbow and wrist, minimizing stress on the tendinous insertion.

COMMON ELBOW AND WRIST INJURIES

De Quervain syndrome: an inflammation or a tendinosis of the sheath or tunnel that surrounds two tendons that control movement of the thumb.

Tendon-related disorders of the elbow and wrist include medial and lateral epicondylitis (Figure 15-14) and **de Quervain syndrome**. Lateral epicondylitis is the most prevalent disorder and is characterized by pain slightly distal to the lateral epicondyle and painful resisted wrist extension. It is important to note that although the common diagnosis continues to be an "-itis," this injury is not an acute inflammatory condition. Current research has clearly shown that in the majority of these patients, a painful extensor

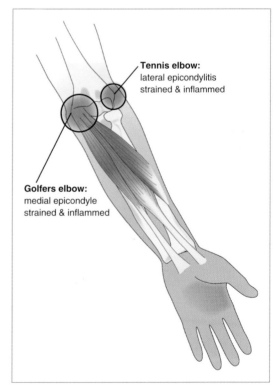

Figure 15.14 Medial and lateral epicondylitis.

tendon has become degenerative, characterized by fibroblastic and vascular changes, and is more accurately described as a tendinopathy (58,61). These changes to the tendon complex are thought to occur as the result of abnormal loading of the extensor tendons, in particular the extensor carpi radialis brevis (57,62). Although not as common or understood, similar processes are thought to take place on the medial elbow about the common flexor tendon. The increased stress on either tendon is likely the result of muscle imbalances about the elbow and wrist. These imbalances may be present as ROM deficits in elbow extension, pronation, and supination, or wrist flexion and extension.

(*Text continues on page 348*)

ASSESSMENT AND CORRECTIVE EXERCISE FOR ELBOW AND WRIST IMPAIRMENTS

➤ SYSTEMATIC PROCESS TO DETERMINE ELBOW AND WRIST IMPAIRMENTS

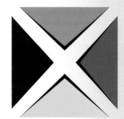

RANGE OF MOTION ASSESSMENT

Assessment of the elbow and wrist to determine the most appropriate corrective exercise strategy can be simplified into two steps: range of motion or flexibility assessment and strength assessment. If limitations in elbow flexion or extension are observed, follow-up assessments of these movements with the shoulder flexed and extended should be conducted to determine which muscles are causing the deficit. If the shoulder is flexed and elbow extension is limited, then the brachialis is the primary muscle involved. If elbow extension is only limited in shoulder extension, then the long head of the biceps is involved. Wrist flexion and extension should similarly be performed with the elbow flexed and extended. If limitations are observed in wrist flexion or extension with the elbow extended, this suggests the common wrist flexors or extensors are limiting the motion. If the motion is limited with the elbow flexed, then this suggests the wrist joint is compromised. A complete examination of the joint by a physical therapist, certified athletic trainer, or physician may be required.

Brachialis Limitation Assessment

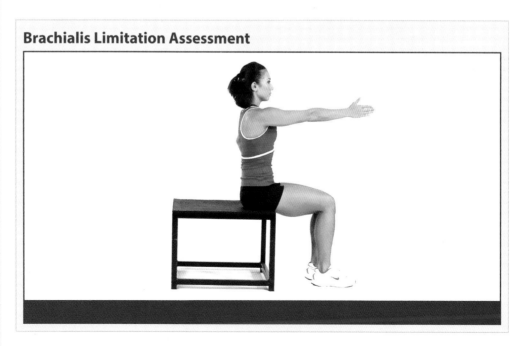

Continued on page 342

Long Head of the Biceps Limitation Assessment

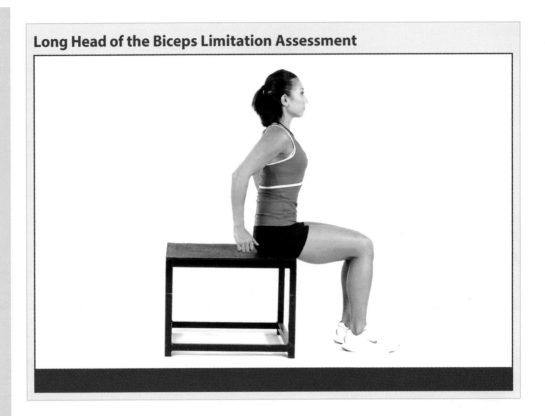

Active Wrist ROM Assessment

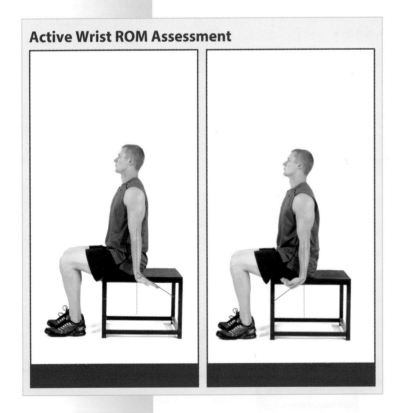

Wrist Limitations

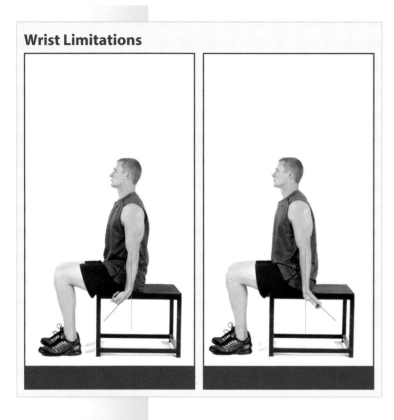

➤ CORRECTIVE EXERCISE STRATEGIES FOR THE ELBOW AND WRIST IMPAIRMENTS

The following section will provide sample programming strategies using the Corrective Exercise Continuum for elbow and wrist limitations (see accompanying table). The photos provided illustrate the exercises that can be done for each component of the continuum to help address these common elbow and wrist impairments.

STEP 1: INHIBIT

Inhibitory techniques can be easily applied by having the individual provide self-applied pressure to regions of tightness and sensitivity on the upper arm and forearm. Maintain that pressure for 30 seconds.

STEP 2: LENGTHEN

A combination of movements that extend the shoulder and elbow are most effective for lengthening the long head of the biceps. Similarly, combined movements of elbow extension and wrist flexion or extension are most effective for lengthening forearm musculature. These techniques should follow lengthening guidelines for bouts of 2 to 3 repetitions for 30 seconds to facilitate a change in length over the course of a few weeks.

Continued on page 344

Static Stretches

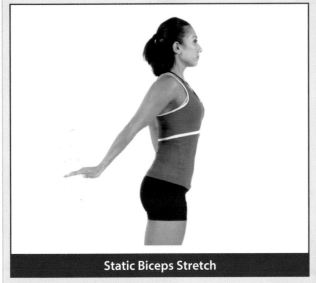

Static Biceps Stretch

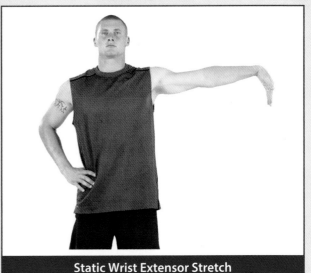

Static Wrist Extensor Stretch

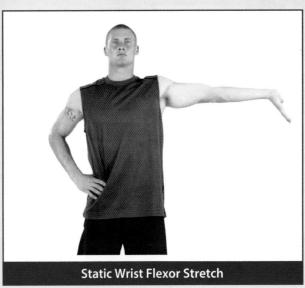

Static Wrist Flexor Stretch

STEP 3: ACTIVATE

Activation exercises to isolate the elbow flexors and extensors as well as the wrist flexors and extensors should follow the selected inhibit or lengthen intervention(s). Effective exercises to isolate both the long and short head of the triceps as well as the long and short head of the biceps are examples of how a traditional strengthening exercise applied in the appropriate progression can obtain optimal results. Similar isolation exercises should be performed for the wrist flexors and extensors.

Isolated Strengthening Exercises for the Elbow and Wrist Musculature

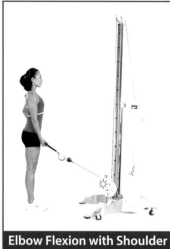

Elbow Flexion with Shoulder Neutral (Start)

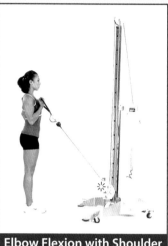

Elbow Flexion with Shoulder Neutral (Finish)

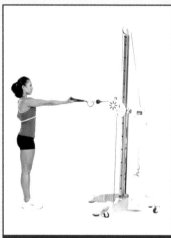

Elbow Flexion with Shoulder Flexed (Start)

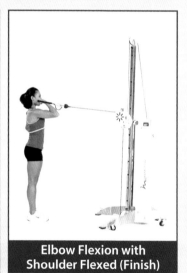

Elbow Flexion with Shoulder Flexed (Finish)

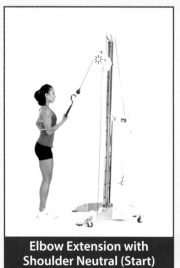

Elbow Extension with Shoulder Neutral (Start)

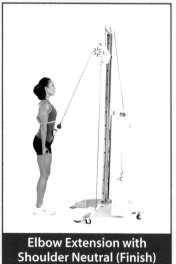

Elbow Extension with Shoulder Neutral (Finish)

Continued on page 346

Isolated Strengthening Exercises for the Elbow and Wrist Musculature

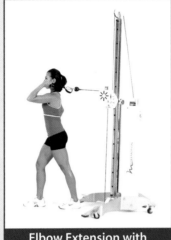

Elbow Extension with Shoulder Flexed (Start)

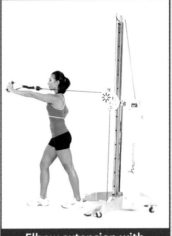

Elbow extension with Shoulder Flexed (Finish)

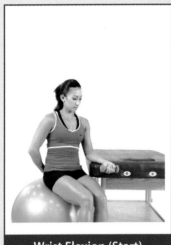

Wrist Flexion (Start)

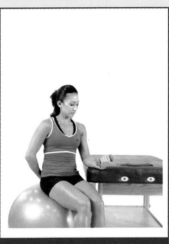

Wrist Flexion (Finish)

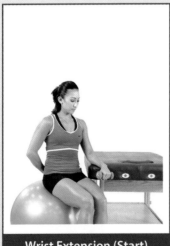

Wrist Extension (Start)

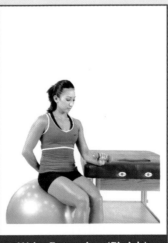

Wrist Extension (Finish)

Isolated Strengthening Exercises for the Elbow and Wrist Musculature

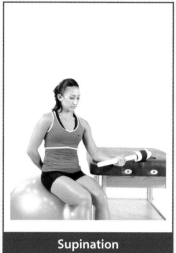

Supination

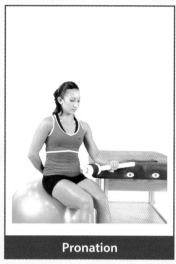

Pronation

STEP 4: INTEGRATION

Integration exercises for the wrist and elbow can include almost any exercise you may currently implement that requires gripping with the hand while performing combined movements of the kinetic chain. The most effective interventions will likely draw on neural principles that couple wrist and elbow flexion with shoulder flexion and wrist extension with elbow extension and shoulder extension. These movements can be incorporated into the full workout during exercise such as a standing latissimus dorsi pulldown (flexor mechanism) or a prone ball triceps extension with cobra (extensor mechanism).

Isolated Integration Exercises for the Elbow and Wrist Musculature

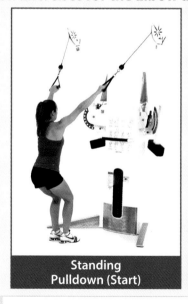

Standing
Pulldown (Start)

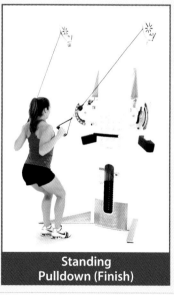

Standing
Pulldown (Finish)

Continued on page 348

Isolated Integration Exercises for the Elbow and Wrist Musculature

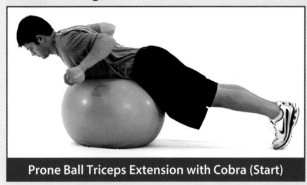

Prone Ball Triceps Extension with Cobra (Start)

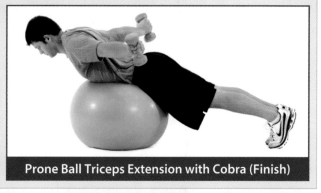

Prone Ball Triceps Extension with Cobra (Finish)

SAMPLE CORRECTIVE EXERCISE PROGRAM FOR ELBOW IMPAIRMENTS AND WRIST IMPAIRMENTS			
Phase	**Modality**	**Muscle(s)**	**Acute Variables**
Inhibit	SMR	Brachialis Biceps brachii Wrist flexors or extensors	Hold on tender area for 30 seconds
Lengthen	Static stretching	Biceps brachii Wrist flexors or extensors	30-seconds hold
Activate	Isolated strengthening	Elbow flexion Elbow extension Wrist flexors or extensors Wrist supination and pronation	10–15 reps with 2-seconds isometric hold and 4-seconds eccentric
Integrate*	Integrated dynamic movement	Standing pulldown Prone ball triceps extension with cobra	10–15 reps under control

*NOTE: If client is not initially capable of performing the integrated dynamic movement exercise listed he or she may need to be regressed to a more suitable exercise.

SUMMARY • Shoulder, elbow and wrist injuries can significantly limit participation in recreational and competitive athletics. Common shoulder injuries such as impingement syndrome and instability are routinely correlated with movement dysfunction. Common elbow injuries include lateral and medial epicondylitis. As with the other regions of the body, identification of movement dysfunction using a battery of simple clinical screens provides an efficient way to address muscle imbalances in many clients. Focused corrective exercise programs progressing from inhibition–lengthen–activate–integrate are likely to address these muscle imbalances of the shoulders, elbow and wrist. Identification of clients with movement dysfunction that does not resolve or produces more pain indicates the need for a more thorough clinical examination by a physical therapist or certified athletic trainer.

References

1. Bongers PM. The cost of shoulder pain at work. *BMJ* 2001;322(7278):64–5.

2. Urwin M, Symmons D, Allison T, et al. Estimating the burden of musculoskeletal disorders in the community: the comparative prevalence of symptoms at different anatomical sites, and the relation to social deprivation. *Ann Rheum Di.* 1998;57(11):649–55.

3. Van der Heijden G. Shoulder disorders: a state of the art review. *Baillieres Best Pract Res Clin Rheumatol* 1999;13(2):287–309.

4. Johnson M, Crosley K, O'Neil M, Al Zakwani I. Estimates of direct health care expenditures among individuals with shoulder dysfunction in the United States. *J Orthop Sports Phys Ther* 2005;35(1):A4–PL8.

5. van der Windt DA, Koes BW, Boeke AJ, Deville W, De Jong BA, Bouter LM. Shoulder disorders in general practice: prognostic indicators of outcome. *Br J Gen Pract* 1996;46(410):519–23.

6. Hovelius L. Shoulder dislocation in Swedish ice hockey players. *Am J Sports Med* 1978;6:373–7.

7. Hovelius L. Incidence of shoulder dislocation in Sweden. *Clin Orthop Relat Res* 1982;166(6):127–31.

8. Simonet WT, Melton J III, Cofield RH, Ilstrup DM. Incidence of anterior shoulder dislocation in Olmsted County, Minnesota. *Clin Ortho Relat Res* 1983;186(6):186–91.

9. Owens BD, Agel J, Mountcastle SB, Cameron KL, Nelson BJ. Incidence of glenohumeral instability in collegiate athletics. *Am J Sports Med* 2009;37(9):1750–4.

10. Owens BD, Duffey ML, Nelson BJ, DeBerardino TM, Taylor DC, Mountcastle SB. The incidence and characteristics of shoulder instability at the United States Military Academy. *Am J Sports Med* 2007;35(7):1168–73.

11. Owens BD, Dawson L, Burks R, Cameron KL. Incidence of shoulder dislocation in the United States military: demographic considerations from a high-risk population. *J Bone Joint Surg Am* 2009;91(4):791–6.

12. Simonet WT, Cofield RH. Prognosis in anterior shoulder dislocation. *Am J Sports Med* 1984;12(1):19–24.

13. Hovelius L, Olofsson A, Sandstrom B, et al. Nonoperative treatment of primary anterior shoulder dislocation in patients forty years of age and younger. A prospective twenty-five-year follow-up. *J Bone Joint Surg Am* 2008;90(5):945–52.

14. Buscayret F, Edwards TB, Szabo I, Adeleine P, Coudane H, Walch G. Glenohumeral arthrosis in anterior instability before and after surgical intervention. *Am J Sports Med* 2004;32(5):1165–72.

15. Cameron ML, Kocher MS, Briggs KK, Horan MP, Hawkins RJ. The prevalence of glenohumeral osteoarthrosis in unstable shoulders. *Am J Sports Med* 2003;31(1):53–5.

16. Carpenter JE, Flanagan CL, Thomopoulos S, Yian EH, Soslowsky LJ. The effects of overuse combined with intrinsic or extrinsic alterations in an animal model of rotator cuff tendinosis. *Am J Sports Med* 1998;26(6):801–7.

17. Soslowsky LJ, Carpenter JE, Bucchieri JS, Flatow EL. Biomechanics of the rotator cuff. *Orthop Clin North Am* 1997;28(1):17–30.

18. Yamaguchi K, Ditsios K, Middleton WD, Hildebolt CF, Galatz LM, Teefey SA. The demographic and morphological features of rotator cuff disease. A comparison of asymptomatic and symptomatic shoulders. *J Bone Joint Surg Am* 2006;88(8):1699–704.

19. Yamaguchi K, Sher JS, Andersen WK, et al. Glenohumeral motion in patients with rotator cuff tears: a comparison of asymptomatic and symptomatic shoulders. *J Shoulder Elbow Surg* 2000;9(1):6–11.

20. Bigliani LU, Levine WN. Subacromial impingement syndrome. *J Bone Joint Surg Am* 1997;79(12):1854–68.

21. NIOSH. Musculoskeletal Disorders (MSDs) and Workplace Factors: A Critical Review of Epidemiologic Evidence for Work-Related Musculoskeletal Disorders of the Neck, Upper Extremity, and Low Back. Cincinnati, OH: Centers for Disease Control and Prevention; 1997.

22. Szeto GPY, Straker L, Raine S. A field comparison of neck and shoulder postures in symptomatic and asymptomatic office workers. *Appl Ergon* 2002;33(1):75–84.

23. Lukasiewicz AC, McClure P, Michener L, Pratt N, Sennett B. Comparison of 3-dimensional scapular position and orientation between subjects with and without shoulder impingement. *J Orthop Sports Phys Ther* 1999;29(10):574–86.

24. Ludewig PM, Cook TM. Alterations in shoulder kinematics and associated muscle activity in people with symptoms of shoulder impingement. *Phys Ther* 2000;80(3):276–91.

25. Thigpen CA, Padua DA, Karas SG. Comparison of scapular kinematics between individuals with and without multidirectional shoulder instability. *J Athl Train* 2005;40(2):15-22

26. Thigpen CA, Padua DA, Xu N, Karas SG. Comparison of scapular muscle activity between individuals with and without multidirectional shoulder instability. *J Orthop Sports Phys Ther* 2005;35(1):A4–PL18.

27. Pink M, Perry J. Athletic Injuries and Rehabilitation. Philadelphia, PA: WB Saunders; 1996.

28. Moore KL. Clinically Oriented Anatomy. 3rd ed. Baltimore, MD: Williams & Wilkins; 1992.

29. Terry G, Chopp T. Functional anatomy of the shoulder. *J Athl Train* 2000;35:248–55.

30. Decker MJ, Tokish JM, Ellis HB, Torry MR, Hawkins RJ. Subscapularis muscle activity during selected rehabilitation exercises. *Am J Sports Med* 2003;31(1):126–34.

31. Hamill J, Knutzen K. Biomechanical Basis of Human Movement. 2nd ed. Philadelphia, PA: Lippincott Williams & Wilkins; 2003.

32. Kibler WB, Sciascia A, Dome D. Evaluation of apparent and absolute supraspinatus strength in patients with shoulder injury using the scapular retraction test. *Am J Sports Med* 2006;34(10):1643–7.

33. Borstad JD. Resting position variables at the shoulder: evidence to support a posture-impairment association. *Phys Ther* 2006;86(4):549–57.

34. Borstad JD, Ludewig PM. The effect of long versus short pectoralis minor resting length on scapular kinematics in healthy individuals. *J Orthop Sports Phys Ther* 2005;35(4):227–38.

35. Michener LA, McClure PW, Karduna AR. Anatomical and biomechanical mechanisms of subacromial impingement syndrome. *Clin Biomech (Bristol, Avon)* 2003;18(5):369–79.

36. Schmitt L, Snyder-Mackler L. Role of scapular stabilizers in etiology and treatment of impingement syndrome. *J Orthop Sports Phys Ther* 1999;29(1):31–8.

37. McClure PW, Michener LA, Karduna AR. Shoulder function and 3-dimensional scapular kinematics in people with and without shoulder impingement syndrome. *Phys Ther* 2006;86(8):1075–90.

38. Hebert LJ, Moffet H, Dufour M. Acromiohumeral distance in a seated position in persons with impingement syndrome. *J Magn Reson Imaging* 2003;18:72–9.

39. Hebert LJ, Moffet H, McFadyen BJ, Dionne CE. Scapular behavior in shoulder impingement syndrome. *Arch Phys Med Rehabil* 2002;83(1):60–9.

40. Finley MA, McQuade KJ, Rodgers MM. Effect of sitting posture on 3-dimensional scapular kinematics measured by skin-mounted electromagnetic tracking sensors. *Arch Phys Med Rehabil* 2003;81:563–8.

41. Thigpen CA, Padua DA, Guskiewicz KM, Michener LA. Three-dimensional shoulder position in individuals with and without forward head and rounded shoulder posture. *J Athl Train* 2006;41(2):-34.

42. Thigpen CA, Padua DA, Michener LA, et al. Head and shoulder posture affect scapular mechanics and muscle activity in overhead tasks. *J Electromyogr Kinesiol* 2010. In press.

43. Janda V. Evaluation of Muscle Imbalances. In: Liebenson C, ed. Rehabilitation of the Spine. Baltimore, MD: Williams & Wilkins; 1996. p 97–112.

44. Meister K. Injuries to the shoulder in the throwing athlete. Part one: biomechanics/pathophysiology/classification of injury. *Am J Sports Med* 2000;28(2):265–75.

45. McCluskey GM, Getz BA. Pathophysiology of anterior shoulder instability. *J Athl Train* 2000;35(3):268–72.

46. Rowe MCR, Harilaos T. Sakellarides M. Factors related to recurrences of anterior dislocations of the shoulder. *Clin Orthop* 1961;20:40–7.

47. Buss DD, Lynch GP, Meyer CP, Huber SM, Freehill MQ. Nonoperative management for in-season athletes with anterior shoulder instability. *Am J Sports Med* 2004;32(6):1430–3.

48. Warner JJ, Micheli LJ, Arslanian LE, Kennedy J, Kennedy R. Patterns of flexibility. laxity, and strength in normal shoulders and shoulders with instability and impingement. *Am J Sports Med* 1990;18(4):366–75.

49. Safran MR, Borsa PA, Lephart SM, Fu FH, Warner JJ. Shoulder proprioception in baseball pitchers. *J Shoulder Elbow Surg* 2001;10(5):438–44.

50. Ozaki J. Glenohumeral movements of the involuntary inferior and multidirectional instability. *Clin Orthop Relat Res* 1989;238:107–11.

51. Davies G, Kraushar D, Brinks K, Jennings J. Neuromuscular Stability of the Shoulder Complex. In: Manske R, ed. Rehabilitation for Post-Surgical Knee and Post-Surgical Shoulder Conditions. Philadelphia, PA. Elsevier Science; 2006. p 133–155

52. Falsone SA, Gross MT, Guskiewicz KM, Schneider RA. One-arm hop test: reliability and effects of arm dominance. *J Orthop Sports Phys Ther* 2002;32(3):98–103.

53. Kibler WB, Sciascia AD, Uhl TL, Tambay N, Cunningham T. Electromyographic analysis of specific exercises for scapular control in early phases of shoulder rehabilitation. *Am J Sports Med* 2008;36(9):1789–98.

54. Maenhout A, Van Praet K, Pizzi L, Van Herzeele M, Cools A. Electromyographic analysis of knee push up plus variations: what's the influence of the kinetic chain on scapular muscle activity? *Br J Sports Med* 2009.

55. Cools AM, Dewitte V, Lanszweert F, et al. Rehabilitation of scapular muscle balance: which exercises to prescribe? *Ame J Sports Med* 2007;35(10):1744–51.

56. Cools AM, Declercq GA, Cambier DC, Mahieu NN, Witvrouw EE. Trapezius activity and intramuscular balance during isokinetic exercise in overhead athletes with impingement symptoms. *Scand J Med Sci Sports* 2007;17(1):25–33.

57. Barr AE, Barbe MF, Clark BD. Work-related musculoskeletal disorders of the hand and wrist: epidemiology, pathophysiology, and sensorimotor changes. *J Orthop Sports Phys Ther* 2004;34(10):610–27.

58. Malliaras P, Maffulli N, Garau G. Eccentric training programmes in the management of lateral elbow tendinopathy. *Disabil Rehabil* 2008;30(20–22):1590–6.

59. Keyserling WM. Workplace risk factors and occupational musculoskeletal disorders, Part 1: a review of biomechanical and psychophysical research on risk factors associated with low-back pain. *Am Ind Hyg Assoc J* 2000;61(1):39–50.

60. Muggleton JM, Allen R, Chappell PH. Hand and arm injuries associated with repetitive manual work in industry: a review of disorders, risk factors and preventive measures. *Ergonomics* 1999;42(5):714–39.

61. Barr AE, Barbe MF. Pathophysiological tissue changes associated with repetitive movement: a review of the evidence. *Phys Ther* 2002;82(2):173–87.

62. Trudel D, Duley J, Zastrow I, Kerr EW, Davidson R, MacDermid JC. Rehabilitation for patients with lateral epicondylitis: a systematic review. *J Hand Ther* 2004;17(2):243–66.

CHAPTER 16

Corrective Strategies for Cervical Spine Impairments

Upon completion of this chapter, you will be able to:

➤ Understand basic functional anatomy for the cervical spine region.

➤ Understand the mechanisms for cervical spine injuries.

➤ Determine common risk factors that can lead to cervical spine injury.

➤ Incorporate a systematic assessment and corrective exercise strategy for cervical spine impairments.

INTRODUCTION

ACCORDING to a survey conducted by the National Institute of Health Statistics (NIHS), neck pain is the third most common type of pain for Americans (1). Roughly two thirds of the population will experience neck pain in their lifetime. Its side effects can be mild or severe, and interfere with normal daily functioning such as sitting, turning, and sleeping. Neck pain can be acute (lasts less than 3 months), or chronic (lasts longer than 3 months). In the NIHS study, the majority of respondents (42%) had suffered neck pain for longer than a year. The survey also showed that women are three times more likely to suffer with this health problem than men and that if you are under severe stress your risk of neck pain increases by one and a half times. However, research has shown that exercise, in the form of neck strengthening, stretching, and proprioceptive exercises, can decrease the risk of neck pain and improve the symptoms of neck pain (2–11).

Like other regions of the body, the cervical spine (CS) is a region that has a massive influence on the structures above and below it. The CS has more than 30 muscles that are located in the cervical spine region and shoulder complex. The neck muscle system is intimately related with reflex systems concerned with vestibular function, proprioceptive systems, stabilization of the head and eyes, postural orientation, and stability of the whole body. Thus, dysfunction in this region can lead to many injuries throughout the body.

REVIEW OF THE CERVICAL SPINE FUNCTIONAL ANATOMY

As previously stated, the CS has a great influence on the rest of the kinetic chain. There are many bones, joints, and muscles involved in the CS; however, the purpose of this section is to provide a general review of the most pertinent structures.

The Neck Region

Looking at the neck specifically (Figure 16-1), the anatomic region from posterior to anterior is from the superior nuchal line to the spine of the scapula. From the side, it extends from the superior nuchal line and external occipital protuberance to the superior border of the clavicle and suprasternal notch.

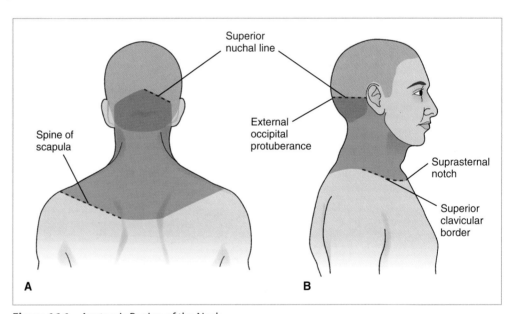

Figure 16.1 Anatomic Region of the Neck.

Bones and Joints

Looking at the cervical spine region specifically (Figure 16-2), the cervical spine begins at the base of the skull and include seven vertebrae. The individual cervical vertebrae are abbreviated C1 (atlas), C2 (axis), C3, C4, C5, C6, and C7. Between C2 and each sequential vertebra are the intervening disks. The cervical spine curvature is termed the cervical lordosis, with the thoracic spine curvature called the thoracic kyphosis.

Each cervical spine vertebra joins the above and below segment with many different types of joints. The base of the skull and C1 (atlas) make up the atlanto-occipital joint. The atlas (C1) and axis (C2) make up the atlanto-odontoid joint and atlantoaxial joints (Figure 16-3). Typical cervical vertebrae have four facet joints: a right and left superior and inferior facet; and two joints that

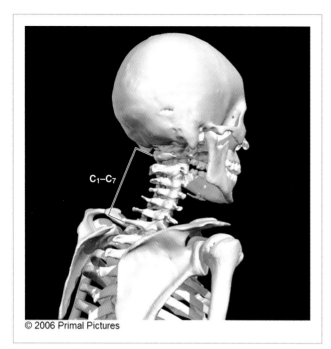

© 2006 Primal Pictures

Figure 16.2 Structure of Cervical Spine.

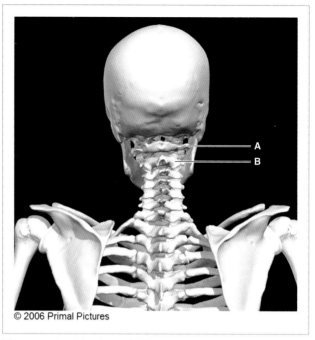

© 2006 Primal Pictures

Figure 16.3 (A) Atlas and (B) Axis.

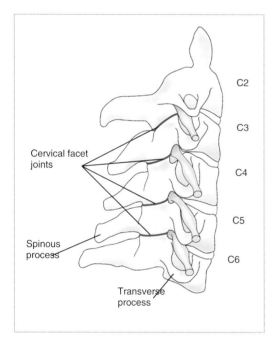

Figure 16-4. Facet Joints.

are called uncovertebral joints (Figure 16-4). Collectively, these structures anchor many of the major myofascial tissues that have a functional impact on the arthrokinematics of the structures above and below.

Above the cervical spine is the skull, including the temporal mandibular joint (TMJ). Below the cervical spine are the thoracic and lumbar spines, rib cage, scapula, humerus, and clavicle. As mentioned in earlier chapters, these structures in combination make up the cervicothoracic and thoracolumbar junctions of the spine, the scapulothoracic, glenohumeral, acromioclavicular (AC), and sternoclavicular (SC) joints (Figure 16-5).

Muscles

Although the CS is a relatively small region of the spine, there are a number of muscles responsible for and contributing to the proper functioning of the CS (Table 16-1). The deep neck flexors (longus colli, longus capitis, rectus capitis anterior and lateralis), lower trapezius, and serratus anterior form the upper oblique subsystem with the pectoralis, upper trapezius, and levator scapula. As a compensatory mechanism for the underactivity and inability of the deep neck flexors and cervical erector spinae to maintain an upright cervical spine position, the upper trapezius, levator scapula, sternocleidomastoid, and pectorals become synergistically dominant (overactive) to provide stability through the core and shoulder girdle complex (12). As mentioned in previous chapters, this imbalance can lead to forward head migration and the rounding of the shoulder (Upper Crossed Syndrome). See chapter two for a detailed review of the location and function of the muscles associated with the CS.

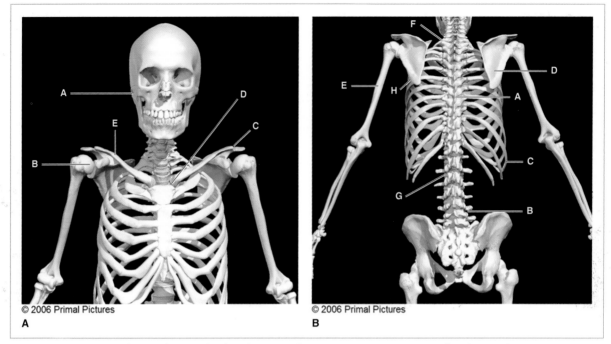

© 2006 Primal Pictures
A

© 2006 Primal Pictures
B

Figure 16.5 Bones and Joint Above and Below the Cervical Spine. **Image A.** (A) TMJ. (B) Glenohumeral joint. (C) Acromio-clavicular joint. (D) Sternoclavicular joint. **Image B.** (A) Thoracic spine. (B) Lumbar spine. (C) Rib cage. (D) Scapula. (E) Humerus. (F) Cervicothoracic junction. (G) Thoracolumbar junction. (H) Scapulothoracic joint.

Table 16.1	**KEY MUSCLES ASSOCIATED WITH THE CERVICAL SPINE**
Levator scapulae	Scalenes
Rhomboids	Cervical erector spinae
Trapezius	Suboccipitals
Sternocleidomastoid	Deep cervical flexors

GETTING YOUR FACTS STRAIGHT

Importance of Cervical Stability during Exercise

The deep neck flexors are primarily made up of the *longus coli* and *longus capitis* muscles. These muscles stabilize the cervical spine in all positions against the effects of gravity. They play a pivotal role in cervical spine conditions, and are often overlooked as a source of locomotor system dysfunction. The anatomic action of the longus capitis and longus colli is to nod the chin. If muscle recruitment is impaired, the balance between the stabilizers on the front and the back of the neck will be disrupted. This will cause loss of proper alignment of the spinal segments and a posture (forward head posture) that could lead to cervical pain (1–4). Thus, maintaining proper cervical alignment (chin tuck) during exercise is crucial to decrease the stress on the cervical spine and the risk of injury.

1. Falla D, Farina D. Neural and muscular factors associated with motor impairment in neck pain. *Curr Rheumatol Rep* 2007;9(6):497–502.
2. Falla D, Jull G, Hodges P. Patients with neck pain demonstrate reduced electromyographic activity of the deep cervical flexor muscles during performance of the craniocervical flexion test. *Spine* 2004;29(19):2108–14.
3. Falla D, Jull G, Dall'Alba P, Rainoldi A, Merletti R. An electromyographic analysis of the deep cervical flexor muscles in performance of craniocervical flexion. *Phys Ther* 2003;83(10):899–906.4. Falla D, Jull G, O'Leary S, Dall'Alba P. Further evaluation of an EMG technique for assessment of the deep cervical flexor muscles. *Exp Brain Res* 2006;16(6):621–8.

COMMON CERVICAL SPINE INJURIES AND ASSOCIATED MOVEMENT DEFICIENCIES

Common complaints above the CS that may stem from dysfunction in the CS are often seen with symptoms associated with the head, including headaches and dizziness or lightheadedness (Table 16-2) (13). Common injuries below the CS toward the shoulder include shoulder pain, trapezius-levator scapula dysfunction, AC impingement, scapulothoracic dysfunction, and thoracic outlet syndrome. At the thoracolumbar spine, low-back pain and sacroiliac joint dysfunction may be seen with various compensations in posture (thoracic extension, anterior pelvic tilt, SIJ translation) as a result of CS dysfunction (Table 16-2).

Each of the typical injuries listed can be problematic for any individual, and the reduction in pain or severity is often the focus of many exercise programs. However, these injuries are primarily symptoms representing a problem in the human movement system.

Table 16.2	COMMON INJURIES ASSOCIATED WITH CS IMPAIRMENT	
Local Injuries	**Injuries Above CS**	**Injuries Below CS**

Neck pain/stiffness
   Trapezius dysfunction
   Levator scapulae dysfunction
Cervical joint dysfunction
Cervical strains
Deep flexor dysfunction
Cervical disk lesions
	Headaches
	Dizziness/lightheadedness
	TMJ-related symptoms
		Upper extremity pain/weakness
		AC impingement
		Scapulothoracic dysfunction
		Thoracic outlet syndrome
		Anterior pelvic tilt/low-back pain
		Sacroiliac joint dysfunction

GETTING YOUR FACTS STRAIGHT

Pelvo-ocular Reflex

The pelvo-ocular reflex is the neuromotor response of the pelvic girdle and lower extremity (1), which serves to orient the body region in response to head position and anticipatory visual reference cues. It is theorized that one's head position can have an effect on one's pelvic position. As one's head migrates forward, the pelvis reflexively rotates anteriorly to readjust one's center of gravity (pelvo-ocular reflex). This rotation of the pelvis with concomitant forward head migration can lead to thoracolumbar pain (1). This example illustrates how a forward head posture could lead to dysfunction and pain in different regions of the body.

1. Lewit K. Muscular and articular factors in movement restriction. *Manual Med* 1985;1:83–5.

(*Text continues on page 367*)

ASSESSMENT AND CORRECTIVE EXERCISES FOR CERVICAL SPINE IMPAIRMENTS

➤ SYSTEMATIC PROCESS TO DETERMINE CERVICAL SPINE IMPAIRMENTS

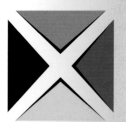

The cervical spine is a focus for investigation of complaints that involve head and upper extremity. Like the other regions of the body, this can be accomplished through the use of static postural assessments, transitional movement assessments, and range of motion assessments. A summary of the assessment process and common findings indicating potential dysfunction is listed in the table.

SAMPLE KNEE ASSESSMENT PROCESS AND OBSERVATIONS	
Assessment	**Observation**
Static posture	Upper crossed syndrome (rounded shoulders and forward head)
Overhead squat	Forward head Asymmetric cervical shift
Sit-up maneuver	Forward head
Pushing, pulling, and pressing assessments	Forward head, elevated, and/or rounded shoulders
Gait assessment	Forward head and rounded shoulders
Range of motion	Decreased cervical posterior translation, lateral flexion, and/or rotation

STATIC POSTURE

Like the shoulder region, a key static postural distortion syndrome to look for to determine potential dysfunction at the CS is the upper crossed postural distortion syndrome. As mentioned in the previous chapter, this is characterized by a rounding of the shoulders and forward head. Every inch of forward displacement of the head requires a tenfold increase of muscular effort to support posture.

Forward Head Posture

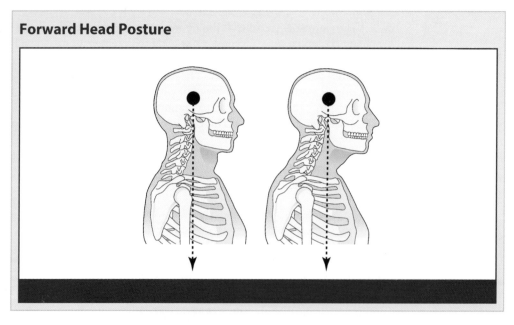

This position can place large stresses on the muscles and connective tissue associated with the CS, leading to injury.

During function, the cervical spine also requires balance between left and right associated musculature to maintain optimal posture. When this does not occur, abnormal asymmetric shifting (lateral flexion, translation, or rotation) can also be seen when assessing one statically. This may be related to an overactive and underactive right and left sternocleidomastoid, scalenes, levator scapulae, and upper trapezius (14–16).

Lateral Flexion, Translation, and Rotation

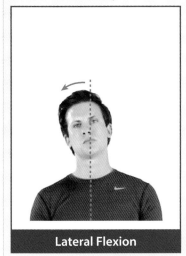 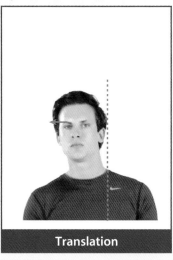 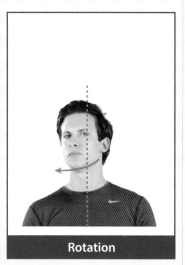

| Lateral Flexion | Translation | Rotation |

TRANSITIONAL MOVEMENT ASSESSMENTS

The overhead squat test can be used to assess multiple movement compensations of the CS. During the overhead squat test, the lower CS may become flexed and the cervicocranial junction hyperextended to keep the eyes level. This may lead to (or be caused by) an overactive sternocleidomastoid producing upper cervical extension and mid-lower cervical flexion (forward head). The suboccipitals may also become overactive and shortened as a result of this neck posture.

Overhead Squat: Forward Head

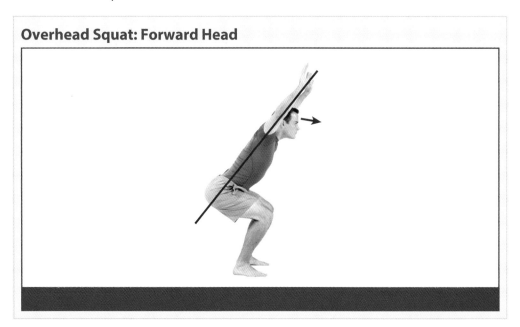

Continued on page 358

Like the static postural assessment, abnormal asymmetric shifting may also be seen during the descent of the overhead squat. As mentioned earlier, this may be related to an overactive and underactive right and left sternocleidomastoid, scalenes, levator scapulae, and upper trapezius (14–16).

Overhead Squat: Asymmetric Shift

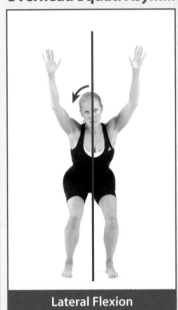 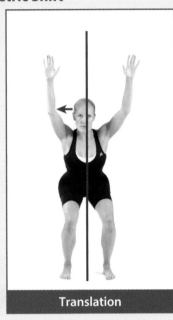 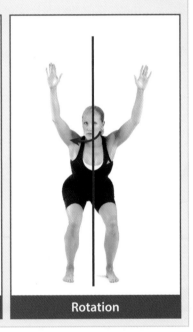

Lateral Flexion	Translation	Rotation

Upper extremity movement and balance have demonstrated an important relationship with CS pain. This may come in the form of shoulder elevation when performing the overhead squat. This is potentially caused by underactivity of the middle and lower trapezius, rhomboid, and rotator cuff with overactivity of the upper trapezius and levator scapulae (13).

Overhead Squat: Shoulder Elevation

Watching for forward head migration and shoulder elevation during pushing, pulling, or pressing movements can also be used to determine potential CS dysfunction.

Cervical Spine Compensation During Pushing, Pulling, and Pressing Movements

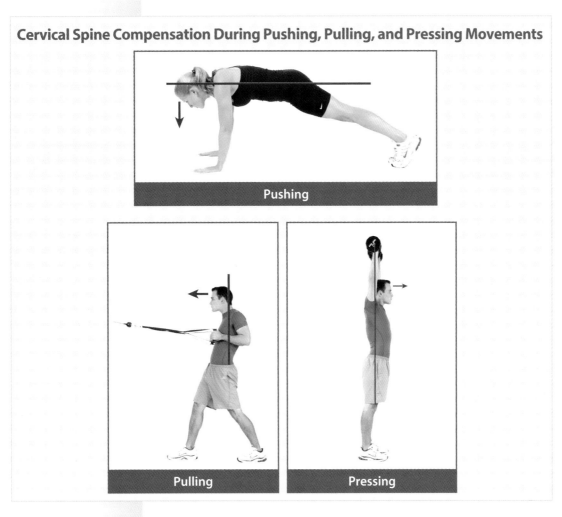

Pushing

Pulling

Pressing

Another transitional movement assessment that can be used to assess cervical spine function is the sit-up maneuver assessment. During this assessment, the chin should tuck first and then the head should smoothly roll off the table while the neck is flexing. If the sternocleidomastoid and suboccipitals are overactive and deep neck flexors are underactive, the head will "jut" forward at the beginning of the movement and will remain protruded throughout the movement.

Sit-up Maneuver: Forward Head

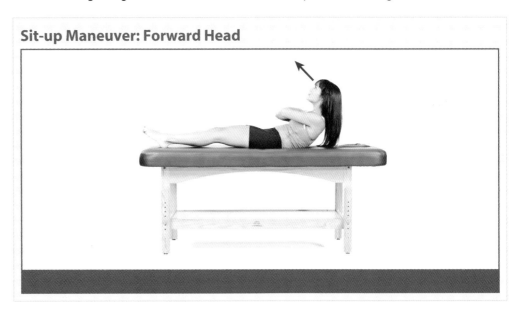

Continued on page 360

DYNAMIC MOVEMENT ASSESSMENT

When performing a dynamic movement assessment, (such as walking on a treadmill), watch for the rounding of the shoulders and a forward head posture (see chapter fifteen).

The table below provides a summary of all of the aforementioned CS compensation and potential overactive and underactive muscles that will need to be addressed in a corrective exercise program.

SUMMARY OF CS MOVEMENT COMPENSATIONS

Compensation	Potential Overactive Muscles	Potential Underactive Muscles	Potential Injuries
Forward head	Sternocleidomastoid Levator scapulae Scalenes Upper trapezius Suboccipitals	Deep cervical flexors Cervical erector spinae Lower trapezius Rhomboids	Headaches Dizziness/ lightheadedness Shoulder pain Trapezius-levator scapulae dysfunction
Asymmetric shift	Sternocleidomastoid (side of shift for lateral flexion and translation; opposite side for rotation) Levator scapulae (side of shift) Scalenes (side of shift) Upper trapezius (side of shift) Suboccipitals (side of shift)	Sternocleidomastoid (opposite side of shift for lateral flexion and translation; same side for rotation) Levator scapulae (opposite side of shift) Scalenes (opposite side of shift) Upper trapezius (opposite side of shift) Suboccipitals (opposite side of shift) Deep cervical stabilizers (opposite side of shift)	AC impingement Scapulothoracic dysfunction Thoracic outlet syndrome Low-back pain SI joint dysfunction
Shoulder elevation	Levator scapulae Upper trapezius	Lower trapezius Rhomboids Serratus anterior Rotator cuff	

RANGE OF MOTION ASSESSMENTS

Cartesian coordinate system: system used for measurements in three-dimensional space.

The **Cartesian coordinate system** is used for analysis of spinal range of motion (17). Degrees of motion refer to the motion of a joint or set of joints taken as a whole. In the cervical spine there is motion in all three axes or planes (x, y, and z), with horizontal motion about the x and y axes, sagittal plane motion about the x and z axes, and frontal motion about the y and z axes. Cervical spine motions include six angular and six in translation. Specific cervical spine active angular motions include:

1. Flexion (y axis)
2. Extension (y axis)
3. Right lateral flexion (x axis)
4. Left lateral flexion (x axis)
5. Right rotation (z axis)
6. Left rotation (z axis)

Cartesian Coordinate System

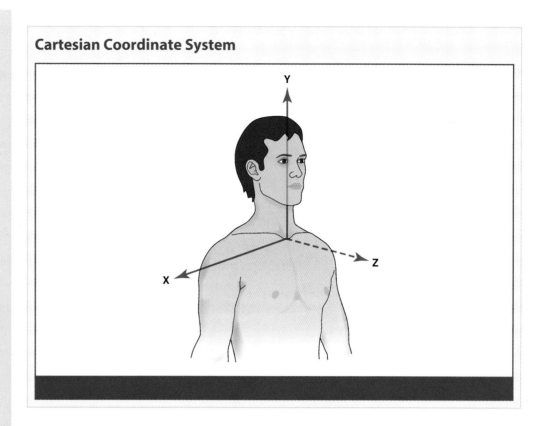

Cervical Spine Active Angular Motions

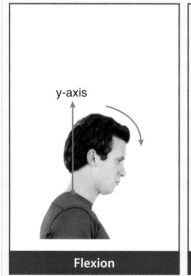

Flexion

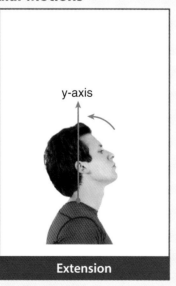

Extension

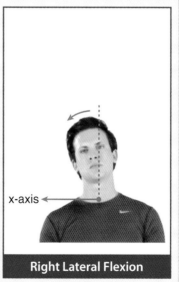

Right Lateral Flexion

Continued on page 362

Cervical Spine Active Angular Motions

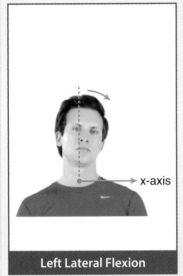
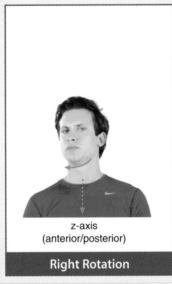
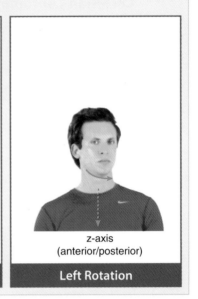

| Left Lateral Flexion | Right Rotation | Left Rotation |

Specific cervical spine active translational motions include:

1. Anterior (*z* axis)
2. Posterior (*z* axis)
3. Right (*x* axis)
4. Left (*x* axis)
5. Superior (*y* axis): assessed passively, must be a qualified licensed professional to perform
6. Inferior (*y* axis): assessed passively, must be a qualified licensed professional to perform

Cervical Spine Active Translational Motions

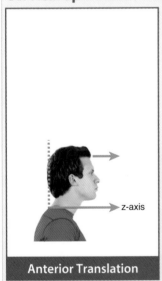
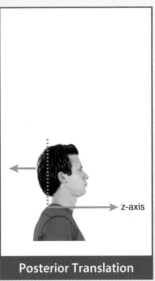
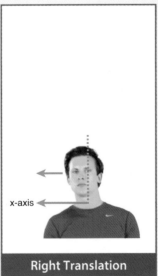
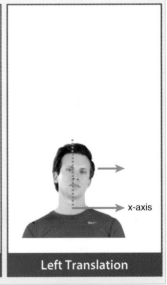

| Anterior Translation | Posterior Translation | Right Translation | Left Translation |

Each of the above is generally assessed actively and passively with care taken to limit the movement to the cervical spine by disassociating the thoracic and trunk region. If movement occurs in other regions while performing these motions (e.g., right shoulder elevation during left lateral flexion, thoracic or lumbar rotation during cervical rotation) can potentially be indicative of limited range of CS motion.

Although manual muscle testing can be a viable means of determining strength and weakness of the cervical spine musculature, it should only be applied by a qualified licensed professional.

➤ SYSTEMATIC CORRECTIVE EXERCISE STRATEGIES FOR CERVICAL SPINE IMPAIRMENTS

The following provides sample programming strategies using the Corrective Exercise Continuum for CS impairments. The photos provided illustrate the exercises that can be done for each component of the continuum to help address the issue of CS impairments as they relate to the compensations mentioned earlier (forward head and asymmetric shift). Shoulder elevation can also lead to CS dysfunction; refer to the corrective strategy provided in chapter fifteen for shoulder elevation to help correct this dysfunction.

CS IMPAIRMENT: FORWARD HEAD

Step 1: Inhibit Key regions to inhibit via foam rolling, self-applied pressure, and instrument-assisted devices include the thoracic spine, sternocleidomastoid, levator scapulae, and upper trapezius.

Self-Myofascial Release

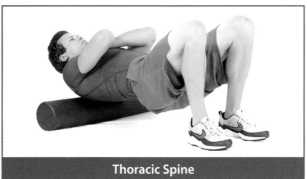

Thoracic Spine

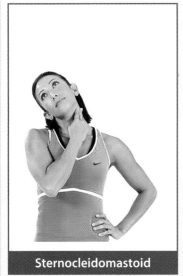

Sternocleidomastoid

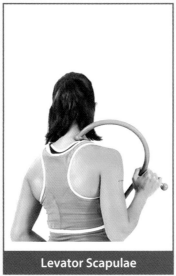

Levator Scapulae

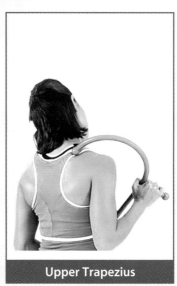

Upper Trapezius

Continued on page 364

Step 2: Lengthen   Key lengthening exercises via static stretching include the sternocleidomastoid, levator scapulae, and upper trapezius.

Static Stretches

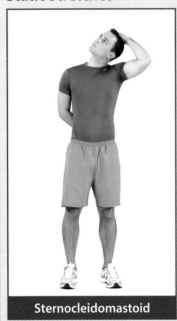

Sternocleidomastoid

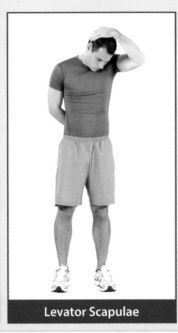

Levator Scapulae

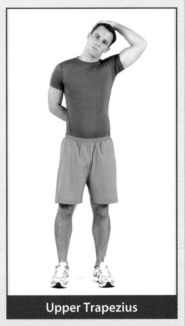

Upper Trapezius

Step 3: Activate   Key activation exercises via isolated strengthening exercises include the deep cervical flexors, cervical-thoracic extensors, and lower trapezius.

Isolated Strengthening Exercises

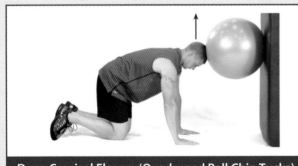

Deep Cervical Flexors (Quadruped Ball Chin Tucks)

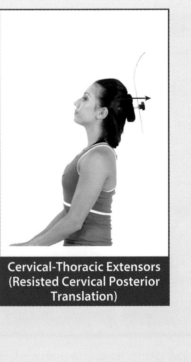

Cervical-Thoracic Extensors (Resisted Cervical Posterior Translation)

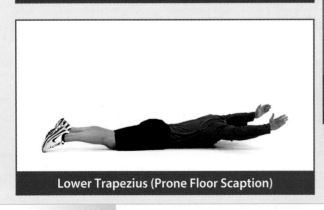

Lower Trapezius (Prone Floor Scaption)

Step 4: Integration An integration exercise that could be implemented could be a ball combo I while maintaining cervical retraction. Although this exercise can also be considered an activation exercise for the shoulder complex, it could be used as an integration exercise for cervical spine impairments to integrate the use of the cervical spine musculature with the shoulder musculature. Performing this movement on a stability ball also forces one to use these muscles in concert with the core and lower extremity musculature to provide stability throughout one's overall structure. This movement can be progressed by incorporating other dynamic functional movements involving the lower extremity (e.g., squat to scaption, step-up to scaption, and lunging to scaption) while maintain proper cervical retraction.

Integrated Dynamic Movement

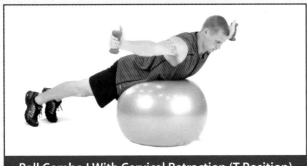

Ball Combo I With Cervical Retraction (Start)

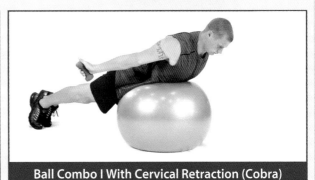

Ball Combo I With Cervical Retraction (Scaption)

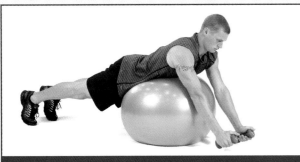

Ball Combo I With Cervical Retraction (T Position)

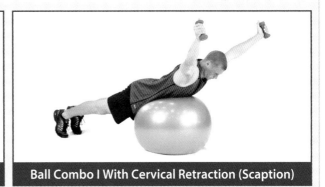

Ball Combo I With Cervical Retraction (Cobra)

SAMPLE CORRECTIVE EXERCISE PROGRAM FOR CS IMPAIRMENT: FORWARD HEAD

Phase	Modality	Muscle(s)	Acute Variables
Inhibit	SMR	Thoracic spine Sternocleidomastoid Levator scapulae Upper trapezius	Hold on tender area for 30 seconds
Lengthen	Static stretching	Sternocleidomastoid Levator scapulae Upper trapezius	30-seconds hold
Activate	Isolated strengthening	Deep cervical flexors Cervical erector spinae Lower trapezius	10–15 reps with 2-seconds isometric hold and 4-seconds eccentric
Integrate	Integrated dynamic movement	Ball combo I with cervical retraction	10–15 reps under control

Continued on page 366

CS IMPAIRMENT: ASYMMETRIC SHIFT (LATERAL FLEXION, TRANSLATION, OR ROTATION)

Step 1: Inhibit   Key regions to inhibit include the upper trapezius/scalenes (side of shift), levator scapulae (side of shift), and sternocleidomastoid (side of shift for lateral flexion or translation; opposite side of shift for rotation, i.e., if the chin rotates to the right, inhibit the left SCM). See photos for the forward head impairment for proper execution.

Step 2: Lengthen   Key lengthening exercises via static stretches include the upper trapezius/scalenes (side of shift), levator scapulae (side of shift), and sternocleidomastoid (side of shift for lateral flexion or translation; opposite side of shift for rotation, i.e., if the chin rotates to the right, lengthen the left SCM). See photos for the forward head impairment for proper execution.

Step 3: Activate   Key activation exercises via isolated strengthening exercises include the rhomboid and lower trapezius (opposite side of shift), upper trapezius (opposite side of shift), and scalene (opposite side of shift).

Isolated Strengthening Exercises

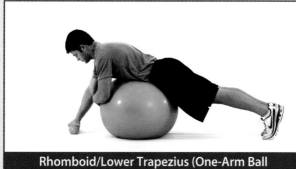

Rhomboid/Lower Trapezius (One-Arm Ball Cobra, Start)

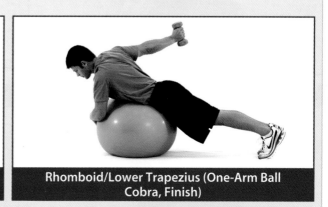

Rhomboid/Lower Trapezius (One-Arm Ball Cobra, Finish)

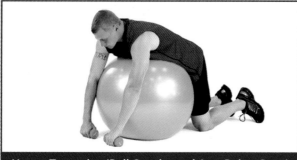

Upper Trapezius (Ball Quadruped Arm Raise, Start)

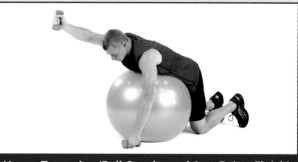

Upper Trapezius (Ball Quadruped Arm Raise, Finish)

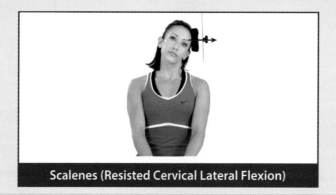

Scalenes (Resisted Cervical Lateral Flexion)

Step 4: Integration An integration exercise that could be implemented for this compensation could also be a ball combo 1 while maintaining cervical retraction (see forward head integration exercise).

SAMPLE CORRECTIVE EXERCISE PROGRAM FOR CS IMPAIRMENT: ASYMMETRIC SHIFT

Phase	Modality	Muscle(s)	Acute Variables
Inhibit	Self-myofascial release	Sternocleidomastoid (side of shift for lateral flexion and translation; opposite side for rotation) Levator scapulae (side of shift) Upper trapezius/scalenes (side of shift)	Hold on tender area for 30 seconds
Lengthen	Static stretching	Sternocleidomastoid (side of shift for lateral flexion and translation; opposite side for rotation) Levator scapulae (side of shift) Upper trapezius/scalenes (side of shift)	30-seconds hold
Activate	Isolated strengthening	Rhomboids/lower trapezius (opposite side of shift) Upper trapezius (opposite side of shift) Scalenes (opposite side of shift)	10–15 reps with 2-seconds isometric hold and 4-seconds eccentric
Integrate	Integrated dynamic movement	Ball combo I with cervical retraction	10–15 reps under control

SUMMARY • As mentioned in the majority of the previous chapters, pain in one region of the body is likely caused by dysfunction in another region of the body. This can be especially true for cervical spine dysfunction owing to the compensatory chain reaction that can occur during human movement dysfunction. Although the cervical spine is a very complex region of the body, having an understanding of functional anatomy, functional biomechanics, and the overall human movement system will greatly assist the health and fitness professional in being able to understand potential causes for cervical spine dysfunction and key elements that must be addressed to help correct these dysfunctions via the Corrective Exercise Continuum.

References
1. National Centers for Health Statistics, Chartbook on Trends in the Health of Americans 2006, Special Feature: Pain. Available at http://www.cdc.gov/nchs/data/hus/hus06.pdf
2. Häkkinen A, Kautiainen H, Hannonen P, Ylinen J. Strength training and stretching versus stretching only in the treatment of patients with chronic neck pain: a randomized one-year follow-up study. Clin Rehabil 2008;22:592–600.
3. Häkkinen A, Salo P, Tarvainen U, Wirén K, Ylinen J. Effect of manual therapy and stretching on neck muscle strength and mobility in chronic neck pain. J Rehabil Med 2007;39:575–9.
4. Ylinen J, Takala EP, Nykänen M, et al. Active neck muscle training in the treatment of chronic neck pain in women: a randomized controlled trial. JAMA 2003;289:2509–16.
5. Cunha AC, Burke TN, França FJ, Marques AP. Effect of global posture reeducation and of static stretching on pain, range of motion, and quality of life in women with chronic neck pain: a randomized clinical trial. Clinics (Sao Paulo) 2008;63:763–70.
6. Taimela S, Takala EP, Asklöf T, Seppälä K, Parviainen S. Active treatment of chronic neck pain: a prospective randomized intervention. Spine 2000;25:1021–7.
7. Nikander R, Mälkiä E, Parkkari J, Heinonen A, Starck H, Ylinen J. Dose-response relationship of specific training to reduce chronic neck pain and disability. Med Sci Sports Exerc 2006;38:2068–74.
8. Ylinen JJ, Häkkinen AH, Takala EP, et al. Effects of neck muscle training in women with chronic neck pain: one-year follow-up study. J Strength Cond Res 2006;20:6–13.

9. Ylinen J, Häkkinen A, Nykänen M, Kautiainen H, Takala EP. Neck muscle training in the treatment of chronic neck pain: a three-year follow-up study. *Eura Medicophys* 2007;43:161–9. Epub 2007 May 28.

10. Ylinen J, Kautiainen H, Wirén K, Häkkinen A. Stretching exercises vs. manual therapy in treatment of chronic neck pain: a randomized, controlled cross-over trial. *J Rehabil Med* 2007;39:126–32.

11. Jull G, Falla D, Treleaven J, Hodges P, Vicenzino B. Retraining cervical joint position sense: the effect of two exercise regimes. *J Orthop Res* 2007;25:404–12.

12. Falla D, Farina D. Neural and muscular factors associated with motor impairment in neck pain. *Curr Rheumatol Rep* 2007;9:497–502.

13. Sahrmann, S. Diagnosis and Treatment of Movement Impairment Syndromes. St. Louis, MO: Mosby; 2001.

14. Falla D, Jull G, Hodges P. Patients with neck pain demonstrate reduced electromyographic activity of the deep cervical flexor muscles during performance of the craniocervical flexion test. *Spine* 2004;29:2108–14.

15. Falla D, Jull G, Dall'Alba P, Rainoldi A, Merletti R. An electromyographic analysis of the deep cervical flexor muscles in performance of craniocervical flexion. *Phys Ther* 2003;83:899–906.

16. Falla D, Jull G, O'Leary S, Dall'Alba P. Further evaluation of an EMG technique for assessment of the deep cervical flexor muscles. *Exp Brain Res* 2006;16:621–8.

17. Kapandji IA. The Physiology of the Joints. The Trunk and the Vertebral Column. Edinburgh: Churchill Livingston; 1974.

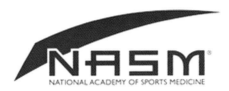

Corrective Exercise Training

MOVEMENT IMPAIRMENT: FEET TURN OUT AND/OR FLATTEN

INHIBIT

Exercise: Self-Myofascial Release	Sets	Duration	Notes
Gastrocnemius Soleus	1	30 sec	Lateral aspect
Biceps Femoris	1	30 sec	
TFL/IT-band	1	30 sec	

LENGTHEN

Exercise: Static Stretch	Sets	Duration	Notes
Gastrocnemius Stretch	1	30 sec	Internally rotate back foot
Soleus Stretch	1	30 sec	
Supine Biceps Femoris Stretch	1	30 sec	
Standing TFL Stretch	1	30 sec	Externally rotate back foot

ACTIVATION

Exercise: Isolated Strengthening	Sets	Reps	Tempo	Rest	Notes
Resisted Ankle Dorsiflexion	1-2	10-15	4/2/2	0	Anterior Tibialis
Resisted Ankle Plantarflexion and Inversion	1-2	10-15	4/2/2	0	Posterior Tibialis
Single-leg Calf Raise	1-2	10-15	4/2/2	0	Medial Gastrocnemius
Resisted Knee Flexion with Hip Internally Rotated	1-2	10-15	4/2/2	0	Medial Hamstring

INTEGRATED DYNAMIC MOVEMENT

Exercise:	Sets	Reps	Tempo	Rest	Notes
Multiplanar Single-leg Balance Reach	1-2	10-15	Slow	30 sec	Maintain proper arch of the foot and knee pointing straight ahead over the second and third toes

Coaching Tips: Activation exercises and integration exercises can be performed in a circuit.

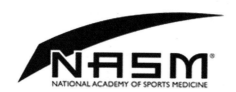

Corrective Exercise Training

MOVEMENT IMPAIRMENT: KNEES MOVE INWARD

INHIBIT

Exercise: Self-Myofascial Release	Sets	Duration	Notes
Gastrocnemius/Soleus	1	30 sec	
Biceps Femoris	1	30 sec	
Adductors	1	30 sec	
TFL/IT-band	1	30 sec	

LENGTHEN

Exercise: Static Stretch	Sets	Duration	Notes
Gastrocnemius/Soleus Stretch	1	30 sec	
Supine Biceps Femoris Stretch	1	30 sec	
Standing Adductor Stretch	1	30 sec	
Standing TFL Stretch	1	30 sec	

ACTIVATION

Exercise: Isolated Strengthening	Sets	Reps	Tempo	Rest	Notes
Resisted Ankle Dorsiflexion	1-2	10-15	4/2/2	0	Anterior Tibialis
Resisted Hip Abduction	1-2	10-15	4/2/2	0	Gluteus Medius
Resisted Hip Extension	1-2	10-15	4/2/2	0	Gluteus Maximus

INTEGRATED DYNAMIC MOVEMENT

Exercise:	Sets	Reps	Tempo	Rest	Notes
Wall Jumps*	1-2	10-15	Controlled	30 sec	

Coaching Tips: *Use the jump task progression only if client can safely demonstrate the wall jumps exercise.

Wall Jumps → Tuck Jumps → Long Jump with Stabilization → Single-leg Hop with Stabilization → Cutting Maneuvers

Use the functional movement progression if the individual cannot perform jumping progressions.

Ball squats → Step ups → Lunges → Single-leg squat

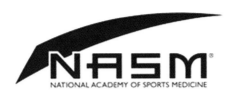

Corrective Exercise Training

MOVEMENT IMPAIRMENT: KNEES MOVE OUTWARD

INHIBIT

Exercise: Self-Myofascial Release	Sets	Duration	Notes
Gastrocnemius/Soleus	1	30 sec	
Biceps Femoris	1	30 sec	
Piriformis	1	30 sec	

LENGTHEN

Exercise: Static Stretch	Sets	Duration	Notes
Gastrocnemius/Soleus Stretch	1	30 sec	
Supine Biceps Femoris Stretch	1	30 sec	
Supine Piriformis Stretch	1	30 sec	

ACTIVATION

Exercise: Isolated Strengthening	Sets	Reps	Tempo	Rest	Notes
Resisted Hip Adduction and Internal Rotation	1-2	10-15	4/2/2	0	Adductors
Resisted Knee Flexion with Hip Internally Rotated	1-2	10-15	4/2/2	0	Medial Hamstring
Resisted Hip Extension	1-2	10-15	4/2/2	0	Gluteus Maximus

INTEGRATED DYNAMIC MOVEMENT

Exercise:	Sets	Reps	Tempo	Rest	Notes
Ball Squats	1-2	10-15	Slow	30 sec	Can place med ball b/w knees

Coaching Tips: Activation exercises and integration exercises can be performed in a circuit.

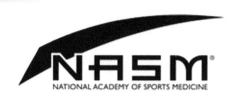

Corrective Exercise Training

MOVEMENT IMPAIRMENT: EXCESSIVE FORWARD LEAN

INHIBIT

Exercise: Self-Myofascial Release	Sets	Duration	Notes
Gastrocnemius/Soleus	1	30 sec	
Quadriceps	1	30 sec	Rectus Femoris

LENGTHEN

Exercise: Static Stretch	Sets	Duration	Notes
Gastrocnemius/Soleus Stretch	1	30 sec	
Kneeling Hip Flexor Stretch	1	30 sec	

ACTIVATION

Exercise: Isolated Strengthening	Sets	Reps	Tempo	Rest	Notes
Resisted Ankle Dorsiflexion	1-2	10-15	4/2/2	0	Anterior Tibialis
Resisted Hip Extension	1-2	10-15	4/2/2	0	Gluteus Maximus
Quadruped Arm/Opposite Leg Raise	1-2	10-15	4/2/2	0	Core Stabilizers
Floor Prone Cobra	1-2	10-15	4/2/2	0	Erector Spinae

INTEGRATED DYNAMIC MOVEMENT

Exercise:	Sets	Reps	Tempo	Rest	Notes
Ball Wall Squat with Overhead Press	1-2	10-15	Slow	30 sec	

Coaching Tips: Activation exercises and integration exercises can be performed in a circuit.

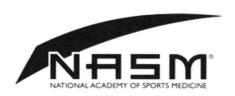

Corrective Exercise Training

MOVEMENT IMPAIRMENT: LOW BACK ARCHES

INHIBIT

Exercise: Self-Myofascial Release	Sets	Duration	Notes
Quadriceps	1	30 sec	Rectus Femoris
Latissimus Dorsi	1	30 sec	

LENGTHEN

Exercise: Static Stretch	Sets	Duration	Notes
Kneeling Hip Flexor Stretch	1	30 sec	
Ball Lat Stretch	1	30 sec	
Erector Spinae Stretch	1	30 sec	

ACTIVATION

Exercise: Isolated Strengthening	Sets	Reps	Tempo	Rest	Notes
Ball Crunch	1-2	10-15	4/2/2	0	Core Stabilizers
Stability Ball Bridge	1-2	10-15	4/2/2	0	Gluteus Maximus

INTEGRATED DYNAMIC MOVEMENT

Exercise:	Sets	Reps	Tempo	Rest	Notes
Ball Wall Squat to Overhead Press	1-2	10-15	Slow	30 sec	

Coaching Tips: Activation exercises and integration exercises can be performed in a circuit.

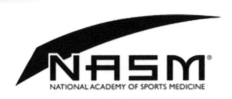

NATIONAL ACADEMY OF SPORTS MEDICINE

Corrective Exercise Training

MOVEMENT IMPAIRMENT: LOW BACK ROUNDS

INHIBIT

Exercise: Self-Myofascial Release	Sets	Duration	Notes
Hamstrings	1	30 sec	
Adductors	1	30 sec	Adductor Magnus

LENGTHEN

Exercise: Static Stretch	Sets	Duration	Notes
Supine Hamstring Stretch	1	30 sec	
Adductor Magnus Stretch	1	30 sec	
Supine Ball Abdominal Stretch	1	30 sec	

ACTIVATION

Exercise: Isolated Strengthening	Sets	Reps	Tempo	Rest	Notes
Floor Cobra	1-2	10-15	4/2/2	0	Erector Spinae
Ball Bridge	1-2	10-15	4/2/2	0	Gluteus Maximus
Resisted Hip Flexion	1-2	10-15	4/2/2	0	Hip Flexors

INTEGRATED DYNAMIC MOVEMENT

Exercise:	Sets	Reps	Tempo	Rest	Notes
Ball Wall Squat with Overhead Press	1-2	10-15	Slow	30 sec	

Coaching Tips: Activation exercises and integration exercises can be performed in a circuit.

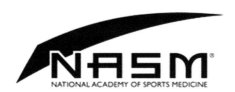

Corrective Exercise Training

MOVEMENT IMPAIRMENT: ASYMMETRICAL WEIGHT SHIFT

INHIBIT

Exercise: Self-Myofascial Release	Sets	Duration	Notes
Adductors	1	30 sec	Same side of shift
Gastrocnemius/Soleus	1	30 sec	Opposite side of shift
Piriformis	1	30 sec	Opposite side of shift
Biceps Femoris	1	30 sec	Opposite side of shift

LENGTHEN

Exercise: Static Stretch	Sets	Duration	Notes
Standing Adductor Stretch	1	30 sec	Same side of shift
Gastrocnemius/Soleus Stretch	1	30 sec	Opposite side of shift
Supine Piriformis Stretch	1	30 sec	Opposite side of shift
Supine Biceps Femoris Stretch	1	30 sec	Opposite side of shift

ACTIVATION

Exercise: Isolated Strengthening	Sets	Reps	Tempo	Rest	Notes
Resisted Hip Abduction (same side of shift)	1-2	10-15	4/2/2	0	Same Side Gluteus Medius
Resisted Hip Adduction and Internal Rotation (opposite side of shift)	1-2	10-15	4/2/2	0	Opposite Side Adductors

INTEGRATED DYNAMIC MOVEMENT

Exercise:	Sets	Reps	Tempo	Rest	Notes
Ball Wall Squat with Overhead Press	1-2	10-15	Slow	30 sec	

Coaching Tips: Activation exercises and integration exercises can be performed in a circuit.

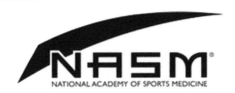

Corrective Exercise Training

MOVEMENT IMPAIRMENT: ARMS FALL FORWARD

INHIBIT

Exercise: Self-Myofascial Release	Sets	Duration	Notes
Latissimus Dorsi	1	30 sec	
Thoracic Spine	1	30 sec	

LENGTHEN

Exercise: Static Stretch	Sets	Duration	Notes
Ball Lat Stretch	1	30 sec	
Standing Pectoral Stretch	1	30 sec	

ACTIVATION

Exercise: Isolated Strengthening	Sets	Reps	Tempo	Rest	Notes
Ball Combo I with Dowel Rod	1-2	10-15	4/2/2	0	

INTEGRATED DYNAMIC MOVEMENT

Exercise:	Sets	Reps	Tempo	Rest	Notes
Squat to Row	1-2	10-15	Slow	30 sec	

Coaching Tips: Activation exercise and integration exercise can be performed in a circuit

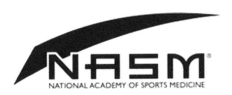

Corrective Exercise Training

MOVEMENT IMPAIRMENT: ELBOW AND/OR WRIST IMPAIRMENT

INHIBIT

Exercise: Self-Myofascial Release	Sets	Duration	Notes
Bicep Brachii	1	30 sec	Self Applied Pressure
Brachialis	1	30 sec	Self Applied Pressure
Wrist Extensor and/or Flexors	1	30 sec	Self Applied Pressure

LENGTHEN

Exercise: Static Stretch	Sets	Duration	Notes
Bicep Brachii Stretch	1	30 sec	With wrist and shoulder extension
Wrist Extensor and/or Flexor Stretch	1	30 sec	

ACTIVATION

Exercise: Isolated Strengthening	Sets	Reps	Tempo	Rest	Notes
Bicep Curl	1-2	10-15	4/2/2	0	
Tricep Extension	1-2	10-15	4/2/2	0	
Wrist Flexion and/or Extension	1-2	10-15	4/2/2	0	
Wrist Supination/Pronation	1-2	10-15	4/2/2	0	

INTEGRATED DYNAMIC MOVEMENT

Exercise:	Sets	Reps	Tempo	Rest	Notes
Standing Lat Pulldown	1-2	10-15	Slow	0	
Prone Ball Tricep Extension with Cobra	1-2	10-15	Slow	30 sec	

Coaching Tips: Activation exercises and integration exercises can be performed in a circuit.

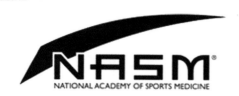

Corrective Exercise Training

MOVEMENT IMPAIRMENT: FORWARD HEAD

INHIBIT

Exercise: Self-Myofascial Release	Sets	Duration	Notes
Thoracic Spine	1	30 sec	Foam roll or Thera Cane
Sternocleidomastoid	1	30 sec	Finger pressure
Levator Scapulae	1	30 sec	Thera Cane
Upper Trapezius	1	30 sec	Thera Cane

LENGTHEN

Exercise: Static Stretch	Sets	Duration	Notes
Sternocleidomastoid Stretch	1	30 sec	
Levator Scapulae Stretch	1	30 sec	
Upper Trapezius Stretch	1	30 sec	

ACTIVATION

Exercise: Isolated Strengthening	Sets	Reps	Tempo	Rest	Notes
Quadruped Ball Chin Tucks	1-2	10-15	4/2/2	0	Deep Cervical Flexors
Resisted Cervical Posterior Translation (chin tucks)	1-2	10-15	4/2/2	0	Cervical-Thoracic Extensors
Floor Prone Scaption	1-2	10-15	4/2/2	0	Lower Trapezius

INTEGRATED DYNAMIC MOVEMENT

Exercise:	Sets	Reps	Tempo	Rest	Notes
Ball Combo I w/Cervical Retraction	1-2	10-15	Slow	30 sec	

Coaching Tips: Activation exercises and integration exercises can be performed in a circuit.

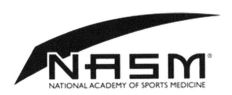

Corrective Exercise Training

SAMPLE PLANTAR FASCIITIS PREVENTION PROGRAM

INHIBIT

Exercise: Self-Myofascial Release	Sets	Duration	Notes
Plantar Fascia	1	30 sec	Use tennis ball or golf ball on sole of foot
Gastrocnemius/Soleus	1	30 sec	
Peroneals	1	30 sec	

LENGTHEN

Exercise: Static Stretch	Sets	Duration	Notes
Gastrocnemius	1	30 sec	
Soleus	1	30 sec	

ACTIVATION

Exercise: Isolated Strengthening	Sets	Reps	Tempo	Rest	Notes
Resisted Ankle Dorsiflexion	1-2	10-15	4/2/0	0	Anterior Tibialis
Single-leg Calf Raise	1-2	10-15	4/2/0	0	Medial Gastrocnemius

INTEGRATED DYNAMIC MOVEMENT

Exercise:	Sets	Reps	Tempo	Rest	Notes
Single-leg Balance Reach	1-2	10-15	Slow	30 sec	

Coaching Tips: Activation exercises and integration exercises can be performed in a circuit.

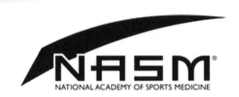

Corrective Exercise Training

SAMPLE PATELLAR TENDONITIS PREVENTION PROGRAM

INHIBIT

Exercise: Self-Myofascial Release	Sets	Duration	Notes
Gastrocnemius/Soleus	1	30 sec	
Adductors	1	30 sec	
TFL/IT-band	1	30 sec	

LENGTHEN

Exercise: Static Stretch	Sets	Duration	Notes
Gastrocnemius/Soleus Stretch	1	30 sec	
Supine Biceps Femoris Stretch	1	30 sec	
Standing Adductor Stretch	1	30 sec	
Kneeling Hip Flexor Stretch	1	30 sec	

ACTIVATION

Exercise: Isolated Strengthening	Sets	Reps	Tempo	Rest	Notes
Resisted Ankle Dorsiflexion	1-2	10-15	4/2/2	0	Anterior Tibialis
Resisted Ankle Plantarflexion and Inversion	1-2	10-15	4/2/2	0	Posterior Tibialis
Resisted Hip Abduction and External Rotation	1-2	10-15	4/2/2	0	Gluteus Medius
Resisted Hip Extension	1-2	10-15	4/2/2	0	Gluteus Maximus

INTEGRATED DYNAMIC MOVEMENT

Exercise:	Sets	Reps	Tempo	Rest	Notes
Ball Squats w/ Resistance Band Around Knees	1-2	10-15	Slow	30 sec	

Coaching Tips: Activation exercises and integration exercises can be performed in a circuit.

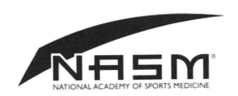

Corrective Exercise Training

SAMPLE LOW BACK PAIN PREVENTION PROGRAM

INHIBIT

Exercise: Self-Myofascial Release	Sets	Duration	Notes
Quadriceps	1	30 sec	Rectus Femoris
TFL/IT-band	1	30 sec	
Adductors	1	30 sec	
Piriformis	1	30 sec	

LENGTHEN

Exercise: Static Stretch	Sets	Duration	Notes
Kneeling Hip Flexor Stretch	1	30 sec	
Seated Ball Adductor Stretch	1	30 sec	
Supine Biceps Femoris Stretch	1	30 sec	
Supine Ball Piriformis Stretch	1	30 sec	

ACTIVATION

Exercise: Isolated Strengthening	Sets	Reps	Tempo	Rest	Notes
Wall Slides	1-2	10-15	4/2/2	0	Gluteus Medius
Quadruped Opposite Arm/Leg Raise	1-2	10-15	4/2/2	0	Core Stabilizers
Stability Ball Bridge	1-2	10-15	4/2/2	0	Gluteus Maximus

INTEGRATED DYNAMIC MOVEMENT

Exercise:	Sets	Reps	Tempo	Rest	Notes
Lateral Tube Walking	1-2	10-15	Slow	30 sec	

Coaching Tips: Activation exercises and integration exercises can be performed in a circuit.

Appendix B A Guide To Common Myofascial Dysfunctions

GASTROCNEMIUS

Referred Pain	Results of Chronic Tightness	Causes of Tightness	Trigger Point Location	Associated Joint Dysfunction
Posterior knee Achilles tendon Medial arch	Achilles tendinitis Low back pain Plantar fasciitis	Subtalar joint dysfunction Tibio-talar joint dysfunction Ankle sprain Poor gait/running mechanics High heels	Proximal medial/lateral border	Subtalar joint Tibio-talar joint Proximal tibio-fibular joint Sacroiliac joint Lumbar spine

SOLEUS

Referred Pain	Results of Chronic Tightness	Causes of Tightness	Trigger Point Location	Associated Joint Dysfunction
Posterior calcaneus Posterior calf	Forefoot pronation Valgus/internal rotation stress at knee Sacroiliac joint stress	Excessive running Ankle/foot arthrokinematic dysfunction Weak posterior tibialis Weak quadriceps	Inferior/medial aspect of muscle	Subtalar joint Tibio-ulnar joint Proximal tibio-fibular joint First metatarsophalangeal joint

ADDUCTORS

Referred Pain	Results of Chronic Tightness	Causes of Tightness	Trigger Point Location	Associated Joint Dysfunction
Antero-lateral hip Groin Medial thigh Medial tibia Anterior knee	Inhibits gluteus medius Decreases frontal plane stability Creates sacroiliac joint dysfunction Creates pubo-symphyseal joint dysfunction Iliotibial band tendinitis Anterior knee pain Pes anserine tendinitis	Weak gluteus medius Sacroiliac joint dysfunction Tibio-talar joint dysfunction Subtalar joint dysfunction Tight pubofemoral ligament Posture Technical inefficiency	Superior muscle belly	Iliofemoral joint Sacroiliac joint Pubic symphyseal joint Thoracic facet joint Subtalar joint Tibio-talar joint First metatarsophalangeal

382

HAMSTRINGS

Referred Pain	Results of Chronic Tightness	Causes of Tightness	Trigger Point Location	Associated Joint Dysfunction
Low back Lower buttock Upper calf Medial/lateral knee	Alters lumbo-pelvic-hip stability Leads to anterior knee pain Alters extensor mechanism function Leads to chronic strains	Substitution for weak abdominals Substitution for weak gluteals Substition for weak gastrocnemius Substitution for weak quadriceps Compensation for tight psoas Subtalar joint dysfunction Tibio-talar joint dysfunction Iliosacral joint dysfunction Sacroiliac joint dysfunction Proximal tibio-fibular joint dysfunction	Mid belly	First metatar-sophalangeal joint Subtalar joint Tibio-talar joint Proximal tibio-fibular joint Tibio-femoral joint Sacroiliac joint Lumbar spine (L5 - S 1)

RECTUS FEMORIS

Referred Pain	Results of Chronic Tightness	Causes of Tightness	Trigger Point Location	Associated Joint Dysfunction
Anterior knee	Sacroiliac joint dysfunction Hamstring strains Patellar tendinitis Posterior tibialis tendinitis Low back pain	Prolonged sitting Compensation for weak lower abdominals Adaptation for weak gluteus medius	Muscle belly	Sacroiliac joint Lumbar spine Tibio-femoral joint Proximal tibio-fibular joint

PIRIFORMIS

Referred Pain	Results of Chronic Tightness	Causes of Tightness	Trigger Point Location	Associated Joint Dysfunction
Posterior thigh Buttock Sacroiliac joint	Low back pain Sacroiliac joint dysfunction Entrapment neuropathy Compressive pathology Iliotibial band tendinitis	Substitution for weak gluteus maximus Substitution for weak gluteus medius Substitution for weak bicep femoris Sacroiliac joint dysfunction Short leg	Muscle belly Sciatic notch	Lumbar spine Sacroiliac joint First metatar-sophalangeal Subtalar joint Tibio-talar joint

PSOAS

Referred Pain	Results of Chronic Tightness	Causes of Tightness	Trigger Point Location	Associated Joint Dysfunction
Low back Sacroiliac joint Patellar tendon	Inhibits multifidus, transverse abdominus, internal oblique, deep erector spinae Inhibits gluteus maximus Leads to extensor mechanism dysfunction Causes patellar tendinitis Causes hamstring strains Leads to piriformis syndrome Leads to sacroiliac joint/lumbar facet syndrome	Weak lower abdominals Weak gluteals Weak Intrinsic lumbo-pelvic-hip complex stabililers Prolonged sitting Prolonged biking Poor neuromuscular control of lumbo-pelvic-hip complex Sacroiliac joint dysfunction	Muscle belly Sacroiliac joint	Lumbar spine (T10 – L1) Sacroiliac joint

TENSOR FASCIA LATAE

Referred Pain	Results of Chronic Tightness	Causes of Tightness	Trigger Point Location	Associated Joint Dysfunction
Lateral aspect of knee	Iliotibial band tendinitis Knee extensor mechanism dysfunction Sacroiliac joint dysfunction Piriformis syndrome Achilles tendinitis Adductor strains Hamstring strains Low back pain Ankle sprains	Substitution for weak gluteus medius Compensation for weak gluteus maximus Adaptation for first metatarsophalangeal, subtalar joint, tibio-talar joint, proximal tibio-fibular joint dysfunction Adaptation for quadratus lumborum dysfunction Adaptation for psoas tightness Prolonged sitting Lateral pelvic shift Forefoot instability	Superior and mid-muscle belly	Sacroiliac joint Lumbar spine (L5 – S1) Proximal tibio-fibular joint Tibio-femoral joint First metatarsophalangeal Subtalar joint Tibio-talar joint

QUADRATUS LUMBORUM

Referred Pain	Results of Chronic Tightness	Causes of Tightness	Trigger Point Location	Associated Joint Dysfunction
Lateral fibers = iliac crest and lateral hip Medial fibers = sacroiliac joint, deep in buttock	Low back pain Sacroiliac joint dysfunction Abnormal frontal plane gait dysfunction	Sacroiliac joint dysfunction Lumbar spine dysfunction Twelfth rib dysfunction Compensation for weak gluteus medius Pattern overload	Inferior to erector spinae and lateral to transverse process of the lumbar spine	Sacroiliac joint Lumbar spine

ERECTOR SPINAE

Referred Pain	Results of Chronic Tightness	Causes of Tightness	Trigger Point Location	Associated Joint Dysfunction
Sacroiliac joint Low back Buttock	Low back pain Sacroiliac joint dysfunction Hamstring strains Inhibition of deep lumbo-pelvic-hip stabilizers	Compensation for weak gluteus maximus Compensation for weak hamstings Compensation for weak abdominals Compensation for weak multifidus Adaptation for tight psoas Postural dysfunction Pattern overload	Muscle belly Spinous process of the spine Transverse process of the spine	Sacroiliac joint Lumbar spine

UPPER TRAPEZIUS

Referred Pain	Results of Chronic Tightness	Causes of Tightness	Trigger Point Location	Associated Joint Dysfunction
Mastoid, along the postero-lateral neck and occiput to the forehead	Headaches Neck pain Altered scapulohumeral rhythm (shoulder impingement)	Occupational stress Compensation for weak lower trapezius Poor posture Carrying heavy purse/bag Compensation for anatomical/functional short leg Emotional stress	Midbelly, anterior; lateral	Cervical facet joints, and cervicothoracic junction

LEVATOR SCAPULAE

Referred Pain	Results of Chronic Tightness	Causes of Tightness	Trigger Point Location	Associated Joint Dysfunction
Vertebral border of the scapula Mid cervical spine	Pain on the same side as rotation Altered scapulohumeral rhythm (shoulder pathology)	Poor posture Occupational stress Compensation for weak lower trapezius and rhomboids	Superomedial border of the scapula	C1-C2, C2-C3 Cervicothoracic dysfunction

STERNOCLEIDOMASTOID

Referred Pain	Results of Chronic Tightness	Causes of Tightness	Trigger Point Location	Associated Joint Dysfunction
Over the eye, frontal area, and mastoid process	Headaches Earaches Decreased neck rotation Inhibition of deep neck flexors	Excessive mechanical overload 1. Painting a ceiling 2. Watching a movie from the front row 3. Riding a bicycle 4. Sleeping with two pillows Poor posture Occupational stress Poor eyesight Compensation for weak deep neck flexors Adaptation for tight suboccipitals	Anywhere along the entire length of the muscle	Cervical facet joints Sternoclavicular joint

SCALENES

Referred Pain	Results of Chronic Tightness	Causes of Tightness	Trigger Point Location	Associated Joint Dysfunction
Pectoralis muscle Upper arm Hand Rhomboids	Cervico-brachial plexopathy	Poor posture (forward head posture) Stress Emotional tension Poor breathing habits	Anywhere along the anterior, medial, or posterior muscle belly Palpate the scalenes cautiously because of the proximity of sensitive neurovascular structures	First rib Flexion dysfunction of the cervical spine

RECTUS CAPITUS (SUB OCCIPITALS)

Referred Pain	Results of Chronic Tightness	Causes of Tightness	Trigger Point Location	Associated Joint Dysfunction
Suboccipitals Forehead Upper shoulders	Headaches Cervical facet syndrome Neck, shoulder, arm pain	Poor posture Trauma Weak deep neck flexors	Base of occiput	C1 to mid cervical

PECTORALIS MINOR

Referred Pain	Results of Chronic Tightness	Causes of Tightness	Trigger Point Location	Associated Joint Dysfunction
Anterior chest Forearm	Creates anterior migration of the humeral head Reciprocal inhibition of the rhomboids	Poor posture Weak scapular stabilizers Pattern overload	Anywhere along the muscle belly	Upper ribs Glenohumeral joint Sternoclavicular joint Acromioclavicular joint

SUBSCAPULARIS

Referred Pain	Results of Chronic Tightness	Causes of Tightness	Trigger Point Location	Associated Joint Dysfunction
Posterior deltoid Posterior arm	Decreased functional range of motion Inhibits posterior rotator cuff Creates an anterior migration of the humeral head, leading to glenohumeral impingement and micro-instability	Pattern overload (throwers) Poor posture Muscle imbalances	Ventral scapula	Glenohumeral joint

INFRASPINATUS/TERES MINOR

Referred Pain	Results of Chronic Tightness	Causes of Tightness	Trigger Point Location	Associated Joint Dysfunction
Anterior deltoid	Difficulty performing functional shoulder movements Pain with overhead activities	Altered scapula-humeral rhythm Pattern overload	Infraspinous fossa	Glenohumeral joint

Glossary

A

A-Band: The region of the sarcomere where myosin filaments are predominantly seen with minor overlap of the actin filaments.

Abduction: A movement in the frontal plane away from the midline of the body.

Acceleration: An ability to rapidly increase running or movement velocity.

Achilles Tendonitis: Irritation and inflammation of the Achilles tendon.

Acidosis: The accumulation of excessive hydrogen that causes increased acidity of the blood and muscle.

Actin: One of the two major myofilaments, actin is the "thin" filament that acts along with myosin to produce muscular contraction.

Action Potential: Nerve impulse that allows neurons to transmit information.

Active Flexibility: Designed to improve soft tissue extensibility in all planes of motion by employing the neurophysiological principle of reciprocal inhibition. Active flexibility utilizes agonists and synergists to actively move a limb through a range of motion, while the functional antagonists are being stretched. Active flexibility incorporates neuromuscular stretching and active isolated stretching.

Active Range of Motion: The amount of motion obtained solely through voluntary contraction from the client.

Activation Techniques: Corrective exercise techniques used to re-educate and/or increase activation of underactive tissues.

Acute Variables: Important components that specify how each exercise is to be performed.

Adaptive: Capable of changing for a specific use.

Adduction: Movement in the frontal plane back toward the midline of the body.

Adenosine Triphospate (ATP): Energy storage and transfer unit within the cells of the body.

Advanced Stage: The second stage of the dynamic pattern perspective theory when learners gain the ability to alter and manipulate the movements more efficiently to adapt to environmental changes.

Afferent Neurons: (Also known as sensory neurons) They gather incoming sensory information from the environment and deliver it to the central nervous system.

Agility: The ability to change direction or orientation of the body based on internal or external information quickly and accurately without significant loss of speed.

Agonist: Muscles that are the primary movers in a joint motion. Also known as prime movers.

Alarm Reaction Stage: The first stage of the GAS syndrome, the initial reaction to a stressor.

Altered Reciprocal Inhibition: The concept of muscle inhibition, caused by a tight agonist, which inhibits its functional antagonist.

Amortization Phase: The electromechanical delay a muscle experiences in the transition from eccentric (reducing force and storing energy) to concentric (producing force) muscle action.

Anatomical Locations: Refers to terms that describe locations on the body.

Annulus Fibrosus: The outer, fibrous, ring-like portion of an intervertebral disc.

Antagonist: Muscles that act in direct opposition to agonists (prime movers).

Anterior: Refers to a position on the front or towards the front of the body.

Appendicular Skeleton: The portion of the skeletal system that includes the upper and lower extremities.

Arthritis: Chronic inflammation of the joints.

Arthrokinematics: The motions of joints in the body.

Articulation: Junctions of bones, muscles and connective tissue where movement occurs. Also known as a joint.

Arthrokinetic Dysfunction: The biomechanical dysfunction in two articular partners that lead to abnormal joint movement (arthrokinematics) and proprioception.

Arthrokinetic Inhibition: The neuromuscular phenomenon that occurs when a joint dysfunction inhibits the muscles that surround the joint.

Association Stage: Fitt's second stage where learners become more consistent with their movement with practice.

Arthrokinematics: Joint motion.

Atrophy: The loss in muscle fiber size.

Augmented Feedback: Information provided by some external source such as a fitness professional, videotape or a heart rate monitor.

Autogenic Inhibition: The process when neural impulses sensing tension are greater than the impulses causing muscle contraction. Stimulation of the Golgi Tendon Organ overrides the muscle spindle.

Autonomous Stage: Fitt's third stage of motor learning where the learner has refined the skill to a level of automation.

Axial Skeleton: The portion of the skeletal system that consists of the skull, rib cage and vertebral column.

Axon: A cylindrical projection from the cell body that transmits nervous impulses to other neurons or effector sites.

B

Balance: The ability to sustain or return the body's center of mass or line of gravity over its base of support.

Balance Threshold: the distance one can squat down on one leg while keeping the knee aligned in a neutral position (in line with the 2nd and 3rd toe).

Ball-and-Socket Joint: Most mobile joints that allow motion in all three planes. Examples would include the shoulder and hip.

Basal Ganglia: A portion of the lower brain that is instrumental in the initiation and control of repetitive voluntary movements such as walking and running.

Biomechanics: Applies the principles of physics to quantitatively study how forces interact within a living body.

Bipenniform Muscle Fibers: Muscle fibers that are arranged with short, oblique fibers that extends from both sides of a long tendon. An example would be the rectus femoris.

Brain Stem: The link between the sensory and motor nerves coming from the brain to the body and vice versa.

Break Test: At the end of available range, or at a point in the range where the muscle is most challenged, the client is asked to hold that position and not allow the examiner to "break" the hold with manual resistance.

C

Cartesian Coordinate System: System used for measurements in 3-D space.

Central Nervous System: The portion of the nervous system that consists of the brain and spinal cord.

Cerebellum: A portion of the lower-brain that compares sensory information from the body and the external environment with motor information from the cerebral cortex to ensure smooth coordinated movement.

Cerebral Cortex: A portion of the central nervous system that consists of the frontal lobe, parietal lobe, occipital lobe and temporal lobe.

Cervical Spine: The area of your spine containing the seven vertebrae that compose the neck.

Chemoreceptors: Sensory receptors that respond to chemical interaction (smell and taste).

Circuit Training System: This consists of a series of exercise that an individual performs one after another with minimal rest.

Chronic Ankle Instability: Repetitive episodes of giving way at the ankle, coupled with feelings of instability.

Circumduction: The circular movement of a limb.

Co-contraction: Muscles contract together in a force couple.

Cognitive Stage: Fitt's first stage of motor learning that describes the learner spends much of the time thinking about what they are about to perform.

Collagen: A protein that is found in connective tissue that provides tensile strength. Collagen unlike elastin is not very elastic.

Compound-Sets: Involve the performance of two exercises for antagonistic muscles. For example a set of bench press followed by cable rows (Chest/Back).

Concentric: When a muscle exerts more force than is being placed upon it, the muscle will shorten. Also known as acceleration or force production.

Condyles: Projections protruding from the bone to which muscles, tendons and ligaments can attach. Also known as a process, epicondyle, tubercle and trochanter.

Condyloid Joint: A joint where the condyle of one bone fits into the elliptical cavity of another bone to form the joint. An example would include the knee joint.

Contralateral: Refers to a position on the opposite side of the body.

Controlled Instability: Training environment that is as unstable as can safely be controlled by an individual.

Coordination: The rate of muscle recruitment and the timing of muscular contractions within the kinetic chain.

Core: The center of the body and the beginning point for movement. The core is considered as the lumbo-pelvic-hip complex that operates as an integrated functional unit providing intersegmental stability, deceleration, and force production during athletic activities.

Core Stability: Neuromuscular efficiency of the lumbo-pelvic-hip complex.

Core Strength: The ability of the lumbo-pelvic-hip complex musculature to control an individual's constantly changing center of gravity.

Coronal Plane: An imaginary plane that bisects the body to create front and back halves. Also known as the Frontal Plane.

Corrective Exercise: A term used to describe the systematic process of identifying a neuromusculoskeletal dysfunction, developing a plan of action and implementing an integrated corrective strategy.

Corrective Exercise Continuum: The systematic programming process used to address neuromusculoskeletal dysfunction through the use of inhibitory, lengthening, activation and integration techniques.

Corrective Flexibility: Designed to correct common postural dysfunctions, muscle imbalances and joint dysfunctions incorporating self-myofascial release, static stretching and neuromuscular stretching.

Cumulative Injury Cycle: A cycle whereby and "injury" will induce inflammation, muscle spasm, adhesions, altered neuromuscular control and muscle imbalances.

D

Davis' Law: States that soft tissue models along the line of stress.

Decelerate: When the muscle is exerting less force than is being placed upon it, the muscle lengthens. Also known as an eccentric muscle action or force reduction.

Deconditioned: Refers to a state in which a person has muscles imbalances, decreased flexibility, and/or a lack of core & joint stability.

Dendrites: A portion of the neuron that is responsible for gathering information from other structures.

Depression: A flattened or indented portion of bone, which could be a muscle attachment site. Also known as a fossa.

DeQuervain's Syndrome: An inflammation or a tendinosis of the sheath or tunnel that surrounds two tendons that control movement of the thumb.

Distal: Refers to a position furthest from the center of the body or point of reference.

Dorsal: Refers to a position on the back or towards the back of the body.

Dorsiflexion: Flexion at the ankle, moving the front of the foot upward.

Drawing-in Maneuver: Activation of the transverse abdominis, multifidus, pelvic floor muscles and diaphragm to provide core stabilization.

Dynamic Functional Flexibility: Multiplanar soft tissue extensibility with optimal neuromuscular efficiency throughout the full range of motion.

Dynamic Movement Assessments: Assessments that involve movement with a change in one's base of support.

Dynamic Pattern Perspective (DPP): The theory that suggests that movement patterns are produced as a result of the combined interactions between many systems (nervous, muscular, skeletal, mechanical, environmental, past experiences, etc.)

Dynamic Joint Stabilization: The ability of the stabilizing muscles of a joint to produce optimum stabilization during functional, multiplanar movements.

Dynamic Posture: How an individual is able to maintain an erect posture while performing functional tasks.

Dynamic Range of Motion: The combination of flexibility and neuromuscular efficiency.

Dynamic Stabilization: When a muscle is exerting force equal to the force being placed upon it. Also known as an isometric contraction.

Dynamic Stretching: Uses the force production of a muscle and the body's momentum to take a joint through the full available range of motion.

Dynamometry: The process of measuring forces at work using a hand held instrument (dynamometer) that measures the force of muscular contraction.

Dyskinesis: An alteration in the normal position or motion of the scapula during coupled scapulohumeral movements.

E

Eccentric: When the muscle is exerting less force than is being placed upon it, the muscle lengthens. Also known as deceleration, or force reduction.

Effectors: Any structure innervated by the nervous system including organs, glands, muscle tissue, connective tissue, blood vessels, bone marrow, etc.

Efferent Neurons: Neurons that transmit nerve impulses from the brain and/or spinal cord to the effector sites such as muscles or glands. Also known as motor neurons.

Elasticity: The spring-like behavior of connective tissue that enables the tissue to return to its original shape or size when forces are removed.

Elastin: A protein that is found in connective tissue that has elastic properties.

Endomysium: The deepest layer of connective tissue that surrounds individual muscle fibers.

Endurance Strength: The ability to produce and maintain force over prolonged periods of time.

Energy: The capacity to do work.

Energy-Utilizing: When energy is gathered from an energy-yielding source by some storage unit (ATP) and then transferred to a site that can utilize this energy.

Epicondyle: Projections protruding from the bone to which muscles, tendons and ligaments can attach. Also known as a condyle, process, tubercle and trochanter.

Epidemiology: Study of the cause and distribution of diseases in human populations.

Epimysium: A layer of connective tissue that is underneath the fascia, and surrounds the muscle.

Equilibrium: A condition of balance between opposed forces, influences or actions.

Eversion: A movement where the inferior calcaneus moves laterally.

Excess Post-Exercise Oxygen Consumption (EPOC): The state where the body's metabolism is elevated following exercise.

Excitation-Contraction Coupling: The process of neural stimulation creating a muscle contraction.

Exhaustion stage: The third stage of the GAS syndrome, when prolonged stress or stress that is intolerable to a client will cause distress.

Expert Stage: The third stage of the dynamic pattern perspective model where as the learner now focuses on recognizing and coordinating their joint motions in the most efficient manner.

Explosive Strength: The ability to develop a sharp rise in force production once a movement pattern has been initiated.

Extensibility: Capability to be elongated or stretched.

Extension: A straightening movement where the relative angle between two adjacent segments increases.

External Feedback: Information provided by some external source such as a fitness professional, videotape or a heart rate monitor.

F

Fan-Shaped Muscle: A muscular fiber arrangement that has muscle fibers span out from a narrow attachment at one end to a broad attachment at the other end. An example would be the pectoralis major.

Fascia: A connective tissue that binds muscles into separate groups.

Fascicle: A grouping of muscle fibers that house myofibrils.

Fast Twitch Fibers: Muscle fibers that can also be characterized by the term Type IIA and IIB. These fibers contain less capillaries, mitochondria and myoglobin. These fibers fatigue faster than Type I fibers.

Feedback: The utilization of sensory information and sensorimotor integration to aid the kinetic chain in the development of permanent neural representations of motor patterns.

Firing rate: The frequency of which a motor unit is activated.

Flat Bones: A classification of bone that is involved in protection and provides attachment sites for muscles. Examples include the sternum and scapulae.

Flexibility: Ability of the human movement system to have optimum range of motion (ROM) as well as neuromuscular control throughout that ROM in order to prevent injury and enhance functional efficiency.

Flexibility Training: Physical training of the body that integrates various stretches in all three planes of motion in order to produce the maximum extensibility of tissues.

Flexion: A bending movement where the relative angle between two adjacent segments decreases.

Force: The interaction between two entities or bodies that result in either the acceleration or deceleration of an object.

Force-Couples: The synergistic action of muscles to produce movement around a joint.

Force Velocity Curve: The ability of muscles to produce force with increasing velocity.

Formed Elements: Refers to the cellular component of blood that includes erythrocytes, leukocytes and thrombocytes.

Fossa: A depression or indented portion of bone, which could be a muscle attachment site. Also known as a depression.

Frontal Lobe: A portion of the cerebral cortex that contains structures necessary for the planning and control of voluntary movement.

Frontal Plane: Bisects the body into front and back halves with frontal plane motion occurring around an anterior-posterior axis.

Functional Efficiency: The ability of the neuromuscular system to monitor and manipulate movement during functional tasks using the least amount of energy, creating the least amount of stress of the kinetic chain.

Functional Flexibility: Designed to improve multi-planar soft tissue extensibility and provide optimum neuromuscular control throughout that full range of motion, while performing functional movements that utilize the body's muscles to control the speed, direction and intensity of the stretch.

Functional Strength: The ability of the neuromuscular system to contract eccentrically, isometrically and concentrically in all three planes of motion.

Fusiform: A muscular fiber arrangement that has a full muscle belly that tapers off at both ends. An example would include the biceps brachii.

G

Gamma Loop: The reflex arc consisting of small anterior horn nerve cells and their small fibers that project to the intrafusal bundle produce its contraction, which initiates the afferent impulses that pass through the posterior root to the anterior horn cells, inducing, in turn, reflex contraction of the entire muscle.

General Adaptation Syndrome (GAS): The human movement systems ability to adapt to stresses placed upon it.

Generalized Motor Program (GMP): A motor program for a distinct category of movements or actions, such as overhand throwing, kicking or running.

General Warm-up: Consists of movements that do not necessarily have any movement specificity to the actual activity to be preformed.

Genu Valgum: Inward or medial curving of the knee; knock-knee.

Glenohumeral Joint: Shoulder joint formed by the articulation between the head of the humerus and the lateral scapula.

Gliding Joint: A non-axial joint that moves back and forth or side to side. Examples would include the carpals of the hand and the facet joints.

Golgi Afferents: High threshold, slowly adapting sensory receptors located in ligaments and menisci. These receptors are mechanically sensitive to tensile loads and are most sensitive at the end ranges of motion.

Golgi Tendon Organs: Located within the musculotendinous junction and are sensitive to changes in muscular tension, and rate of tension change.

Goniometric Assessment: Technique measuring angular measurement, and joint range of motion.

Gravity: The attraction between earth and the objects on earth.

Ground Reaction Force (GRF): The equal and opposite force that is exerted back onto the body every step that is taken.

H

Hierarchical Theories: Theories that propose all planning and implementation of movement results from one or more higher brain centers.

High Ankle Sprain: A syndesmotic sprain involving the distal tibiofibular joint just proximal to the ankle.

High-load Speed Strength: The muscles ability to contract with high force at high speed with a heavy resistance and quantified by power output.

Hinge Joint: A uniaxial joint that allows movement in one plane of motion. Examples would include the elbow and ankle.

Homeostasis: The ability or tendency of an organism or a cell to maintain internal equilibrium by adjusting its physiological processes.

Human Movement Science: The study of functional anatomy, functional biomechanics, motion learning and motor control.

Hypertrophy: Enlargement of skeletal muscle fibers in response to overcoming force from high volumes of tension.

Hypertrophy Training: The third phase of the OPT™ Model.

Hypomobility: Restricted motion.

H-Zone: The area of the sarcomere where only myosin filaments are present.

I

I-Band: The area of the sarcomere that only actin filaments are present.

Inferior: Refers to a position below a reference point.

Inhibitory Techniques: Corrective exercise techniques used to release tension, and/or decrease activity of overactive neuro-myofascial tissues in the body.

Inner Unit: Provides inter-segmental stabilization of the lumbo-pelvic-hip complex and generally consists of the transverse abdominus, multifidus, internal oblique and pelvic floor musculature.

Insertion: The part of a muscle by which it is attached to the part to be moved—compare to origin.

Integrated Flexibility Training: A multi-faceted approach integrating various flexibility techniques to achieve optimum soft tissue extensibility in all planes of motion.

Integrated Functional Unit: Muscle synergies

Integrated Performance Paradigm: This paradigm states that in order to move with precision; forces must be reduced (eccentrically), stabilized (isometrically), and then produced (concentrically).

Integrative (Function of Nervous System): The ability of the nervous system to analyze and interpret the sensory information to allow for proper decision making to produce the appropriate response.

Integration Techniques: Corrective exercise techniques used to re-train the collective synergistic function of all muscles through functionally progressive movements.

Integrated Training: A comprehensive approach that attempts to improve all components necessary for an athlete to perform at the highest level and prevent injury.

Intensity: The level of demand that a given activity places on the body. A level of muscular activity quantified by power output.

Internal Feedback: The process whereby sensory information is utilized to reactively monitor movement and the environment.

Internal Rotation: Rotation of a joint toward the middle of the body.

Interneurons: Transmit nerve impulses from one neuron to another.

Inter-Muscular Coordination: The ability of the entire human movement system and each muscular subsystem to work interdependently to improve movement efficiency.

Intervertebral Foramen: The lateral opening through which spinal nerve roots exit on each side of the spinal column; formed by the bony and soft tissues at each spinal joint.

Intra-Muscular Coordination: The ability of the neuromuscular system to allow optimal levels of motor unit recruitment and synchronization within a muscle.

Intrapulmonary Pressure: Pressure within the thoracic cavity.

Inversion: A movement where the inferior calcaneus moves medially.

Ipsilateral: Refers to a position on the same side of the body.

Irregular Bones: A classification of bone that has its own unique shape and function, which does not fit the characteristics of the other categories. Examples include the vertebrae and pelvic bones.

Isokinetic Testing: Muscle strength testing performed with a specialized apparatus that provides variable resistance to a movement, so that no matter how much effort is exerted, the movement takes place at a constant speed. Such testing is used to assess and improve muscular strength and endurance, especially after injury.

Isometric: When a muscle is exerting force equal to the force being placed upon it. Also known as dynamic stabilization.

IT-Band Syndrome: Continual rubbing of the IT-band over the *lateral femoral epicondyle* leading to the area becoming inflamed.

J

Joint: Junctions of bones, muscles and connective tissue where movement occurs. Also known as an articulation.

Joint Mechanoreceptors: Receptors located in joints throughout the fibrous capsule and ligaments. These receptors signal joint position, movement, and pressure changes.

Joint Mobility: The ability of a joint to move through its natural, effective range of motion and is further characterized as the balance of strength and flexibility regulating contrasting motions around a joint (i.e. flexion and extension).

Joint Motion: Movement in a plane occurs about an axis running perpendicular to the plane.

Joint Stiffness: Resistance to unwanted movement.

K

Kinesthesia: The conscious awareness of joint movement and joint position sense that results from proprioceptive input sent to the central nervous system.

Kinetic: Force.

Kinetic Chain: The combination and interrelation of the nervous, muscular and skeletal systems.

Knee Valgus: Femur internally rotated, and tibia externally rotated; knock-knee.

Knowledge of Performance (KP): A method of feedback that provides information about the quality of the movement pattern performed.

Knowledge of Results (KR): A method of feedback after the completion of a movement to inform the client about the outcome of their performance.

Kyphosis: Exaggerated outward curvature of the thoracic region of the spinal column resulting in a rounded upper back.

L

Lateral: Refers to a position relatively farther away from the midline of the body or toward the outside of the body.

Lateral Ankle Sprain: Any of the lateral ligaments including the anterior talofibular ligament (ATFL), calcaneofibular ligament (CFL), and posterior talofibular ligament (PTFL) may be injured often caused by forced plantar flexion and inversion of the ankle during landing on an unstable or uneven surface.

Lateral Flexion: The bending of the spine (cervical, thoracic and/or lumbar) from side to side.

Law of Acceleration: Acceleration of an object is directly proportional to the size of the force causing it, in the same direction as the force and inversely proportional to the size of the object.

Law of Action-Reaction: Every force produced by one object onto another produces an opposite force of equal magnitude.

Law of Gravitation: Two bodies have an attraction to each other that is directly proportional to their masses and inversely proportional to the square of their distance from each other.

Lengthening Techniques: Corrective exercise techniques used to increase the extensibility, length and range of motion (ROM) of neuro-myofascial tissues in the body.

Length-Tension Relationship: Refers to the resting length of a muscle and the tension the muscle can produce at this resting length.

Ligament: Primary connective tissue that connects bone-to-bone to provide stability, proprioception, guide and limit joint motion.

Limit Strength: The maximum force a muscle can produce in a single contraction.

Linear Speed: The ability to move the body in one intended direction as fast as possible.

Load: The amount of weight prescribed to an exercise set.

Long Bones: A characteristic of bone that has a long cylindrical body with irregular or widened bony ends. Examples include the clavicle and humerus.

Longitudinal Muscle Fiber: A muscle fiber arrangement, that's fibers run parallel to the line of pull. An example would include the sartorius.

Lordosis: Low back frounding.

Low-load Speed Strength: The muscles ability to contract with high force at high speed with low resistance and quantified by power output.

Lower-Brain: The portion of the brain that includes the brain stem, the basal ganglia and the cerebellum.

Lower Crossed Syndrome: A dysfunctional muscle pattern characterized by an anterior tilt to the pelvis and lower extremity muscle imbalances.

Lower-Extremity Postural Distortion: Usually characterized by excessive foot pronation (flat feet), increased knee valgus (tibia externally rotated and femur internally rotated and adducted or knock-kneed) and increased movement at the LPHC (extension and/or flexion) during functional movements.

Lumbar Spine: The portion of the spine, commonly referred to as the small of the back. The lumbar portion of the spine is located between the thorax (chest) and the pelvis.

Lumbo-Pelvic-Hip Complex: Involves the anatomical structures of the lumbar, thoracic and cervical spine, the pelvic girdle, and the hip joint.

Lumbo-Pelvic-Hip Postural Distortion: Altered joint mechanics in an individual which lead to increased lumbar extension and decreased hip extension.

M

Maximal Speed: The maximal running speed one is able to attain.

Maximal Strength: The maximum force an individual's muscle can produce in a single voluntary effort, regardless of the rate of force production.

Mechanical Specificity: The specific muscular exercises using different weights and movements that are performed to increase strength or endurance in certain body parts. Refers to the weight and movements placed on the body.

Mechanoreceptors: Sensory receptors that respond to mechanical forces. Specialized neural receptors embedded in connective tissue that converts mechanical distortions of the tissue into neural codes to be conveyed to the central nervous system.

Medial: Refers to a position relatively closer to the midline of the body.

Medial Ankle Sprain: Ankle sprains involving the deltoid ligament of the ankle, and may include avulsion fractures of the tibia or other foot bones.

Medial Tibial Stress Syndrome (Shin Splints): Pain in the front of the tibia caused by an overload to the tibia and the associated musculature.

Metabolic Specificity: The specific muscular exercises using different levels of energy that are performed to increase endurance, strength or power. Refers to the energy demand required for a specific activity.

Metatarsal Stress Fracture: Fractures that occur to the metatarsals; the long bones of the foot between the phalanges (the toes) and the tarsals.

Mitochondria: The mitochondria are the principal energy source of the cell. Mitochondria convert nutrients into energy as well as doing many other specialized tasks.

M-Line: The portion of the sarcomere where the myosin filaments connect with very thin filaments called titin and create an anchor for the structures of the sarcomere.

Momentum: The product of the size of the object (mass) and its velocity (speed with which it is moving).

Mortise: A common name for the talocrual (ankle) joint because of the similarity of shape of the talocrual joint and a carpenter's mortise.

Motor Behavior: The collective study of motor control, motor learning and motor development. Motor response to internal and external environmental stimuli.

Motor Control: The study of posture and movements with the involved structures and mechanisms used by the central nervous system to assimilate and integrate sensory information with previous experiences. How the central nervous system integrates internal and external sensory information with previous experiences to produce a motor response.

Motor Development: The change in motor behavior over time throughout the lifespan.

Motor (Function of Nervous System): The neuromuscular response to sensory information.

Motor Learning: The integration of motor control processes with practice and experience that lead to relatively permanent changes in the capacity to produced skilled movements.

Motor Neurons: Neurons that transmit nerve impulses from the brain and/or spinal cord to the effector sites such as muscles or glands. Also known as efferent neurons.

Motor Unit: A motor neuron and the muscle fibers that it innervates.

Motor Unit Activation: The progressive activation of a muscle by successive recruitment of contractile units (motor units) to accomplish increasing gradations of contractile strength.

Movement Impairment Syndromes: Refer to the state in which the structural integrity of the HMS is compromised because the components are out of alignment.

Multipenniform: Muscles that have multiple tendons with obliquely running muscle fibers.

Multisensory Condition: Training environment that provides heightened stimulation to proprioceptors and mechanoreceptors.

Muscle Action Spectrum: The range of muscle actions that include concentric, eccentric and isometric actions.

Muscle Balance: Establishing normal length-tension relationships, which ensures proper length and strength of each muscle around a joint.

Muscle Imbalance: Alteration of muscle length surrounding a joint.

Muscle Fiber Arrangement: Refers to the manner in which the fibers are situated in relation to the tendon.

Muscle Fiber Recruitment: Refers to the recruitment pattern of muscle fiber/motor units in response to creating force for a specific movement.

Muscle Spindles: Microscopic intrafusal fibers that are sensitive to change in length and rate of length change.

Muscular Endurance: The ability of the body to produce low levels of force and maintain them for extended periods of time.

Muscle Hypertrophy: Characterized by the increase in the cross sectional area of individual muscle fibers and is believed to result from an increase in the myofibril proteins.

Muscle Synergies: The ability of muscles to work as an integrated functional unit.

Multi-directional Speed: Being able to create speed in any direction or body orientation (forward, backward, lateral, diagonal, etc).

Myofascial: The connective tissue in and around muscles and tendons.

Myofibrils: A portion of muscle that contains myofilaments.

Myofilaments: The contractile components of muscle, actin and myosin.

Myosin: One of the two major myofilaments known as the "thick" filament that works with actin to produce muscular contraction.

Myotatic Stretch Reflex: When a muscle is stretched very quickly, the muscle spindle contracts, which in turn stimulates the primary afferent fibers that causes the extrafusal fibers to fire, and tension increases in the muscle.

N

Nervous System: A conglomeration of billions of cells specifically designed to provide a communication network within the human body.

Neural Adaptation: An adaptation to strength training where muscles are under the direct command of the nervous system.

Neuromuscular Efficiency: The ability of the central nervous system (CNS) to allow agonists, antagonists, synergists, stabilizers, and neutralizers to work interdependently during dynamic athletic activities.

Neuromuscular Junction: The point where the neuron meets the muscle, to allow the action potential to continue its impulse.

Neuromuscular Specificity: The specific muscular exercises using different speeds and styles that are performed to increase neuromuscular efficiency. Refers to the speed of contraction and exercise selection.

Neuron: The functional unit of the nervous system.

Neurotransmitters: Chemical messengers that cross the neuromuscular junction to trigger the appropriate receptor sites.

Neutral Spine: The natural position of the spine when all three curves of the spine cervical, thoracic and lumbar are present and in good alignment. This is the safest position to perform movement.

Nocioceptors: Sensory receptors that respond to mechanical deformation and pain.

Novice Stage: The first stage of the dynamic pattern perspective model, the learner simplifies movements by minimizing the specific timing of joint motions, which tends to result in movement that is rigid and jerky.

Nucleus Pulposus: A semi-fluid mass of fine white and elastic fibers that form the central portion of an intervertebral disc.

O

Objective Information: Measurable data about a client's physical state such as body composition, movement and cardiovascular ability.

Occipital Lobe: A portion of the cerebral cortex that deals with vision.

Optimal Strength: The ideal level of strength that an individual needs to perform functional activities.

Origin: The more fixed, central, or larger attachment of a muscle- compare to insertion.

Osteoarthritis: Arthritis in which cartilage becomes soft, frayed or thins out, due to trauma or other conditions.

Osteopenia: A decrease in the calcification or density of bone as well as reduced bone mass.

Osteoporosis: Condition in which there is a decrease in bone mass and density as well as an increase in the space between bones, resulting in porosity and fragility.

Overtraining: Excessive frequency, volume, or intensity of training, resulting in fatigue (which is due also to a lack of proper rest and recover).

P

Paciniform Afferents: Large, cylindrical, thinly encapsulated, multi-cellular end organ structures. These receptors are widely distributed around the joint capsule and surrounding peri-articular tissue that are mechanically sensitive to local compression and tensile loading, especially at extreme ranges of motion. These receptors are associated with the detection of acceleration, deceleration, or sudden changes in the deformation of the mechanoreceptors.

Parietal Lobe: A portion of the cerebral cortex that is involved with sensory information.

Passive Range of Motion: The amount obtained by the examiner without any assistance by the client.

Patellofemoral Pain: Pain in the knee region that is provoked or accentuated by actions that involve motion at the patellofemoral joint and/or increase pressure of patella against the femoral condyles.

Patellofemoral Syndrome: Vague discomfort of the inner knee area and may be caused by abnormal tracking of the patella within the femoral trochlea.

Pattern Overload: Repetitive physical activity that moves through the same patterns of motion, placing the same stresses on the body over a period of time.

Perception: The integrating of sensory information with past experiences or memories.

Perimysium: The connective tissue that surrounds fascicles.

Periosteum: A membrane that lines the outer surface of all bones.

Pes Cavus: A high medial arch when weight bearing.

Pes Plantus: A flattened medial arch during weight bearing.

Physical Activity Readiness Questionnaire (PAR-Q): A questionnaire that has been designed to help qualify a person for low-to-moderate-to-high activity levels.

Pivot Joint: Allow movement in predominately the transverse plane, examples would include the alantoaxial joint at the base of the skull and between the radioulnar joint.

Plane of Motion: Refers to the plane (sagittal, frontal and/or transverse) in which the exercise is performed.

Plantar Fasciitis: An inflamed and irritated plantar fascia.

Plantarflexion: Ankle extension such that the toes are pointed toward the ground.

Plasticity: The unrecoverable or permanent elongation of soft tissue.

Plyometric Training: Exercises that utilize quick, powerful movements involving an eccentric contraction immediately followed by an explosive concentric contraction.

Posterior: Refers to a position on the back or towards the back of the body.

Posterior Pelvic Tilt: A movement in which the pelvis rotates backward.

Postural Distortion Patterns: Predictable patterns of muscle imbalances.

Postural Equilibrium: The ability to efficiently maintain balance throughout the body segments.

Posture: Position and bearing of the body for alignment and function of the kinetic chain.

Power: The ability to exert maximal force in the shortest amount of time.

Power Endurance: The repetitive execution of explosive movement.

Pre-Programmed: Activation of muscles in healthy people that occurs automatically and independently of other muscles prior to movement.

Principle of Individualism: Refers to the uniqueness of a program to the client for whom it is designed.

Principle of Overload: Implies that there must be a training stimulus provided that exceeds the current capabilities of the kinetic chain to elicit the optimal physical, physiological, and performance adaptations.

Principle of Progression: Refers to the intentional manner in which a program is designed to progress according to the physiological capabilities of the kinetic chain and the goals of the client.

Principle of Specificity: The kinetic chain will specifically adapt to the type of demand placed upon it. Also known as the SAID principle.

Processes: Projections protruding from the bone to which muscles, tendons and ligaments can attach. Also known as condyle, epicondyle, tubercle, and trochanter.

Program Design: A purposeful system or plan put together to help an individual achieve a specific goal.

Pronation: A multi-planar, synchronized joint motion that occurs with eccentric muscle function.

Pronation Distortion Syndrome: A dysfunctional muscle pattern characterized by foot pronation and lower extremity muscle imbalances.

Proprioception: The cumulative neural input to the central nervous system from all mechanoreceptors that sense position and limb movement.

Proprioceptively Enriched Environment: An environment that challenges the internal balance and stabilization mechanisms of the body.

Proximal: Refers to a position nearest the center of the body or point of reference.

Q

Q-angle: The angle formed by lines representing the pull of the quadriceps muscle and the axis of the patellar tendon.

Quadrilateral Muscle Fiber: An arrangement of muscle fibers that are usually flat and four-sided. An example would include the rhomboid.

Quickness: The ability to react and change body position with maximum rate of force production, in all planes of motion, from all body positions, during functional activities. Also defined as the ability to execute movement skill in a comparatively brief amount of time.

R

Range of Motion: Refers to the range that the body or bodily segments move during and exercise.

Rate Coding: Muscular force can be amplified by increasing the rate of incoming impulses from the motor neuron after all prospective motor units have been activated.

Rate of Force Development: The time it takes to generate a particular force.

Rate of Force Production: Ability of muscles to exert maximal force output in a minimal amount of time.

Reaction Time: The time elapsed between the athlete's recognizing the need to act and initiating the appropriate action.

Reactive Strength: The ability of the neuromuscular system to switch from an eccentric contraction to a concentric contraction quickly and efficiently.

Reactive Training: Exercises that utilize quick, powerful movements involving an eccentric contraction immediately followed by an explosive concentric contraction.

Reciprocal Inhibition: Muscles on one side of a joint relaxing to accommodate contraction of antagonist muscles on the other side of that joint.

Recruitment: An impulse transmitted simultaneously over an increasing number of nerve fibers pulling in increasingly more muscle fibers for the task. This is sensitive to the stretch intensity and the number of fibers recruited.

Recurrent Inhibition: A feedback circuit that can decrease the excitability of motor neurons via the interneuron called the Renshaw cell.

Relative Flexibility: When the body seeks the path of least resistance during functional movement patterns.

Relative Strength: The maximum force that an individual can generate per unit of body weight, regardless of the time of force development.

Repetition Tempo: The speed with which each repetition is performed.

Resistance Development Stage: The second stage of the GAS syndrome, when the body increases it functional capacity to adapt to the stressor.

Rest Interval: The time taken to recuperate between sets and/or exercises.

Roll: The joint motion that depicts the rolling of one joint surface on another. Examples would include that of the femoral condyles over the tibial condyles during a squat.

Rotary Motion: Movement of an object or segment around a fixed axis in a curved path.

Ruffini Afferents: Large, encapsulated, multi-cellular end organ structures located within the collagenous network of the joint's fibrous capsule. These receptors are mechanically sensitive to tissue stresses that are activated during extremes of extension and rotation.

S

Sacroiliac Joint: The joint connecting the tail bone (sacrum) and pelvic bone (ilium).

Sacroiliac Joint Dysfunction: Dysfunction of the sacroiliac joint due to trauma or degenerative changes.

Saddle Joint: One bone is shaped as a saddle, the other bone is shaped as the rider, the only example is in the carpometacarpal joint in the thumb.

Sagittal Plane: An imaginary plane that bisects the body into right and left halves. Sagittal plane motion occurs around a frontal axis.

Sarcomere: The functional unit of muscle, repeating sections of actin and myosin.

Sarcolemma: A plasma membrane that surrounds muscle fibers.

Sarcopenia: A decrease in muscle fiber numbers.

Sarcoplasm: Cell components that contain glycogen, fats, minerals and oxygen that are found in the sarcolemma.

Self-Myofascial Release: A flexibility technique that focuses on the neural and fascial systems in the body. Self-myofascial release concentrates on alleviating myofascial trigger points and areas of hyper-irritability located within a band of muscle. This form of stretching incorporates the concept of autogenic inhibition to improve soft tissue extensibility.

Self-Organization: This theory, which is based on the dynamic pattern perspective, provides the body with the ability to overcome changes that are placed upon it.

Sensation: The process whereby sensory information is received by the receptor and transferred to the spinal cord for either reflexive motor behavior and/or to higher cortical areas for processing.

Sensorimotor Integration: The ability of the nervous system to gather and interpret sensory information to anticipate, select and execute the proper motor response.

Sensors: Provide feedback from the effectors to the central controller and cardiovascular control system. They include baroreceptors, chemoreceptors, and muscle afferents.

Sensory Feedback: The process whereby sensory information is utilized to reactively monitor movement and the environment.

Sensory Information: The data that the central nervous system receives from sensory receptors to determine such things as the body's position in space, limb orientation as well as information to the environment, temperature, texture, etc.

Sensory Neurons: Neurons that gather incoming sensory information from the environment delivered to the central nervous system. Also known as afferent neurons.

Short Bones: A classification of bone that appears cubical in shape. Examples include the carpals and tarsals.

Slide: The joint motion that depicts the sliding of a joint surface across another. Examples would include the tibial condyles moving across the femoral condyles during a knee extension.

Sliding Filament Theory: The proposed process of the contraction of the filaments within the sarcomere takes place.

Slow Twitch Fibers: Another term for Type I muscle fibers, fibers that are characterized by a higher amount of capillaries, mitochondria and myoglobin. These fibers are usually found to have a higher endurance capacity than fast twitch fibers.

Specific Adaptations to Imposed Demands (SAID Principle): Principle that states the body will adapt to the specific demands placed upon it.

Specific Warm-Up: Consists of movements that more closely mimic those of the actual activity.

Speed Strength: The ability of the neuromuscular system to produce the greatest possible force in the shortest possible time.

Spin: Joint motion that depicts the rotation of one joint surface on another. Examples would include the head of the radius rotating on the end of the humerus during pronation and supination of the forearm.

Sprain: A partial or complete tear of a ligament.

Stability: The ability of the body to maintain postural equilibrium and support joints during movement.

Stabilizer: Muscles that support or stabilize the body while the prime movers and the synergists perform the movement patterns.

Stabilization Endurance: The ability of the stabilization mechanisms of the kinetic chain to sustain proper levels of stabilization to allow for prolonged neuromuscular efficiency.

Stabilization Strength: Ability of the stabilizing muscles to provide dynamic joint stabilization and postural equilibrium during functional activities.

Starting Strength: The ability to produce high levels of force at the beginning of a movement.

Static Posture: How an individual physically presents themselves in stance. It is reflected in the alignment of the body.

Static Stretching: Combines low force and long duration movements utilizing the neurophysiological principles of autogenic inhibition to improve soft tissue extensibility, allowing for relaxation and concomitant elongation of muscle. Static stretching requires holding the stretch at the first point of tension or resistance barrier for 30 seconds.

Strength: The ability of the neuromuscular system to produce internal tension in order to overcome an external force.

Strength Endurance: The ability of the body to repeatedly produce high levels of force, over prolonged periods of time.

Stretch Reflex: A muscle contraction in response to stretching within the muscle.

Stretch-Shortening Cycle: An active stretch (eccentric contraction) of a muscle followed by an immediate shortening (concentric contraction) of that same muscle. Also defined as the process of the forced, rapid lengthening of a muscle immediately followed by a shortening, creating a release of energy.

Structural Efficiency: The alignment of the musculoskeletal system, which allows our center of gravity to be maintained over a base of support.

Subacromial Impingement Syndrome (SAIS): A common diagnosis broadly defined as compression of the structures (tendons) that run beneath the coracoacromial arch, most often from a decrease in the subacromial space. The impinged structures include the supraspinatus and infraspinatus tendons, the subacromial bursa, and the long head of the biceps tendon.

Subjective Information: Information that is provided by a client regarding personal history such as occupation, lifestyle and medical history.

Sulcus: A groove in a bone that allows a soft structure to pass through.

Superior: Refers to a position above a reference point.

Superset System: Utilizes a couple of exercises performed in rapid succession of one another.

Supination: A multi-planar, synchronized joint motion that occurs with concentric muscle function.

Supine: Lying on one's back.

Synarthrosis Joint: A joint without any joint cavity and fibrous connective tissue. Examples would include the sutures of the skull and the symphysis pubis.

Syndesmosis: A joint where two bones are joined by a ligament or membrane. An example is the distal tibiofibular joint.

Synchronization: The synergistic activation of multiple motor units.

Synergist: Muscles that assist prime movers during functional movement patterns.

Synergistic Dominance: When synergists compensate for a weak or inhibited prime mover in an attempt to maintain force production and functional movement patterns.

Synovial Joints: This type of joint is characterized by the absence of fibrous or cartilaginous tissue connecting the bones. Examples would include the ball-and-socket joint, the hinge joint and the saddle joint.

T

Temporal Lobe: A portion of the cerebral cortex that deals with hearing.

Tendon: Connective tissue that attaches muscle to bone and provides an anchor for muscles to exert force.

Tendinopathy: A combination of pain, swelling, and impaired performance commonly associated with the Achilles tendon.

Tendinosis: Damage to a tendon at a cellular level, but does not present to inflammation.

Thoracic Spine: The twelve vertebrae in mid-torso that are attached to the rib cage.

Torque: The ability of any force to cause rotation around an axis. A force that produces rotation. Common unit of torque is the Newton-Meter or Nm.

Total Response Time: The total summation of time it takes to execute a reactionary movement.

Transitional Movement Assessments: Assessments that involve movement without a change in one's base of support.

Transverse Plane: An imaginary plane that bisects the body to create upper and lower halves. Transverse plane motion occurs around a longitudinal or a vertical axis.

Transfer-of-Training Effect: The more similar the exercise is to the actual activity, the greater the carryover into real-life settings.

Trochanter: Projections protruding from the bone to which muscles, tendons and ligaments can attach. Also known as a condyle, process, tubercle and epicondyle.

Trochlea: A groove in front of the femur where the patella moves as the knee bends and straightens.

Tubercle: Projections protruding from the bone to which muscles, tendons and ligaments can attach. Also known as a condyle, process, epicondyle and trochanter.

U

Unipenniform Muscle Fiber: Muscle fibers that are arranged with short, oblique fibers that extend from one side of a long tendon. An example would include the tibialis posterior.

Upper Crossed Syndrome: A dysfunctional muscle pattern characterized by a forward head and rounded shoulders with upper extremity muscle imbalances.

Upper-Extremity Postural Distortion: Usually characterized as having rounded shoulders, a forward head posture and/or improper scapulothoracic and/or glenohumeral kinematics during functional movements.

Universal Athletic Position: Standing in a ¼ squat with flat feet, hands in front, hips back, knees over the shoulders, shoulders over the knees and neutral spine.

V

Ventral: Refers to a position on the front or towards the front of the body.

Vertical Loading: A variation of circuit training alternating body parts trained from set to set, starting from the upper extremity and moving to the lower extremity.

Viscoelasticity: The fluid-like property of connective tissue that allows slow deformation with an imperfect recovery after the deforming forces are removed.

Volume: The total amount of weight lifted in a session or week and quantified by repetitions times weight.

W

Wolff's Law: The principle that every change in the form and the function of a bone or in the function of the bone alone, leads to changes in its internal architecture and in its external form.

Work Capacity: The ability to endure high workloads within various intensities and durations utilizing a range of energy systems and displaying the ability to recover for the next bout of exercise.

Index

DATE DUE